Hepato-Biliary-Pancreatic Surgery and Liver Transplantation

Hee Chul Yu
Editor

Hepato-Biliary-Pancreatic Surgery and Liver Transplantation

A Comprehensive Guide, with Video Clips

The Korean Association of
Hepato-Biliary-Pancreatic Surgery

Springer

Editor
Hee Chul Yu
Chairman of the Korean Association of HBP Surgery
Jeonbuk National University Medical School
Jeonbuk National University Hospital
Jeonju, Korea (Republic of)

ISBN 978-981-16-1995-3 ISBN 978-981-16-1996-0 (eBook)
https://doi.org/10.1007/978-981-16-1996-0

This Springer imprint is published by the registered company Springer Nature Singapore Pte Ltd.
The registered company address is: 152 Beach Road, #21-01/04 Gateway East, Singapore 189721, Singapore

Preface

Established in 1992, the Korean Association of Hepato-Biliary-Pancreatic Surgery (KAHBPS) has a history of more than 20 years and improved its status in terms of quality, as well as quantitative growth, including liver transplantation, beyond Asia to the global level.

Hepatobiliary and pancreatic (HBP) surgery requires a lot of expertise. Safe surgical practices can minimize complications after surgery and are directly related to the patient's prognosis. In particular, KAHBPS began to contemplate the need for surgical guidelines that could be referenced by young HBP surgeons who were currently developing their skills. Therefore, we worked for two years with about 50 HBP experts in Korea and completed the Korean version of the *Hepatobiliary and Pancreatic Surgery Master collection* in 2015.

Currently, many Korean HBP surgeons are leading global research members in international research and academic fields. Therefore, since KAHBPS felt the responsibility not only to focus on the education of Korean surgeons but to provide extensive help to young HBP surgeons across the world and beyond the language barrier, we decided to publish an English version.

The contents of the book were divided into three parts: the liver, biliary tract, and pancreas. We tried to write the surgical techniques as simply and concisely as possible and attached pictures and videos for easy understanding. In particular, as the worlds' leading group in the field of liver transplantation, we added relatively more content on transplantation.

We would like to thank the authors for their hard work in writing from time to time while performing long hours of surgery and medical practice. We remain grateful to the planning director, the committee members, and the publishers who put their entire hearts and souls into publishing a beautiful book with meticulous effort.

We trust that this book will contribute to improving the surgical skills of HBP surgeons and hope it will be widely used as a valuable material in the training process of young surgeons. Based on this book, we hope that standard surgical procedures will be established in the field of HBP surgery and progressively developed worldwide.

Jeonju, Republic of Korea — Hee Chul Yu

Contents

List of Videos

Part I

Operative Technique of Hepatectomy

1 Use of Intraoperative Ultrasonography

Il-Young Park

Abstract

Intraoperative ultrasonography is an important technique to find, resect, and treat lesions. Laparoscopic ultrasound is a useful tool for laparoscopic surgery. Hepato-pancreato-biliary surgeons have to be familiar with ultrasonography during operations.

Keywords

Intraoperative ultrasonography
Laparoscopic ultrasound

Ultrasound is an essential technique for surgeons. Particularly, hepato-pancreato-biliary (HPB) surgeons should be familiar with ultrasound when diagnosing, treating, or operating a patient. This chapter will focus on intraoperative ultrasound techniques, with the intent to allow HPB surgeons to perform ultrasound more easily during surgery.

Intraoperative ultrasonography (IOUS) was first performed in 1979 by Makuuchi during hepatectomy and, thereafter, continued to improve following the development of B-mode ultrasound. The detection rate of liver mass with IOUS is superior to that of CT, MRI, and even laparotomy. IOUS can detect lesions as small as 1 mm stones and 3–5 mm masses [1]. Thus, HPB surgeons greatly benefit from IOUS by integrating their anatomical knowledge with ultrasound techniques.

IOUS consists of a body and probes of different types. The ultrasound frequencies used in probes range from 5 MHz to 10 MHz, and 7.5 MHz probe is most commonly used. These probes can penetrate around 6–10 cm in depth. IOUS probes include linear, T-shape, I-shape, convex, and sector-type probes, similar to general ultrasound probes. When examining the anatomical structures, methods such as sliding, rotating, tilting, and rocking are used in IOUS, similar to the techniques used in abdominal ultrasound. IOUS not only enables surgeons to screen for diseases involving liver, gallbladder, and pancreas, but also diseases involving retroperitoneal space consisting of kidney, adrenal gland, spleen, and aorta.

Lesions of the liver are easily detected and compared with surrounding structures with ultrasound. The division of the anatomical structure of liver is based on hepatic vein according to the Couinaud classification. In addition to the normal anatomical structures, HBP surgeons are advised to be familiar with different variations of the

Supplementary Information The online version contains supplementary material available at https://doi.org/10.1007/978-981-16-1996-0_1.

I.-Y. Park (✉)
Department of Surgery, Bucheon St. Mary's Hospital, The Catholic University of Korea College of Medicine, Bucheon, South Korea
e-mail: parkiy@catholic.ac.kr

H. C. Yu (ed.), *Hepato-Biliary-Pancreatic Surgery and Liver Transplantation*,
https://doi.org/10.1007/978-981-16-1996-0_1

HBP structures [2–4]. When performing IOUS, T-type probes are most commonly used; the probe is placed between the index and middle fingers during the examination of liver surface. When examining the liver, the left and the right lobes should be scanned transversely and then longitudinally. Next, the probe should be slid, rotated, tilted, and rocked in all four ways in order to identify the anatomical structures of liver. Finally, the bottom of liver should also be scanned for any existing lesions (Fig. 1.1, Video 1.1). Images using stand-off method can be obtained by pressing the probe against the liver surface or by placing saline solution in between the probe and the skin (Fig. 1.2). Common benign lesions of the liver include low-echogenic liver cyst and high-echogenic hemangioma; malignant lesions of liver include hepatocellular carcinoma and metastatic cancer with low-echogenic halo surrounding the mass.

In addition to localization of liver lesions, IOUS allows the surgeon to constantly evaluate whether the lesion is accurately resected during surgery. Further, IOUS is used to inject the dye into the portal vein, after which the liver is anatomically resected along the dye-stained area. Even during liver transplantation, IOUS is necessary for identifying the blood flow before and after the transplantation. In cases where the hepatic lesions cannot be resected, IOUS is used to perform ultrasound-guided radio-frequency ablation (RFA) (Fig. 1.3, Video 1.4).

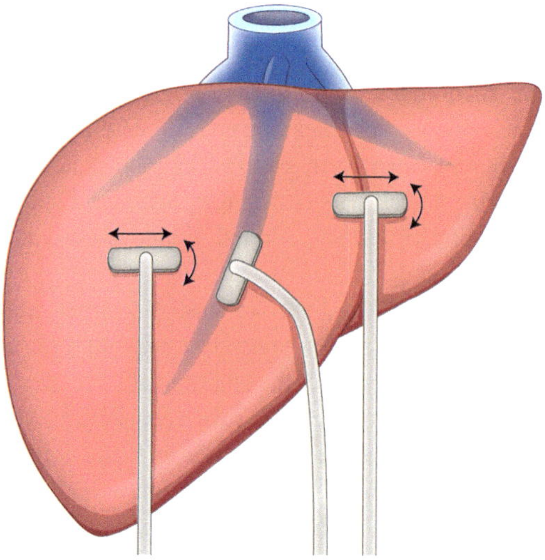

Fig. 1.1 Intraoperative liver scanning

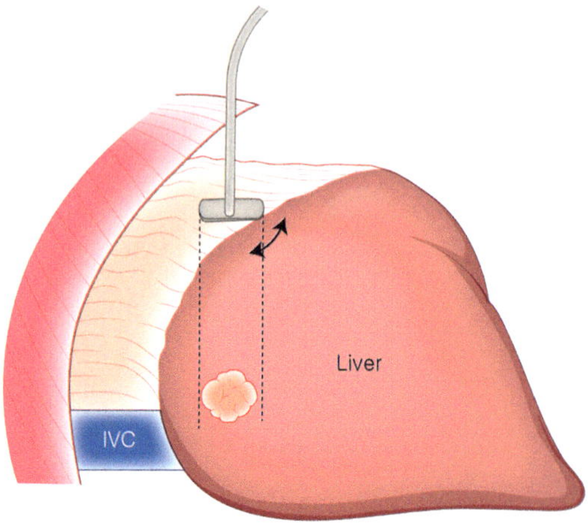

Fig. 1.2 Standoff scanning

Compared to intraoperative cholangiography, IOUS can be used to detect biliary stones more easily and quickly, owing to its superior detection rate. Bile duct is visualized by scanning the cystic duct and common bile duct transversely and longitudinally. However, in cases where bile duct cannot be reached directly, a stand-off technique can be used: saline is poured in between the liver and the peritoneum, and the probe is placed within the saline during IOUS (the shape of bile duct, portal vein, and hepatic artery during ultrasound resembles the face of Mickey Mouse). The color Doppler allows a surgeon to easily distinguish bile ducts from arteries, and biliary stones are found along with a posterior shadowing.

Before performing IOUS, the pancreas should first be scanned transversely and longitudinally, followed by sliding, rocking, rotating, and tilting to identify the lesion and the nearby structures (Fig. 1.4). In order to better visualize the pancreatic head, the Kocher maneuver can be performed before IOUS. IOUS is useful in detecting acute pancreatitis, pancreatic pseudocysts, pancreatic stones and pancreatic duct dilation in chronic pancreatitis, benign pancreatic tumors such as insulinoma, and pancreatic cancer. Splenic vein and pancreatic duct can be visualized by directly applying the probe onto the pancreas. In cases where direct contact is difficult, the stand-off tech-

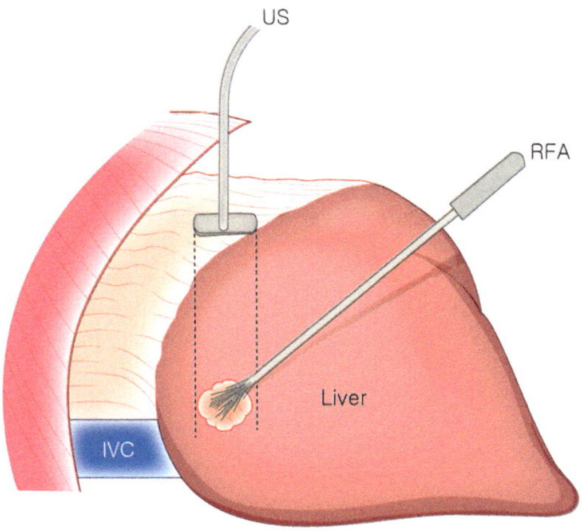

Fig. 1.3 Radio-frequency ablation method

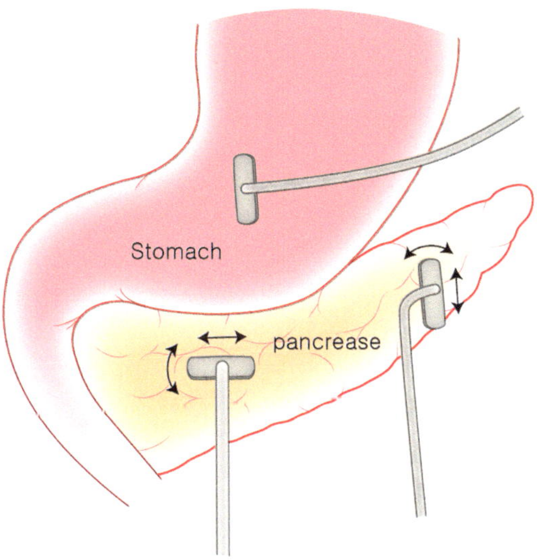

Fig. 1.4 Intraoperative pancreatic scanning

nique can be performed by pouring saline into the lesser sac. In patients with chronic pancreatitis, IOUS facilitates surgery by allowing the surgeons to locate pancreatic duct and pancreatic stones.

With increasing number of laparoscopic operations, direct palpation of internal organs during laparoscopic surgery has become less accessible. To overcome these shortcomings, laparoscopic ultrasound (LUS) can be inserted into the abdomen via the port to visualize anatomical structures, find lesions, and perform biopsy or RFA [1, 5]. LUS is similar to other ultrasound devices,

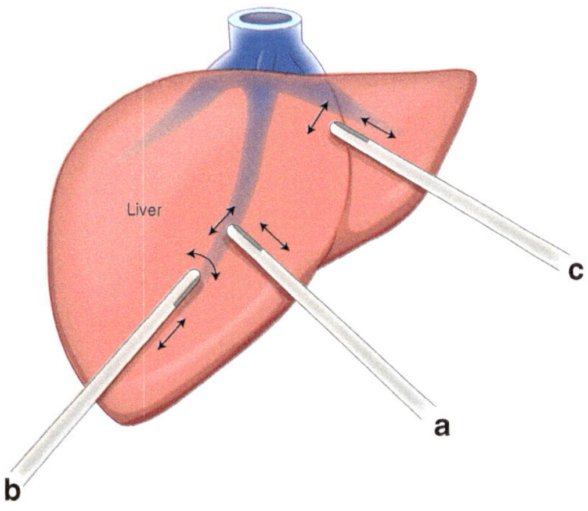

Fig. 1.5 Laparoscopic ultrasound scan of the liver (**a**) umbilical port, (**b**) right lower abdominal port, (**c**) left abdominal port

but is distinct in that its distal end is equipped with a sector, rigid, flexible linear array probe of 4 cm in size, which bends to a maximum of 90° in most cases. When performing LUS, the device is inserted into the umbilical port or upper abdominal quadrant port via 10 mm trocar, and the liver is examined longitudinally and transversely (Fig. 1.5, Video 1.5). Similarly, the common bile duct is scanned longitudinally and transversely to visualize portal vein and hepatic artery, which are the landmarks that allow the surgeon to detect bile duct and lesions such as biliary stones and cysts. In case of pancreas, the LUS probe is inserted into the upper abdominal or umbilical port. Laparoscopic ultrasonography is either performed via stomach after removing the gastric gas or on the pancreas directly (Fig. 1.6). Performing LUS during laparoscopic surgery not only allows the surgeon to obtain intraoperative images and localize the lesion, but also enables the surgeon to perform ultrasound-guided biopsies and provide treatments such as RFA.

To summarize, IOUS plays an important role in HPB surgery. It is highly sensitive for detecting HPB lesions and guiding biopsies, resections, and ablation therapies. Thus, HPB surgeons should become familiar with IOUS techniques so as to explore all its advantages during surgery.

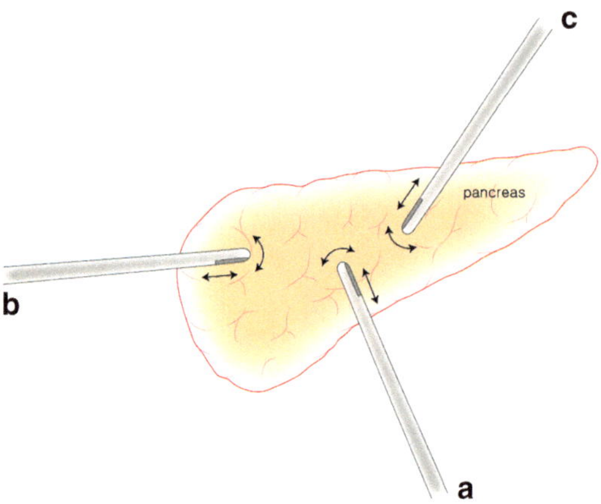

Fig. 1.6 Laparoscopic ultrasound scan of the pancreas (**a**) umbilical port, (**b**) right abdominal port, (**c**) left abdominal port

References

1. Benson MD, Gandhi MR. Ultrasound of the hepatobiliary-pancreatic system. World J Surg. 2000;24(2):166–70.
2. Kruskal JB, Kane RA. Intraoperative US of the liver: techniques and clinical applications. Radiographics. 2006;26(4):1067–84.
3. Patel NA, Roh MS. Utility of intraoperative ultrasound. Surg Clin North Am. 2004;84(2):513–24.
4. Schrope B. Surgical and interventional ultrasound. McGraw-Hill Education; 2014.
5. Machi J, et al. Technique of laparoscopic ultrasound examination of the liver and pancreas. Surg Endosc. 1996;10(6):684–9.

2 The Techniques and Instruments for Minimizing Bleeding During Parenchymal Dissection

Dong-Sik Kim

Abstract

Because the liver is an organ with high-blood flow, liver resection is accompanied by significant bleeding unless adequate surgical techniques and appropriate instruments are not prepared. In this chapter, commonly used surgical techniques and instruments to minimize bleeding during liver resection are introduced. Understanding and application of appropriate techniques and instruments are essential components of safe and efficient surgery.

Keywords

Inflow control · Pringle method · Total vascular exclusion · Liver resection Parenchymal transection · CUSA

Methods routinely used to reduce bleeding during hepatectomy include blocking of blood inflow to the liver to reduce bleeding from the portal vein or hepatic artery, placing the liver higher than natural position after mobilization to reduce the bleeding from the hepatic vein, lowering the central venous pressure, and minimizing the time required for transection of the parenchyma.

D.-S. Kim (✉)
Division of HBP Surgery and Liver Transplantation, Department of Surgery, Korea University College of Medicine, Seoul, South Korea
e-mail: kimds1@korea.ac.kr

2.1 Methods to Control Blood Flow

Although it is a natural process to occlude the blood supply to the site for partial resection of the liver, unexpected bleeding may occur frequently due to abundant blood flow in the liver during the process of parenchymal transection. Because the liver is relatively resistant to ischemia, blood flow to the liver can be frequently controlled to reduce bleeding during transection of the parenchyma.

2.1.1 Inflow Control, Pringle Maneuver

It is the most commonly used and convenient method to block blood flow to the liver using a simple instrument across hepatoduodenal ligament, which contains the common hepatic artery and the main portal vein (Fig. 2.1).

First, the transparent portion in the lesser omentum on the left side of the hepatoduodenal ligament should be identified and opened via electrocautery. The hepatoduodenal ligament can be easily wrapped and evaluated using the left-hand middle

H. C. Yu (ed.), *Hepato-Biliary-Pancreatic Surgery and Liver Transplantation*,
https://doi.org/10.1007/978-981-16-1996-0_2

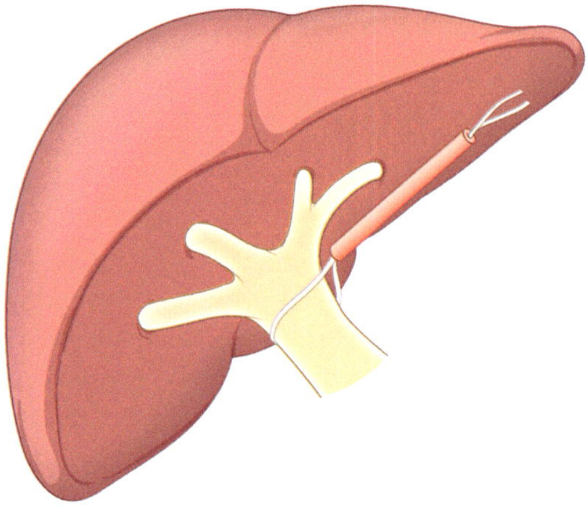

Fig. 2.1 When the hepatoduodenal ligament is wound with a nylon tape and the Rummel catheter is inserted, and the Rummel catheter is tightened using a Kelley clamp, blood flow to the liver can be blocked

finger through the foramen of Winslow. A nylon tape with a Rummel catheter or an angled vascular clamp covered with rubber can be used to occlude blood inflow to the liver. In general, intermittent inflow occlusion is frequently used by alternating 15 min of blockade with 5 min of release. Parenchymal transection can be performed during 15 min of inflow occlusion. However, in some cases, a continuous blockade is inevitable. It should be noted that prolonged blockage of the portal vein can lead to intestinal congestion.

The duration of safe inflow occlusion has yet to be determined, but it is clear that the higher the liver dysfunction, the shorter is the tolerance limit [1]. If the structures of the hepatic hilum are individually dissected, the hepatic artery and the portal vein may be separately blocked using a Bull-dog clamp. Even in cases of adhesion involving the hepatic hilum or in relatively simple cases of resection, it is important to always prepare for the inflow control to reduce bleeding and prepare for unexpected situations.

If it is possible to achieve the desired purpose by blocking bloodstream only on the right or left side at a time due to tumor location or in cases of central bisectionectomy, it is also possible to use hemihepatic inflow occlusion, via hanging nylon tape separately on the right and left sides after dissection of hilar plate. In this case, only half of the liver becomes ischemic and intestinal congestion can be avoided.

2.1.2 Total Vascular Exclusion

In contrast to the Pringle maneuver in which only the blood flow to the liver is blocked, total vascular exclusion is a method used to simultaneously block the hepatic vein or both the upper and lower vena cava to block the reflux through the hepatic vein in addition to blocking the inflow. Theoretically, reduction in bleeding may be more effective, but in practice, it can be applied only after the liver is completely mobilized or the hepatic veins are isolated, which takes more time and effort. Compared with inflow control, additional benefits are not clear for conventional liver resections and there is a potential risk of hemodynamic instability. However, it is used selectively when surgery is performed in the proximity of the hepatic veins or when resection or reconstruction of the cava is required.

If the duration of total vascular exclusion is expected to be prolonged, perfusion of a cold organ preservation solution such as histidine–tryptophan–ketoglutarate (HTK) solution may be considered through the portal vein to minimize ischemic damage to the liver (total vascular exclusion with hypothermic perfusion). In this case, to prevent congestion of the intestine and help hemodynamic stability, it is common to bypass blood circulation in the portal vein and the inferior vena cava to superior vena cava using a centrifugal pump (Fig. 2.2).

In the case of a normal liver, it is known that this method can be used for up to 2 h, and it is reported that it has advantages in hemodynamics during surgery or renal function after surgery compared to simple total vascular exclusion [2].

In alternative cases, a method of excision of the inferior vena cava while bypassing hepatic venous blood flow extracorporeally, rather than portal blood flow, has also been reported [3].

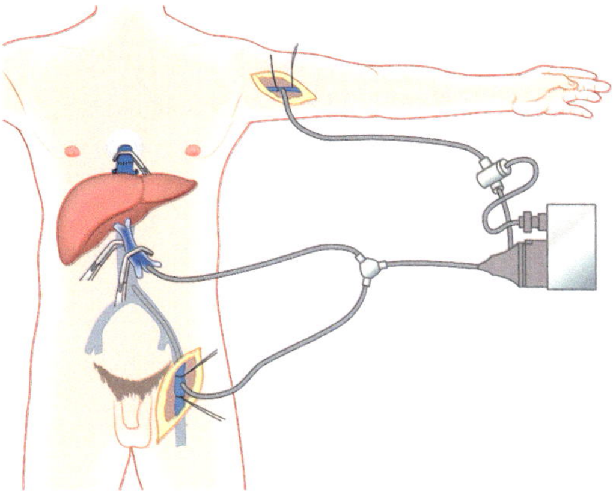

Fig. 2.2 Total vascular exclusion with veno-venous bypass using a centrifugal pump

2.2 Methods and Instruments for Parenchymal Transection

Resection of the liver parenchyma entails crushing the parenchymal tissues while effectively ligating and resecting the blood vessels or biliary ducts inside the liver, which are distributed along the desired resection line. To this end, instruments (Fig. 2.3) using various mechanisms of operation have been developed. However, an important principle to always keep in mind, regardless of the instrument used, is that there must be adequate physical traction on both the sides of the cut surface so that the transection is facilitated by effective functioning of the instruments. The surgeon and the first assistant should be careful to maintain this traction effectively throughout the entire process so that the transection can progress quickly and effectively. To this end, sutures can be placed on both sides of the transection surface to pull the parenchyma (Fig. 2.4), or the cut surface is spread to both sides using a forceps or malleable retractor. In some cases, the transection surface may be spread using the left hand of the operator or even gravity based on liver weight.

2.2.1 Clamp Crushing Method

It is the oldest, but the most basic and universally used method. Common instruments used are Kelly clamp and Pean hemostat. Comparative studies with other recently developed instruments reported that the superiority of the latest instruments could not be observed in conventional hepatic resection [4].

First, the cutting line of the liver surface is marked with electrocautery. At this time, it is important to cauterize the capsules on the liver surface completely, so that they can be easily separated by the device. To facilitate the cutting of the parenchyma and to control the cutting direction, a suture-tie at the edge is placed to pull the liver to both sides of the cutting surface and evenly about 45° each with an assistant. In the beginning, it is better to start with a small bite of the liver that is crushed at a time and determine the tendency to bleed from the cut surface. When breaking the parenchyma, only the tubular structures remain, which are ligated using a clip or tie and then cut.

Very small blood vessels or connective tissues resulting from liver fibrosis can also be cut via electrocautery. In some cases, the first assistant may save time by cauterizing small blood vessels with an instrument such as a bipolar coagulator. When the vasculature is not clear due to crushed parenchymal tissues, it can be seen more clearly by squirting from a spoid. At this time, placing the capped suction in the lower or behind of the right lobe of the liver helps to keep the surgical field clear.

2.2.2 Cavitron Ultrasonic Surgical Aspirator (CUSA)

This is a device that pulverizes the parenchyma while leaving only the vasculature of the interstitial tissue using ultrasonic vibration, and at the same time aspirates and removes the crushed tissue. It is most widely used in hepatectomies for live donors or hilar cholangiocarcinoma. Depending on the model, the electrocautery is integrally combined to facilitate the use. Because the physical properties of the liver may vary depending on the presence or absence of fatty liver or the degree of fibrosis, the intensity of ultrasonic vibration needs to be adjusted.

While moving the tip of the instrument perpendicular to the cut surface, the tissue is crushed

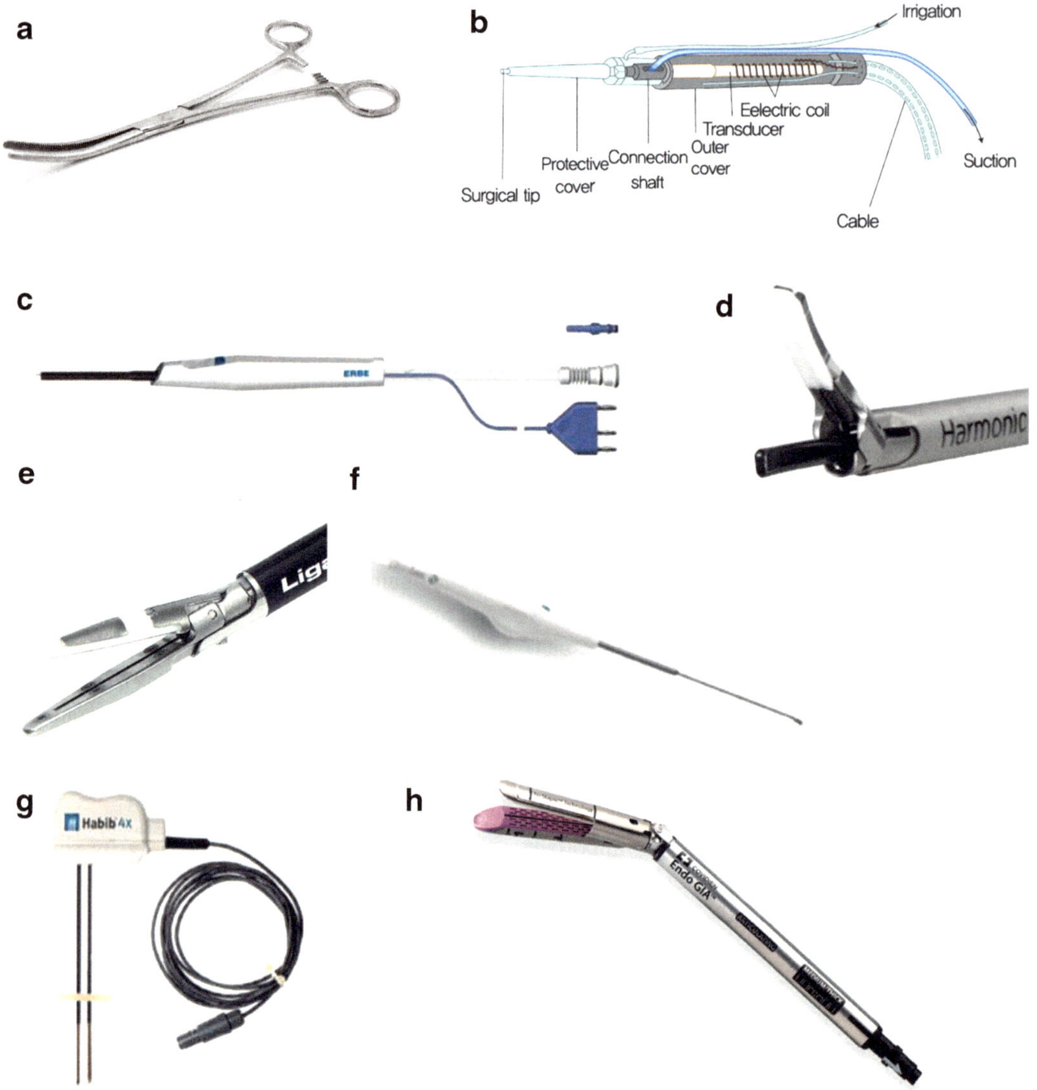

Fig. 2.3 Instruments for parenchymal transection using (**a**) Kelley Clamp, (**b**) CUSA (Cavitron Ultrasonic Surgical Aspirator), (**c**) Water-jet, (**d**) Harmonic Scalpel, (**e**) Ligasure, (**f**) Tissue-Link, (**g**) Habib, (**h**) Stapler

by contact with the parenchyma and the remaining tubular structures are cauterized or ligated using clips or ties. If Glisson pedicles appear, they should be ligated, taking care not to destroy the capsule of pedicle by the tip of the instrument. If the hepatic vein is exposed to the cutting surface, bleeding should be avoided because the branch is cut off due to excessive traction.

2.2.3 Water Jet

It is a mechanism that destroys the parenchyma and leaves only the tubular structures using a high-pressure stream of water, which acts similar to CUSA.

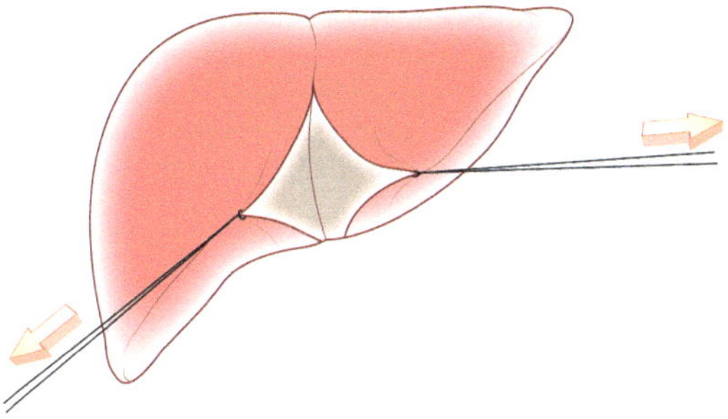

Fig. 2.4 Traction of the liver during parenchymal transection. Suture-tie using thick sutures on both sides of the liver parenchyma. It can be reinforced using a pledget to avoid tearing of the liver from traction. The traction forces from the operator and the assistant should be balanced so that they are not biased on either side

2.2.4 Harmonic Scalpel

It is a device that cuts while cauterizing the parenchyma using thermal energy generated by ultrasonic vibration and is often used in laparoscopic liver resection surgery. The harmonic scalpel can easily proceed up to 1 cm from the surface of the liver, where few important vasculatures are located, but care must be taken not to damage the vasculature that requires ligation when proceeding deeper. Therefore, do not cauterize large amounts of tissue at a time, but proceed gradually to determine if there are major structures to be ligated.

2.2.5 Ligasure

Originally developed as a concept of the vessel-sealing device, it is a bipolar energy device that is sometimes used for liver resection. It is used similar to the harmonic scalpel, and it is safer to ligate separately rather than to seal important vasculature thermally.

2.2.6 Tissue-Link

The principle is to mechanically ablate using a hook at the end of the instrument after solidifying the tissue by dripping saline, which has been heated by high-frequency energy, on the ablation surface.

2.2.7 Habib

This is a method of solidifying the liver tissue of the cut surface using microwave energy and then cutting with scissors and clips. The liver can be resected relatively quick, but care must be taken due to the risk of unexpected damage when important vasculature exists on the coagulated cut surface. In addition, the extent of coagulation should be predicted adequately so that only the site to be excised is coagulated.

2.2.8 Stapler

Staplers can be selectively used when rapid resection is required in trauma patients with unstable hemodynamics or when the parenchymal thickness is thin, such as in the left lateral section by passing the stapler blades along the expected resection plane and cutting the parenchyma. Adequate knowledge about the blood vessels and biliary tract structure inside the liver can ensure safe use. Otherwise, it may cause severe bleeding or leakage of the bile. It is recommended to wait about 10 s after closing the jaw before firing. Insufficient vascular seal is suggested when the excessive parenchyma is included between the jaws. In most cases, only the left or right Glisson or hepatic vein is selectively separated and cut using a stapler.

References

1. Torzilli G, Procopio F, Donadon M, Del Fabbro D, Cimino M, Montorsi M. Safety of intermittent Pringle maneuver cumulative time exceeding 120 minutes in liver resection: a further step in favor of the "radical but conservative" policy. Ann Surg. 2012;255(2):270–80.
2. Azoulay D, Eshkenazy R, Andreani P, Castaing D, Adam R, Ichai P, et al. In situ hypothermic perfusion of the liver versus standard total vascular exclusion for complex liver resection. Ann Surg. 2005;241(2):277–85.

3. Kim DS, Yu YD, Jung SW, Ji W, Suh SO. Extracorporeal hepatic venous bypass during en bloc resection of right trisection, caudate lobe, and inferior vena cava: a novel technique to avoid hypothermic perfusion. J Am Coll Surg. 2013;216(5):e47–50.
4. Rahbari NN, Koch M, Schmidt T, Motschall E, Bruckner T, Weidmann K, et al. Meta-analysis of the clamp-crushing technique for transection of the parenchyma in elective hepatic resection: back to where we started? Ann Surg Oncol. 2009;16(3):630–9.

3 The Safe Application of Hanging Maneuver

Seoung Hoon Kim

Abstract

The liver can be divided into three sections depending on the area supplied by the right anterior, right posterior, and left Glissonian pedicles. It can also be divided into three sections according to the area drained by the right, middle, and left hepatic veins. A hanging tape can be applied along the anteromedian surface of the retrohepatic inferior vena cava or the ligamentum venosum with its upper end among the three hepatic veins and its lower end among the three Glissonian pedicles. The advantages of the liver hanging maneuver and the anatomic characteristics inherent to the liver enable hepatic surgeons to make safe and effective use of a hanging technique in a variety of anatomic liver resections.

Keywords

Hanging maneuver · Liver resection
Hepatectomy · Liver anatomy · Liver surgery

Supplementary Information The online version contains supplementary material available at https://doi.org/10.1007/978-981-16-1996-0_3.

S. H. Kim (✉)
Department of Surgery, National Cancer Center, Goyang-si, Gyeonggi-do, South Korea
e-mail: kshlj@hanmail.net

3.1 Liver Anatomy Based on Three Glisson's Pedicles and Three Hepatic Veins

Portal vein, hepatic artery, and bile duct, which are encased in a sheath, constitute the Glissonian pedicle, which is divided into the right and the left Glissonian pedicles at the liver hilum. The right Glissonian pedicle branches into the anterior and posterior Glissonian pedicles (Fig. 3.1). Accordingly, liver can be divided into three sections that are supplied by the three Glissonian pedicles, respectively. The liver can also be divided into three sections that are drained by each of the three major hepatic veins: right hepatic vein (RHV), middle hepatic vein (MHV), and left hepatic vein (LHV) (Fig. 3.2).

Variations such as anomalous branching of the three Glissonian pedicles or the three major hepatic veins can occur, sometimes accompanied by large inferior hepatic veins.

The preoperative dynamic CT scan can be used to elucidate the anatomy, to enable surgical dissection of the three Glissonian pedicles or the three major hepatic veins during operation.

H. C. Yu (ed.), *Hepato-Biliary-Pancreatic Surgery and Liver Transplantation*,
https://doi.org/10.1007/978-981-16-1996-0_3

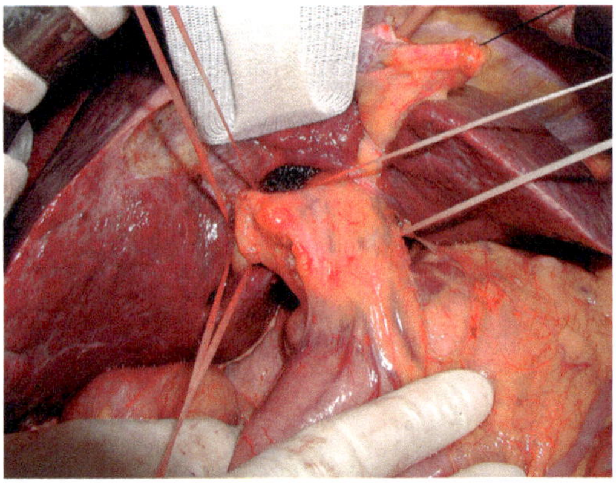

Fig. 3.1 Hilar dissection of three Glissonian pedicles. The anterior, posterior, and left Glissonian pedicles are dissected and encircled by a sling, respectively

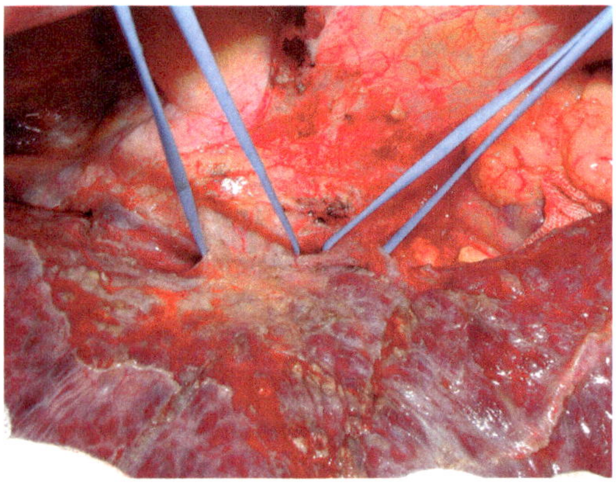

Fig. 3.2 Three hepatic veins at the suprahepatic confluence around IVC. The MHV and LHV are dissected and encircled by a sling, respectively

3.2 Hanging Maneuver

The hanging maneuver proposed by Belghiti et al. during right hepatectomy using a tape passing between the anterior surface of the inferior vena cava (IVC) and the liver parenchyma has several advantages in major hepatic resection [1]. The tape used in this procedure plays two important roles: first, as a guide to the transection plane, and second, as a means to control the liver. Pulling and aiming at the tape surrounding the transection plane facilitate the exposure and bleeding control of the deep portion of the parenchyma, protecting the retrohepatic IVC and the main Glissonian pedicle and hepatic vein of the remaining liver, and maintain the transection plane effectively without other auxiliary techniques, so that the parenchyma can be safely divided without compression of the remaining liver. Glissonian approach using hanging maneuver was also reported in various kinds of hepatectomy in which the simple and effective technique yielded good outcomes [2].

A single plane of transection yields two complementary types of anatomic liver resection. For example, right posterior sectionectomy with RHV carries the same transection plane as left trisectionectomy with the caudate lobe. All the transection planes discussed in this article are longitudinal, parallel to, and oriented to the IVC or the ligamentum venosum along which the tape is located. The resected parenchyma has an inverted pyramid shape.

3.3 Surgical Techniques

A J-shaped incision with or without a left extension is generally used to enter the abdomen, depending on the specific circumstances. Large tumors of the right liver, especially those lying posteriorly and possibly involving the IVC, may require extension via the right thoracoabdominal approach. However, the upper midline incision above the umbilicus can be used in living donors or patients with tumors measuring less than 5 cm [3]. After dissection at the liver hilum and hepatic venous confluence near IVC, the hanging tape can be located along the anteromedian surface of the retrohepatic IVC or the ligamentum venosum with its upper end among the three hepatic veins and its lower end among the three Glisson's pedicles. The tape on the retrohepatic IVC can be positioned not only via retrohepatic tunneling but also after liver mobilization (Fig. 3.3).

Occlusion of one to two of the three Glissonian pedicles, which supply the resected hepatic section, reveals the demarcation line on the liver surface that corresponds to a transection plane. The parenchymal transection is performed with the ultrasonic dissection device and usually proceeds from the bottom to the top and from the front to the back along the line with both ends of the tape

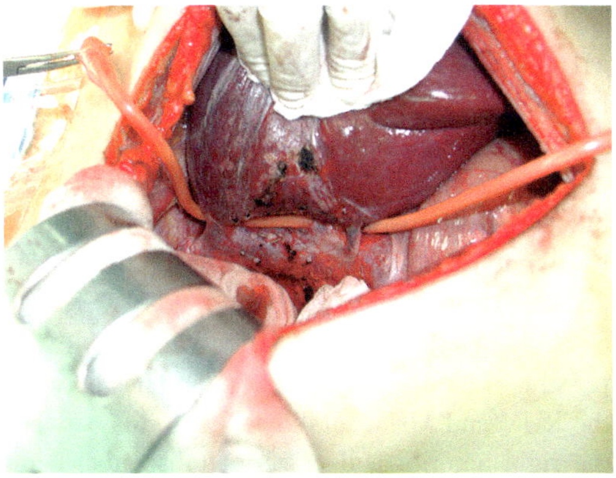

Fig. 3.3 After liver mobilization, a tape for the hanging maneuver is positioned along the IVC with its upper end located between the RHV and MHV and its lower end on the left side of the two right inferior hepatic veins

oriented and pulled up for the transection plane, if necessary, using the Pringle maneuver and continued cephalad and posteriorly aiming at the tape until the tape is exposed. The maneuver should not be attempted in case of tumors invading or abutting the retrohepatic IVC, the extrahepatic three Glissonian pedicles, or the three hepatic veins because the dissection to locate a hanging tape at the live hilum or hepatic venous confluence may induce profuse bleeding or tumor spillage.

In case of living donor right hepatectomy, in the presence of sizable venous branches of the anterior section, the parenchymal transection is performed until those venous branches, and the hanging tape can be repositioned in order to preserve the venous branches.

Anatomic major liver resection requires four major steps entailing mobilization of the resected hepatic section, dissection of hilar Glissonian pedicles, parenchymal transection, and dissection of hepatic venous confluence around suprahepatic IVC.

During the hanging maneuver, the other three steps are performed before parenchymal transection. However, the parenchymal transection may precede or follow the mobilization of the resected liver section similar to the anterior approach hepatectomy or living donor surgery, respectively.

The division of hilar Glissonian pedicle and hepatic vein around IVC of the resected section of liver can be done before or after parenchymal transection. However, the author prefers cutting after parenchymal transection, because only after complete parenchymal transection is the Glissonian pedicle or hepatic vein exposed widely to secure sufficient space for stapling or clamping, and division to prevent injuries such as strictures or occlusions involving artery, portal vein, or bile duct within the Glissonian sheath or hepatic vein of the remaining liver. The Glissonian pedicle can be divided not only en masse but also individually after dissection into its artery, portal vein, and bile duct similar to surgeries involving hilar cholangiocarcinoma or living donors [4].

To enhance the application of the hanging maneuver, the inferior portion of caudate lobe under the hepatic hilum is transected until the branch point of the main Glissonian pedicle. The lower end of the tape located on the anteromedial surface of the IVC is repositioned between the three Glissonian pedicles already dissected. Only after this transection can the hanging tape encircle the transection plane smoothly to facilitate pulling up of the hanging catheter [5].

3.4 Single Tape along the Anterior Surface of Retrohepatic IVC

Right posterior sectionectomy without the RHV is possible if its upper end is on the right side of the RHV and its lower end lies between the right anterior and posterior Glissonian pedicles.

Right posterior sectionectomy with the RHV or left trisectionectomy with the caudate lobe is facilitated by the location of its upper end between the RHV and MHV, and its lower end between the right anterior and posterior Glissonian pedicles (Fig. 3.4a).

Right hepatectomy without MHV or left hepatectomy with the caudate lobe and MHV is enabled if its upper end lies between the RHV and MHV, and its lower end is between the right and left Glissonian pedicles (Fig. 3.4b).

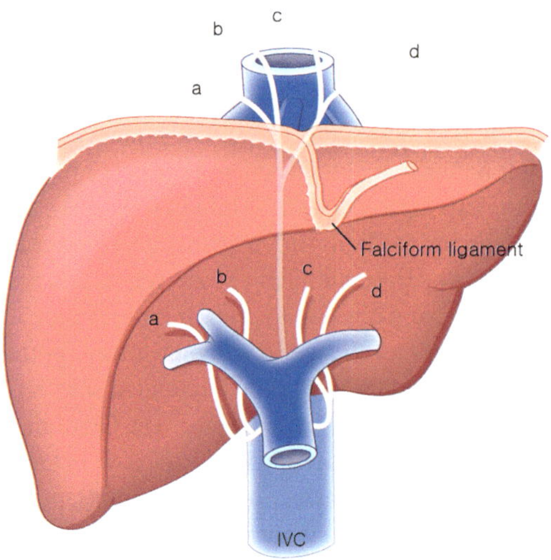

Fig. 3.4 Locations of the hanging tape along the antero-median surface of the retrohepatic IVC

Right hepatectomy with the MHV or left hepatectomy with the caudate lobe is possible if its upper end lies between the MHV and LHV, and its lower end between the right and left Glissonian pedicles (Fig. 3.4c).

Right trisectionectomy is indicated if the upper end of the tape is between the MHV and LHV, and its lower end is between the right and left Glissonian pedicles, and both the ends are pulled up close to the right side of the umbilical portion of the left Glissonian pedicle (Fig. 3.4d).

3.5 Two Tapes along the Anterior Surface of Retrohepatic IVC

Central bisectionectomy is favored if the upper end of one tape is between the RHV and MHV and its lower end is located between the right anterior and posterior Glissonian pedicles, and the upper end of the other tape is between the MHV and LHV and its lower end is between the right and left Glissonian pedicles with both the ends oriented clockwise close to the right side of the umbilical portion of the left Glissonian pedicle and pulled up in the direction (Fig. 3.4a–d).

Right anterior sectionectomy without the MHV is possible if the upper end of one tape lies between the RHV and the MHV, and its lower end is between the right anterior and posterior Glissonian pedicles, and the upper end of the other tape is between the RHV and MHV, and its lower end is between the right and left Glissonian pedicles (Fig. 3.4a, b).

Right anterior sectionectomy with the MHV is possible if the upper end of one tape lies between the RHV and MHV, and its lower end is between the right anterior and posterior Glissonian pedicles, and the upper end of the other tape is between the MHV and LHV and its lower end is between the right and left Glissonian pedicles (Fig. 3.4a–c).

Left medial sectionectomy without the MHV is possible if the upper end of one tape lies between the MHV and LHV, and its lower end is between the right and left Glissonian pedicles with both the ends oriented towards the border of the right and left liver, and the upper end of the other tape is between the MHV and LHV, and its lower end is between the right and left Glissonian pedicles with both the ends oriented clockwise close to the right side of the umbilical portion of the left Glissonian pedicle and pulled up in the direction (Fig. 3.4c, d).

Left medial sectionectomy with the MHV is facilitated if the upper end of one tape lies between the RHV and MHV, and its lower end is located between the right and left Glissonian pedicles, and the upper end of the other tape is between the MHV and LHV, and its lower end is between the right and left Glissonian pedicles (Fig. 3.4b–d).

3.6 One Tape along the Ligamentum Venosum

The prerequisites for a successful liver hanging maneuver are accurate positioning of tape based on liver anatomy and surgical feasibility. For left hepatectomy, if the lower end of the hanging tape is placed between the right and left Glissonian pedicles similar to dissection of the right Glissonian pedicle during right hepatectomy, the caudate pedicle branching from the left Glissonian pedicle may be subject to injury because it lies on the transection plane, which can trigger atrophy or bile duct dilatation of the caudate lobe (Fig. 3.5a). This problem can be avoided by dissecting the left Glissonian pedicle along with the ligamentum venosum and using a hanging tape dorsally on the ligamentum venosum (Fig. 3.5b) [6].

Left hepatectomy via MHV or right hepatectomy with the caudate lobe is facilitated if the upper end of the tape is between the RHV and MHV and its lower end is located between the right and left Glissonian pedicles (Fig. 3.6a–o).

Left hepatectomy without MHV or right hepatectomy with the caudate lobe and MHV is enabled when the upper end of tape lies between the MHV and LHV and its lower end is located between the right and left Glissonian pedicles. Right trisectionectomy with the caudate lobe or living donor left lateral sectionectomy is indicated when the tape lies in the same position and both the ends of the tape pulled up close to the right side of the umbilical portion of the left Glissonian pedicle (Fig. 3.6b–o).

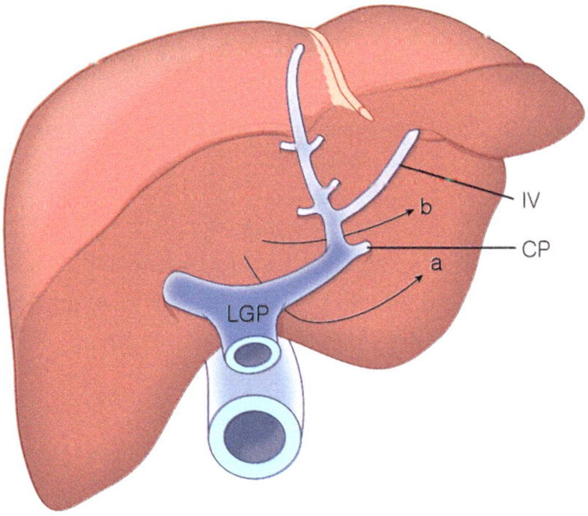

Fig. 3.5 Methods of dissection of the left Glissonian pedicle for positioning a hanging tape in left hepatectomy. *LGP* left Glissonian pedicle. *LV* ligamentum venosum, *CP* caudate pedicle

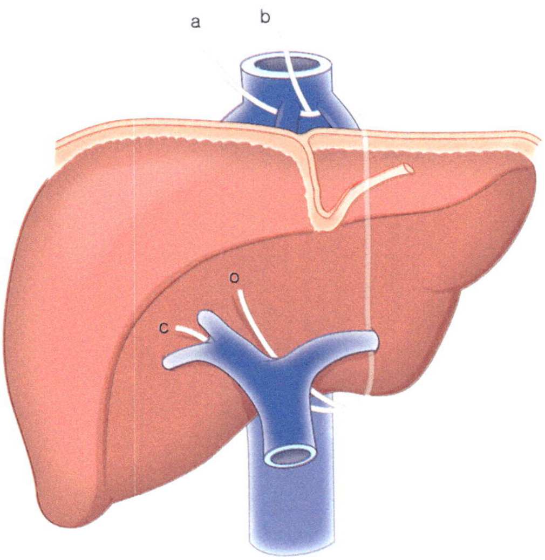

Fig. 3.6 Locations of the hanging tape along the ligamentum venosum

Left trisectionectomy without the caudate lobe or right posterior sectionectomy with the caudate lobe is facilitated if its upper end is located between the RHV and MHV, and its lower end is between the right anterior and posterior Glissonian pedicles (Fig. 3.6a–c).

Left lateral sectionectomy is possible if its upper end is between the MHV and LHV and its lower end is in the left side of the umbilical portion of the left Glissonian pedicles.

3.7 One Tape along the Anterior Surface of the Retrohepatic IVC and Ligamentum Venosum

Isolated caudate lobectomy is facilitated if the upper end of the tape located between the RHV and MHV along the IVC is passed through a tunnel behind the common trunk of the MHV and LHV, pulled down along the ligamentum venosum, and laid under the hepatic hilum (Fig. 3.7) [7].

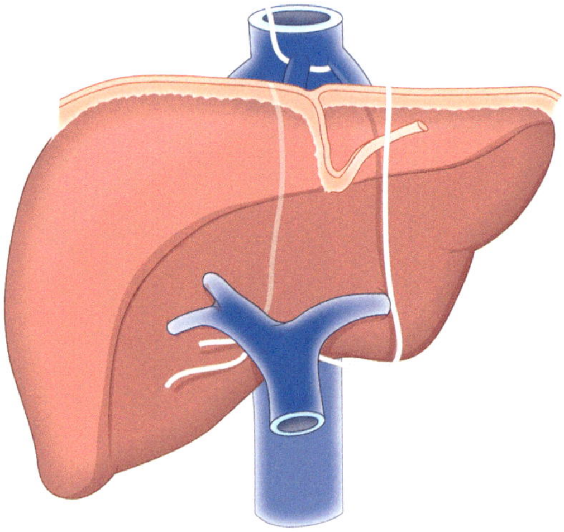

Fig. 3.7 Location of the tape for hanging maneuver in the isolated caudate lobectomy

3.8 Other Types of Liver Resection by Hanging Maneuver

Right inferior sectionectomy (resection of segments 5 and 6) is indicated after the right liver is partially mobilized, and some parenchymal transection along the inferior side of right Glissonian pedicle shows Glissonian branches of segments 5 and 6. The dissection and temporary occlusion of the Glissonian branches reveals the demarcation line of segments 5 and 6 on the liver surface. The hanging tape is used to surround the transection plane and the parenchymal transection is performed with both ends of the tape pulled up (Fig. 3.8).

Extended right posterior sectionectomy is facilitated when both ends of the tape positioned at the border of right anterior and posterior sections are rotated clockwise toward the right anterior Glissonian pedicle. Parenchymal transection occurs via division of the right-sided branches of the right anterior Glissonian pedicle so that the remaining liver can carry intact Glissonian pedicle and draining vein.

Resection of segments 4b and 5 is also feasible. This type of liver resection has three transection planes. The hanging maneuver can be applied during parenchymal transection partially or totally with the tape pulled up in line with each transection plane. It may be useful in extended cholecystectomy (Fig. 3.9).

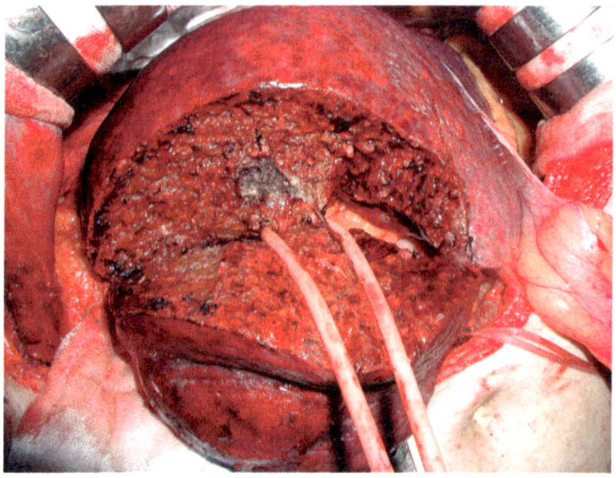

Fig. 3.8 Hanging maneuver for parenchymal transection during right inferior sectionectomy (resection of segments 5 and 6)

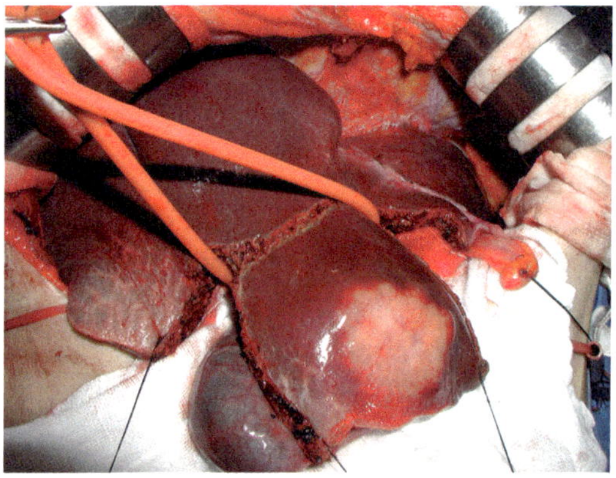

Fig. 3.9 Hanging maneuver during resection of segment 4b and 5 for gallbladder cancer

References

1. Belghiti J, Guevara OA, Noun R, Saldinger PF, Kianmanesh R. Liver hanging maneuver: a safe approach to right hepatectomy without liver mobilization. J Am Coll Surg. 2001;193(1):109–11.
2. Kim SH, Park SJ, Lee SA, Lee WJ, Park JW, Hong EK, et al. Various liver resections using hanging maneuver by three glisson's pedicles and three hepatic veins. Ann Surg. 2007;245(2):201–5.
3. Kim SH, Kim YK. Upper midline incision for liver resection. HPB (Oxford). 2013;15(4):273–8.

4. Kim SH, Cho SY, Lee KW, Park SJ, Han SS. Upper midline incision for living donor right hepatectomy. Liver Transpl. 2009;15(2):193–8.
5. Kim SH, Kim YK. Living donor right hepatectomy using the hanging maneuver by Glisson's approach under the upper midline incision. World J Surg. 2012;36(2):401–6.
6. Kim SH, Kim YK. Hanging manoeuver for a left hepatectomy using Glisson's approach with a focus on tape position in liver hilum. HPB (Oxford). 2013;15(9):681–6.
7. Kim SH, Park SJ, Lee SA, Lee WJ, Park JW, Kim CM. Isolated caudate lobectomy using the hanging maneuver. Surgery. 2006;139(6):847–50.

4 Left Hemihepatectomy

Jin Sub Choi

Abstract

Left hemi-hepatectomy is a relatively easier surgical procedure than the other major hepatectomies. However, an indolent approach to left hemi-liver may result in fatal complications. Accurate understanding of hepatic hilum, biliary system, and hepatic vein is essential for acceptable surgical outcomes.

Keywords

Left hemihepatectomy · Liver hilum · Bile duct anatomy · Cantlie line

Left hemihepatectomy entails resection of the left hemi-liver, which is supplied by the left portal vein and left hepatic artery (segments 2, 3, and 4 according to the Couinaud classification). This area is located on the left side of Cantlie line and simply identified after occlusion of the left portal vein and the left hepatic artery. The left and middle hepatic veins drain vessels from left hemi-liver.

The indications for this type of resection are various benign or malignant tumors, direct invasion of the gastric malignant tumor, complex liver cystic diseases or intrahepatic duct stones and finally traumatic liver injury involving segments 2, 3 and 4.

Patients with severe cardiopulmonary impairment that cannot tolerate general anesthesia as well as those with distant metastasis or intraperitoneal seeding of malignant tumor are contraindicated for surgery.

The patient is held on an operative table in supine position, with the left arm attached to the body.

The generally used xiphoumbilical median incision is adequate to resect left hemi-liver but occasionally other large incisions may be needed depending on tumor size: a transverse incision may be combined with the median incision, or a bilateral subcostal incision alongside upper median extension (Fig. 4.1).

Mobilization of left hemi-liver is the first step in this surgery and is completed by division of the umbilical, the falciform, the left coronary, and the left triangular ligaments (Fig. 4.2).

Division of the falciform ligament occurs along the anterior surface of IVC to expose the right hepatic, the left hepatic, and the middle hepatic vein inlets into the IVC (Fig. 4.3).

Supplementary Information The online version contains supplementary material available at https://doi.org/10.1007/978-981-16-1996-0_4.

J. S. Choi (✉)
Division of Hepatopancreaticobiliary Surgery, Department of Surgery, Yonsei University College of Medicine, Seoul, South Korea
e-mail: choi5491@yuhs.ac

H. C. Yu (ed.), *Hepato-Biliary-Pancreatic Surgery and Liver Transplantation*,
https://doi.org/10.1007/978-981-16-1996-0_4

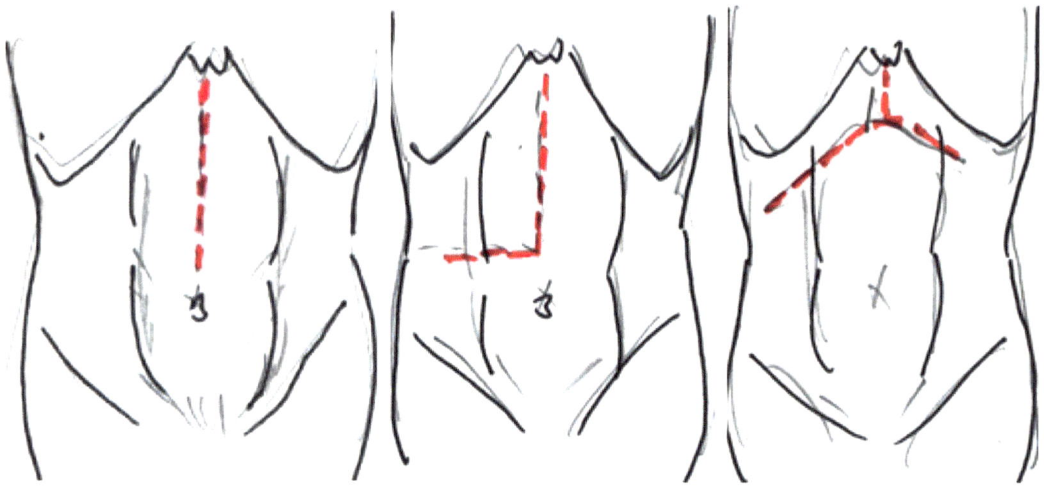

Fig. 4.1 Various types of skin incision

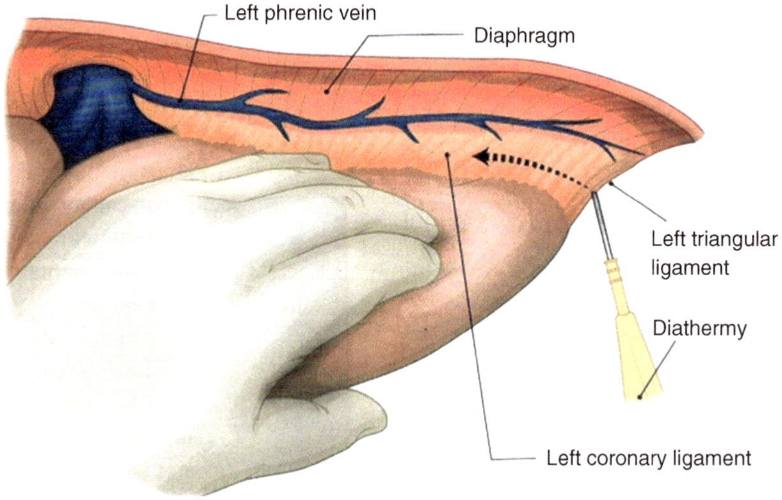

Fig. 4.2 Dissection of the left coronary and the left triangular ligaments

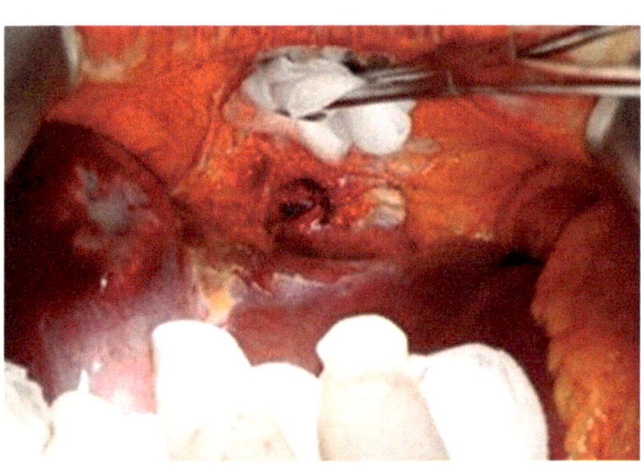

Fig. 4.3 Dissection of the falciform ligament exposes the anterior wall of inferior vena cava and common trunk of the middle and left hepatic veins

The anterior leaflet of the left coronary ligament is divided from the left side of the left hepatic vein and IVC, and proceeds to the left side. Occasionally, the left diaphragmatic vein crosses the left coronary ligament, and it should be ligated and divided. The left triangular vein also must be ligated and divided to avoid unnecessary bleeding.

Division of the lesser omentum is the next step in liver mobilization. The lesser omentum should be divided close to the liver parenchyma with great care to identify accessory or aberrant left hepatic artery from the left gastric artery or celiac trunk (Fig. 4.4).

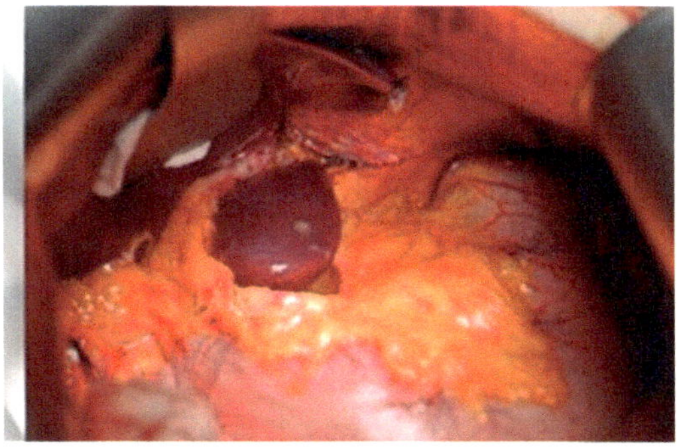

Fig. 4.4 The lesser omentum often contains aberrant left hepatic artery

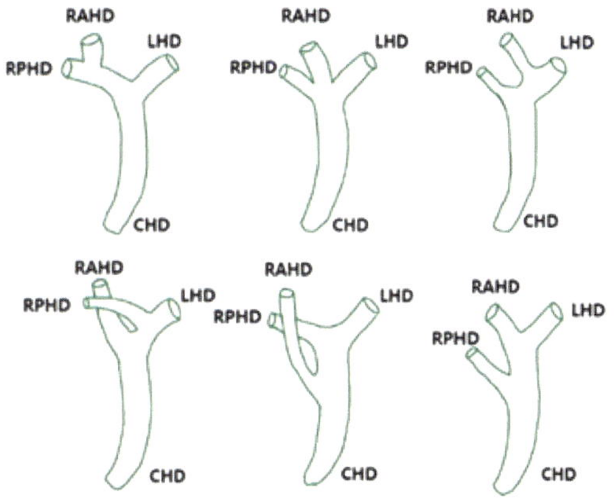

Fig. 4.5 Variation of the biliary system

The hilar dissection is performed after completion of liver mobilization. The umbilical ligament is pulled upward, and the cholecystectomy is carried out initially. The anatomy of bile duct should be identified by MRCP before operation or via intraoperative cholangiography to identify any bile duct variant (Fig. 4.5).

The anterior peritoneum of hepatoduodenal ligament is divided transversely. The common hepatic, right hepatic, middle hepatic, and left hepatic arteries are identified via careful dissection of loose connective tissue and neural plexus in the hepatoduodenal ligament (Fig. 4.6).

The left and middle hepatic arteries are divided after double or fixed ligatures. Below the artery, the left surface of the main or left portal vein is exposed following further dissection of loose connective tissue and neural plexus along the left side of hepatoduodenal ligament. The left portal vein is identified after further cranial dissection (Fig. 4.7).

A few small caudate branches are found on the posterior aspect of the left portal vein, 1–2 cm from the main portal bifurcation, and saved to preserve caudate blood flow (Fig. 4.8).

The left portal vein is divided above the caudate branch between double or transfixed ligatures. The left bile duct is not handled during this stage and will be managed during parenchymal division.

The left hemi-liver becomes ischemic after the left portal vein ligation. The ischemic demarcated area is easily identified, and the Glisson

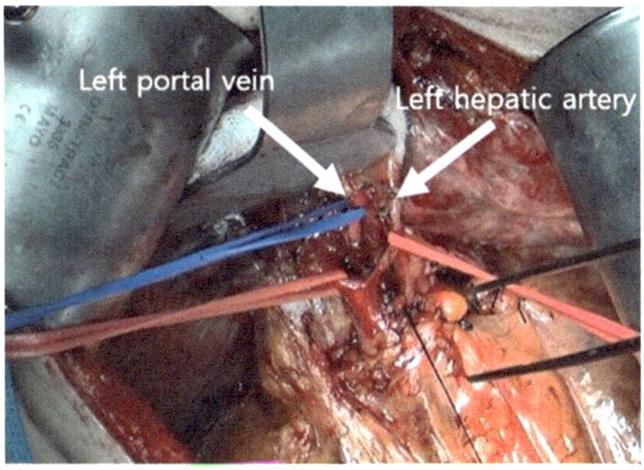

Fig. 4.6 Dissection of liver hilum

capsule on the anterior surface is incised via electrocautery as the parenchyma division line (Fig. 4.9).

The parenchymal division is conducted via classical Kelly clamp crushing or with an ultrasonic device or other energy devices. The parenchymal division proceeds from the caudal area to the cranial side between the right side of sagittal hepatic vein and the left side of middle hepatic vein along the Cantlie line. The left hilar plate should not be damaged during parenchymal division to protect the right posterior bile duct, which runs into the left hepatic duct. The left hepatic duct encountered during parenchyma division is divided as far as possible from main duct bifurcation via en-bloc ligature or transfixed stitch using a 4-0 monofilament suture (Fig. 4.10).

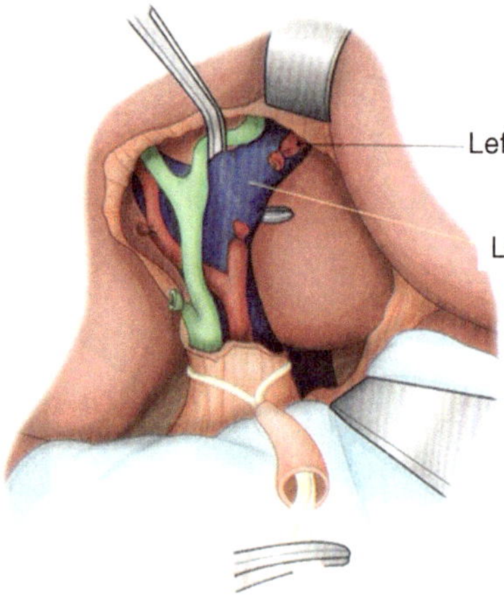

Fig. 4.7 Dissection of the left portal vein

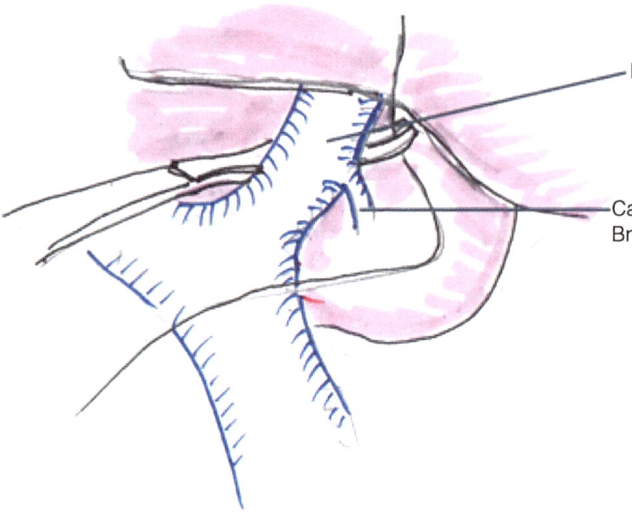

Fig. 4.8 Caudate branch of the left portal vein

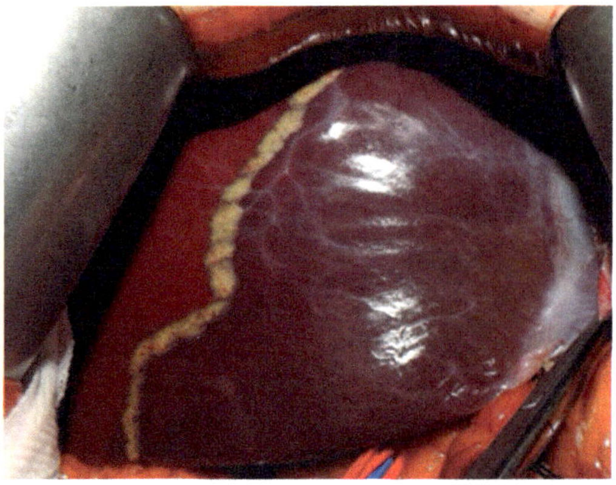

Fig. 4.9 Discoloration of the left liver along the Cantlie line

The parenchymal division into common trunk of the middle and left hepatic veins continues after division of the medial branch of the middle hepatic vein. The left hepatic vein is clamped and divided, and the stump of the left hepatic vein is sutured with 5-0 monofilament running stitches.

Any bleeding must be controlled via electrocautery, sutures, or topical agents. Any bile leakage or bile duct damage must be controlled appropriately.

The operation is completed after positioning the closed suction drain in the dead space.

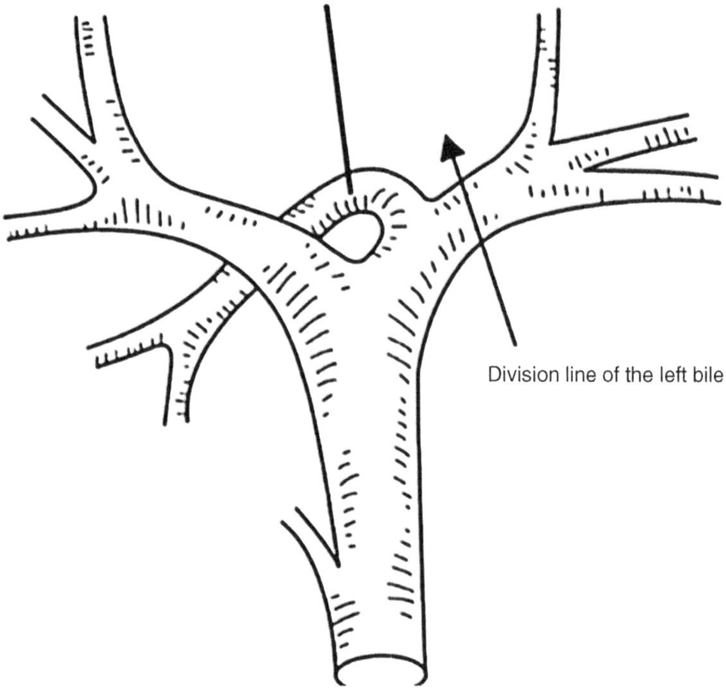

Fig. 4.10 Division of the left bile duct avoiding injury to the right posterior bile duct

5 Right Hemihepatectomy

Yoon Jin Hwang and Hyung Jun Kwon

Abstract

The right hemihepatectomy is a standardized procedure. It entails resection of liver parenchyma on the right side of the Cantlie line towards the right of the middle hepatic vein. According to the new classification proposed by the International Hepato-Pancreato-Biliary Association in 2000, the right hepatectomy entails resection of segments V, VI, VII, and VIII. The right hepatectomy is mostly indicated for primary liver or biliary malignancies involving metastatic tumors, particularly metastatic colorectal cancer. Less frequently, this operation is indicated for large, symptomatic benign tumors or for large retroperitoneal tumors involving the right liver. Rarely, liver or biliary infections or bile duct injuries are an indication for the right hepatectomy. Tumors involving the main inflow pedicle and/or outflow venous drainage to the right liver typically require right hepatectomy for removal. Similarly, this procedure is required for diffuse tumors involving most of the parenchyma or all segments of the right liver. The right hepatectomy is a major liver resection that requires preoperative liver function, resectability, and assessment of future liver remnant (FLR) volume.

Keywords

Liver · Surgery · Resection · Right Hepatectomy

Supplementary Information The online version contains supplementary material available at https://doi.org/10.1007/978-981-16-1996-0_5.

Y. J. Hwang (✉) · H. J. Kwon
Department of Surgery, School of Medicine, Kyungpook National University, Daegu, South Korea
e-mail: yjhwang@knu.ac.kr

5.1 Position

The patient is placed in supine position with the right arm at 90° of abduction.

5.2 Laparotomy

Although various laparotomy approaches can be used, generally, an inverted L-incision is made as a median incision extending to the right at a 90° angle. The incision to the right can be extended as needed, and the incision should be at least 2–3 cm away from the costal margin. The xiphoid process can be removed to secure the surgical field of view, and the round ligament at the bottom of the median incision is used to pull the liver during liver resection. After the falciform ligament is dissected in a cephalad direction, two retractors are used to retract both the costal margins to expose the right upper quadrant.

H. C. Yu (ed.), *Hepato-Biliary-Pancreatic Surgery and Liver Transplantation*,
https://doi.org/10.1007/978-981-16-1996-0_5

5.3 Mobilization of Right Liver and Identification of Right Hepatic Vein

A longitudinal incision is made on the right side of the hepatoduodenal ligament for ligation, and cutting of the cystic artery and duct. After resection of the gallbladder, as the right liver is wrapped with gauze and retracted downward left in a rolling motion, the falciform and the right coronary ligaments are dissected. The falciform ligament is first dissected from the abdominal wall until the inferior vena cava of the upper liver is exposed. The right coronary ligament is then dissected as close to the liver as possible to prevent bleeding from damage to diaphragm and its vessels. At this time, the connective tissue between the middle hepatic vein and the right hepatic vein is dissected, and the right hepatic vein is identified. The right liver is then retracted upwards left to dissect the right triangular ligament to advance into the bare area. As the right liver is retracted in a cephalad direction, the hepatorenal ligament is dissected to expose the anterior wall and the right wall of the inferior vena cava. As the right liver is retracted upwards left once again, the dissection of the bare area dissection downwards exposes the anterior side of the right adrenal gland. In some cases, the right adrenal gland is firmly adhered to the right liver, causing excessive bleeding during the dissection. In these cases, instead of dissecting the adrenal gland from the liver, after inserting tonsil forceps in a cephalad direction from the caudal side between the adrenal gland and the right wall of the inferior vena cava, vascular clamps are applied to the sides of the liver and the adrenal gland, cut between them, and the cut surfaces are continuously sutured with Prolene. On the cranial side, the right wall of the inferior vena cava is exposed after the ligation and cutting of the firm inferior vena cava ligament. Occasionally, short hepatic veins or right posterior hepatic veins are located close to the inferior vena cava ligament. In such cases, the tonsil forceps must be inserted in a cephalad direction from the caudal side, ensuring that the veins are not injured during the ligation and cutting of the ligament. After exposing the right wall of the inferior vena cava, the right liver is retracted and elevated left anteriorly to dissect between the inferior vena cava and the liver, and short hepatic veins may be exposed in the process. Short hepatic veins are sequentially ligated and cut to reach the left side of the inferior vena cava, cautious about occasional re-bleeding from ligation sites. If necessary, the stump on the inferior vena cava side can be ligated once or twice and additionally clipped above the ligation site to prevent loss of the ligation. Larger short hepatic veins may be continuously sutured with Prolene to prevent bleeding. After ligation of the short hepatic veins, the gap between the middle hepatic vein and the right hepatic vein along the anterior side of the inferior vena cava on the cranial side can be identified. Kelly forceps are inserted along the gap from the caudal to the cranial sides, and the Penrose drainage tube is passed around the right hepatic vein for elevation during the hanging maneuver.

5.4 Hepatic Hilum Manipulation

5.4.1 Hepatic Hilar Vessel Manipulation

The bile duct is first located, and the cystic duct stump suture is pulled with tonsil forceps, followed by longitudinal dissection of the connective tissue below the bile duct on the right side towards the hilum. The right hepatic artery is identified. The right hepatic artery is blocked by pulling the previously inserted Penrose drainage tube and using the Bulldog vascular clamp. The course and the blood flow of the left hepatic artery is then determined. Note that the aberrant right hepatic artery can be identified at a frequency of 10–15%. Once the left hepatic artery has been evaluated, the right hepatic artery is ligated twice and cut (Fig. 5.1). The right wall of the portal vein is exposed by dissecting connective tissue on the dorsal side of the right hepatic artery while pulling the extrahepatic bile duct and the right hepatic artery to the left with vein retractors. When the right wall of the portal vein is exposed, the anterior wall of the right portal vein

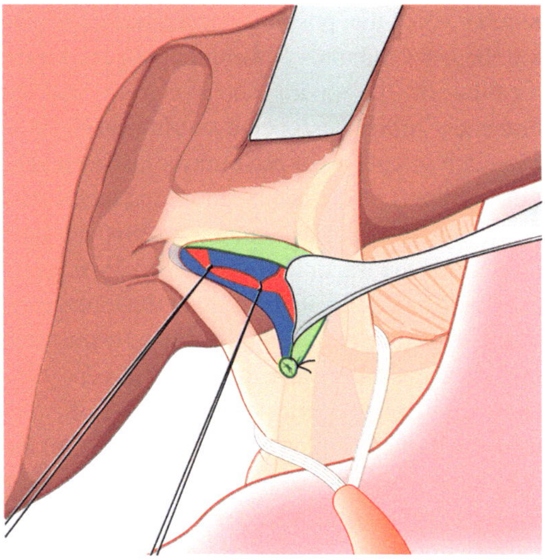

Fig. 5.1 Ligation of the right hepatic artery. The right hepatic artery can be identified via longitudinal dissection of the connective tissue towards the portal vein, followed by retraction

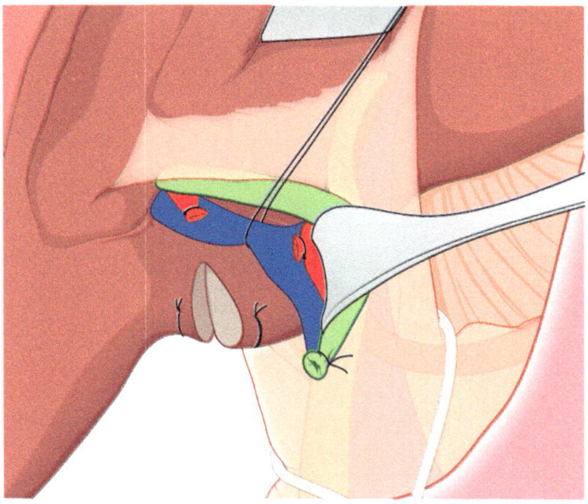

Fig. 5.2 Identification of the right portal vein. The right wall of the portal vein is exposed as the extrahepatic duct, and the right portal vein is retracted to the left with the vein retractors. The connective tissue dorsal to the right hepatic duct is dissected

is dissected to expose the root of anterior and posterior branches. The anterior side of the portal vein is then exposed. After evaluating the root of the left and right portal veins, pulling the right portal vein in the caudad direction with the Debakey forceps at the root of the right portal vein, the dissection is advanced dorsally from the cranial side. Any caudate branch encountered should be ligated and cut carefully to prevent tears. The same dissection is performed in a cephalad direction from the ventrodorsal side, hang the right portal vein with the vessel loop using the Mixter forceps (Fig. 5.2). After the above dissection is completed, the blood flow of the right hepatic artery and the right portal vein is blocked temporarily using the Bulldog vascular clamp, and the area of blood flow blockage along the Cantlie line is determined. The ligation of the right hepatic artery and the right portal vein may be performed before or after the parenchymal transection as needed. Using the vein retractor, the hepatoduodenal ligament is pulled to the left at a 45° angle, to identify the caudate lobe below the right hepatic portal vein. After the demarcation line is drawn using an electric cautery machine on the right margin of the inferior vena cava at the boundary of the right lobe and the caudate lobe, each side of the demarcation line is suture-ligated with 3-0 Prolene. While retracting the sutures, the liver parenchyma is transected to a depth of 2–3 cm.

5.4.2 Manipulation of Glisson Pedicle

The Glisson capsule covering the left and right branches of the Glisson pedicle is cut horizontally at the lower margin of quadrate lobe, with an electric cautery machine, and the hilar plate is dissected from the liver parenchyma using the suction tip. In the process, a thin Glisson pedicle may be encountered, which is ligated and cut with care. After the dissection is completed adequately 1 cm to the left and the right, it is advanced dorsally. Even if bleeding occurs in the liver parenchyma, it can be easily controlled by applying pressure and proceed to the next step. While inserting Mixter forceps from the dorsal to the caudal side, penetrating the space between the Glisson capsule and the liver parenchyma, the hepatoduodenal ligament is pulled using the vein retractor at a 45° angle to the left, to evaluate below the ligament. If resistance is felt at the end of the Mixter forceps, it is important not to force the insertion, instead, the area with the least resis-

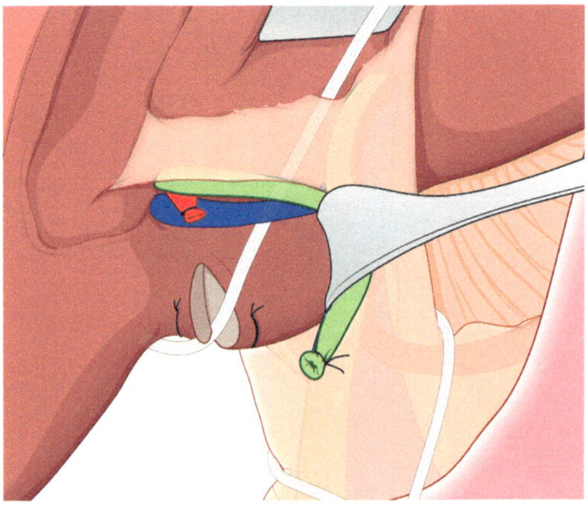

Fig. 5.3 Manipulation of the Glisson pedicle and the Penrose drainage tube insertion. The hepatic hilum is dissected from the liver parenchyma, and the Penrose drainage tube is inserted between the Glisson capsule and the liver parenchyma

tance should be selected, in order to avoid damage to the Glisson pedicle. After dissection, the previously inserted Penrose drainage tube is passed along the transection site of the caudate lobe and placed at the back of the treated Glisson pedicle (Fig. 5.3).

5.5 Liver Resection

For liver transection, it is recommended to lower the central venous pressure to 5 cm H_2O or less. In order to reduce the amount of bleeding during liver transection, the Pringle technique, which intermittently blocks and reperfuses the liver via hepatic artery and the portal vein as needed, is used. After making an incision in the avascular area of the lesser omentum on the left side of the hepatoduodenal ligament, the right-angle clamp is passed under the hepatoduodenal ligament and covered with the umbilical tape. The blood circulation is regulated by the tape on the tourniquet. Until the liver transection is completed, the blood flow is repeatedly blocked for 15 min, and then reperfused for 5 min. The liver transection is carried out considering the tumor location and the demarcation line on the liver surface. The liver transection is performed after identifying the size, number, and the positional relationship of the intrahepatic structures of the tumor, especially the location of the middle hepatic vein and its branches, using intraoperative ultrasound. It is more advantageous to perform the liver transection 1 cm left of the demarcation line on the surface of the liver. A stay suture with No.0 chromic is used for the traction of the imaginary transection line to the left and the right at the lower edge of the liver. The two methods of liver transection include the CUSA® and the Kelly forceps. The liver parenchyma is crushed using the CUSA® or the Kelly forceps, followed by cauterization of the remaining Glisson pedicle and hepatic vein branches with an electrocautery machine, and the larger branches are clipped or ligated. The goal of liver transection is to proceed broadly and thinly in order to easily stop the bleeding of the hepatic vein. The liver transection proceeds along the right margin of the middle hepatic vein. When more than 50% of liver transection is completed, including the liver parenchyma in the hilar direction, the liver transection is continued after elevating the Penrose drainage tube that was previously passed through the gap between the right hepatic vein and the middle hepatic vein for the hanging maneuver (Fig. 5.4). Hanging maneuver reduces

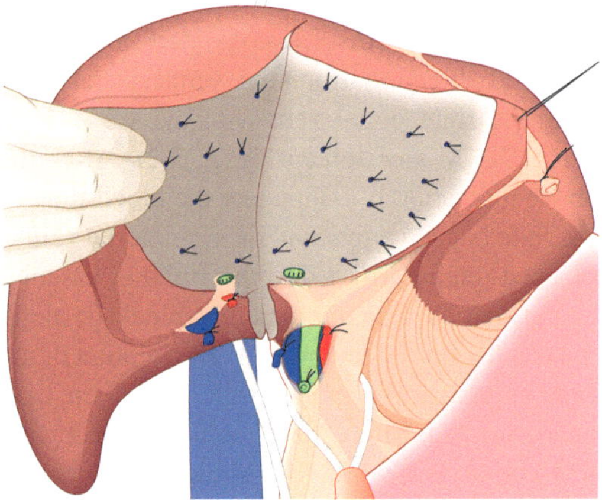

Fig. 5.4 Transection of the liver parenchyma. After crushing the liver parenchyma, the remaining Glisson pedicle and hepatic vein branches are cauterized with an electrocautery machine, and the larger branches are clipped or ligated

the anterior dissection area of the inferior vena cava which is invisible. It also reduces bleeding by compressing the transection surface. Also, it is possible to maintain the parenchymal transection direction along the straight plane of transection. If the right hepatic artery and the right portal vein branches are not ligated before the liver transection, the right hepatic duct, the right hepatic artery, and then the right portal vein branches are ligated, cut, and elevated. After the transection of the liver parenchyma, the right hepatic vein is ligated in the last step using the vascular TA®.

5.6 Drainage Tube Insertion, Closure

The Jackson-Pratt drainage tube is placed below the right diaphragm, in the direction of the transection surface and the abdomen is closed.

5.7 Bleeding Control, Bile Leakage Test and Fixation of Falciform Ligament

In the event of bleeding from the liver transection surface, the bleeding site is cautcrized using tools like argon beam coagulator or sutures if the bleeding cannot be controlled. When the leak test is performed, a tube with a small diameter is inserted through the cystic duct, indigo carmine pigment mixed with normal saline is injected to evaluate leakage, and the leaked area is closed with sutures.

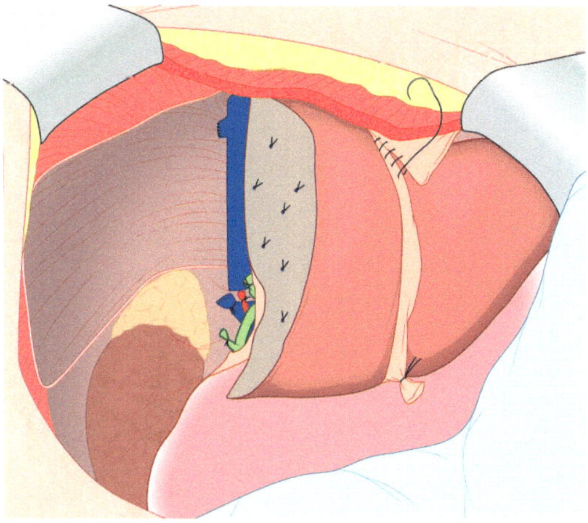

Fig. 5.5 Evaluation of the transection surface and fixation of the falciform ligament. The liver transection surface, ligated bile duct, and vessels are evaluated for bleeding and leakage, and the falciform ligament is fixed

The falciform ligament should be fixed to the abdominal wall in its original position to prevent the rotation of the remaining left liver (Fig. 5.5).

Central Bisectionectomy

6

Kyung Sik Kim

Abstract

Central bisectionectomy (mesohepatectomy) is a procedure used to resect the central region of the liver (IVA, IVB, V, and VIII) that drains into the middle hepatic vein. It can be used to overcome the challenges due to insufficient residual liver volume by reducing the volume of resected liver. The safety procedure has been established after improvement in the understanding of liver anatomy and the development of surgical equipment.

Keywords

Central bisectionectomy · Mesohepatectomy Middle hepatic vein · Extensive hepatic resection · Insufficient residual liver volume Liver failure

Extended hepatectomy or non-anatomical liver resection is indicated for tumors located in the Couinaud segments 4, 5, and 8 (Fig. 6.1a). However, in the case of extensive hepatic resection, a large portion of the liver parenchyma is removed, and the remaining liver volume is small, leading to liver failure and mortality. Therefore, there are limitations in surgical approach for patients with liver cancer accompanied by liver cirrhosis.

Central bisectionectomy (mesohepatectomy) is a procedure used to remove the central region of the liver (IVA, IVB, V, and VIII) that drains into the middle hepatic vein [1]. This procedure was first attempted in 1972 with a patient with gallbladder cancer. It has been applied in patients with bile duct and liver cancer. It can be used to overcome the challenges due to insufficient residual liver volume by reducing the volume of resected liver. The safety of the procedure has been established with the advancement in understanding of liver anatomy and the development of surgical equipment. It can also be performed as a laparoscopic surgery [2].

Supplementary Information The online version contains supplementary material available at https://doi.org/10.1007/978-981-16-1996-0_6.

K. S. Kim (✉)
Department of Hepatobiliary and Pancreatic Surgery, Severance Hospital, Yonsei University College of Medicine, Seoul, South Korea
e-mail: kskim88@yuhs.ac

H. C. Yu (ed.), *Hepato-Biliary-Pancreatic Surgery and Liver Transplantation*,
https://doi.org/10.1007/978-981-16-1996-0_6

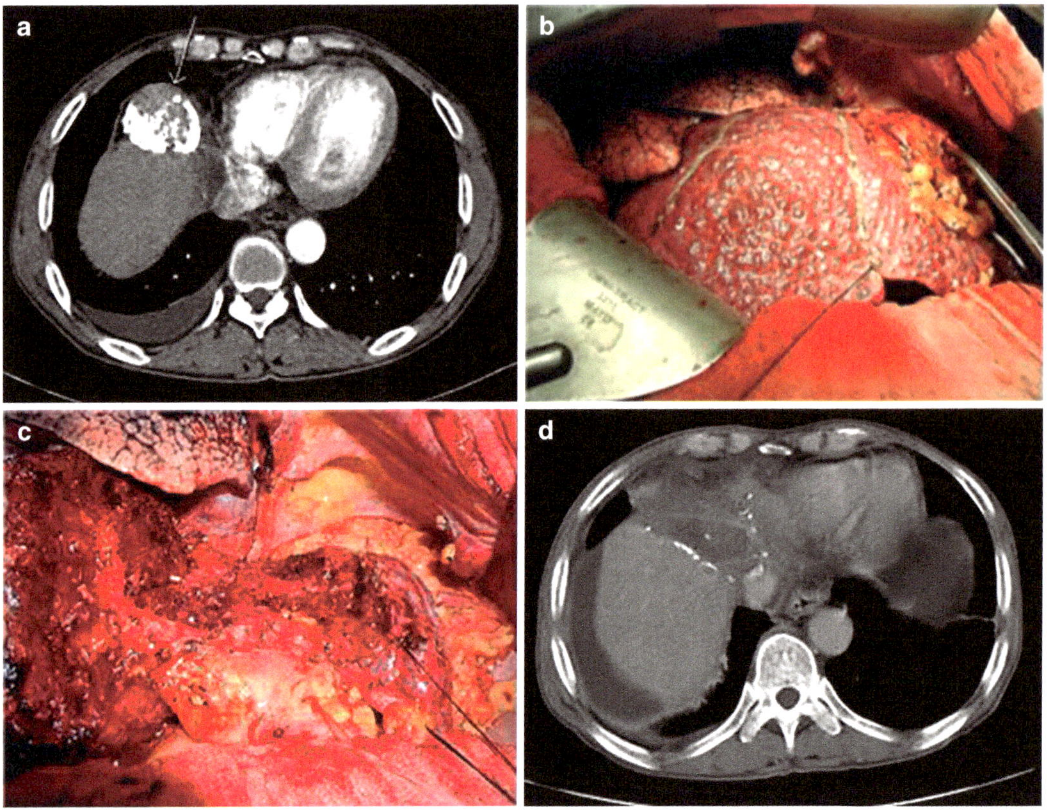

Fig. 6.1 (**a**) The CT scan showed the uptake of lipiodol in the hepatocellular carcinoma located in Segment VIII. (**b**) The dissection planes determined by intraoperative ultrasonography were marked along the medial side of the falciform ligament and right anterior fissure. (**c**) The raw surfaces of the residual liver following delivery of the specimen exposing portal and hepatic veins. (**d**) The follow-up CT scan taken at postoperative seventh day. *RHV* right hepatic vein, *LHV* left hepatic vein, *RPV* right portal vein, *LPV* left portal vein

6.1 Preoperative Preparation

Liver function must be evaluated based on the Child-Pugh score and the ICG R15 test. Computed tomography (CT) and abdominal magnetic resonance imaging (MRI) are performed prior to surgery to evaluate the resectability and the anatomy of blood vessels and bile ducts. Recently, it has been possible to obtain increasingly accurate information via 3D image reconstruction using CT or MRI data. Also, the estimation of the resecting and remaining volume of the liver is very important in preparation for possible liver failure after surgery.

6.2 Operative Procedures [3]

Skin incision can be made in several ways, but in my experience, the skin incision is made right under the sternum along with a midline of about 4 cm, spanning the ribs until the right anterior axillary line. A subcostal transverse skin incision is made. A part of the falciform ligament and the left and right coronary ligaments are divided to expose the whole liver. The left triangular ligament is not resected to prevent the instability of the remaining hepatic parenchyma after the resection of the central zones. Later, the retractor is applied to ensure the operative field.

The two blades of the retractor are used in the left and the right sides of the median incision and one blade of the retractor is applied at the end of the right subcostal incision. If necessary, an additional retractor blade compressing the gastrointestinal tract is used to prevent protrusion. Intraoperative ultrasonography is performed to confirm the location of tumor and the course of surrounding vessels and bile duct. The location of the tumor, its spread to the surrounding area, liver metastasis, and tumor embolism in the portal vein or hepatic vein are also evaluated. At this time, the three-dimensional relationship between the tumor and the related veins like portal vein and hepatic vein is confirmed to establish the resection boundary. A mark is made between the driving direction of the right hepatic vein and the left and inner and outer regions (Fig. 6.1b).

Next, the cystic duct and the cystic artery are divided to expose the hepatic hilum, and the left side of the right hepatic artery, the left side of the right hepatic portal vein, and the common hepatic duct are detached and taped. Vascular isolation techniques are used to minimize bleeding during parenchymal resection, to reduce residual liver ischemic damage, and to delineate the resection boundary. In particular, it is necessary to note the direction of the pathway of the middle hepatic artery while performing a meticulous hepatic dissection. Parenchymal resection is carried out by pulling the round ligament upward, lifting the left liver upward, and starting the parenchymal resection at the right side of the umbilical fissure first, then heading to the medial region. The liver parenchyma is divided with CUSA®. The arterial branch, portal branch, and bile duct entering the liver area 4 from the front are ligated, but in the event of extensive bleeding, the blood circulation should be temporarily blocked to the left hepatic artery and portal vein, which were previously isolated and looped, to induce ischemia. Hemostasis is induced by packing gauze on the resected surface to treat the middle vein when the hepatic parenchymal resection reached the middle venous root under a good field of view. Hepatic parenchymal resection of the right anterior segment is initiated to the left along the direction of the right hepatic vein marked in advance, exposing the root of the right hepatic vein, and simultaneously continuing to cut toward the hepatic portal, cutting the parenchyma on the left. When the right anterior Glisson's sheath is exposed, double-ligation or hemlock is used to cut. After lifting the center 2 area liver parenchyma, the middle vein is ligated using an automatic vascular suture (Fig. 6.1c).

A schematic diagram of the central bisectionectomy is shown in Fig. 6.2.

Since biloma formation is the most common complication in central bisectionectomy, it is very important to confirm the absence of biliary fistula in the branches of the bile duct. In the past, biliary tract imaging was performed during surgery, but recently, injection into the cystic duct using air and saline or a fluid containing lipid has been used to confirm damage to the bile duct. In the case of methylene blue, it can be seen clearly at first, but is not recommended because the surrounding tissue is stained, thus disabling further identification. When no further bleeding from the resection surface or damage to the biliary tract is detected, the drainage tube is mounted on the resection surface similar to the conventional procedure, and the abdominal wall is closed.

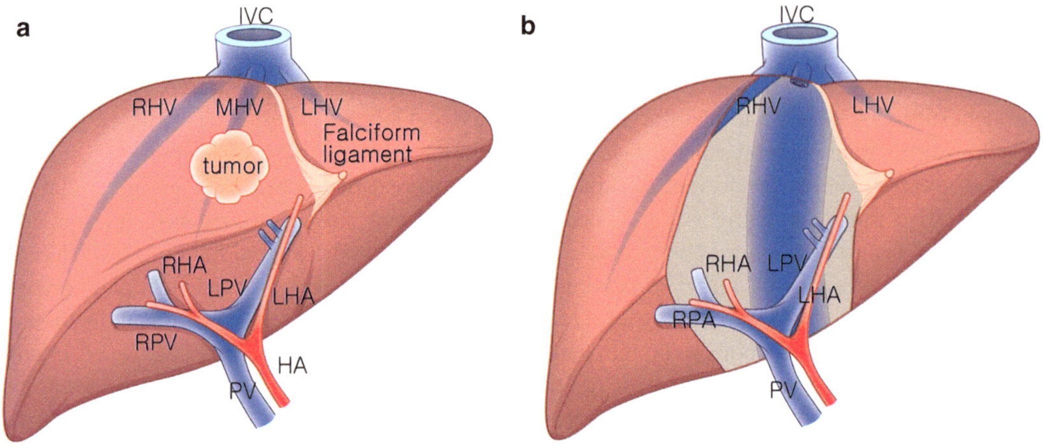

Fig. 6.2 (**a**) Schematic figures of the central bisectionectomy. The tumor is located at segments 4 and 5 of the liver above the middle hepatic vein (MHV). (**b**) The medial aspect of the falciform ligament is transected firstly, and right anterior section is transected. After the specimen is delivered, MHV, RHV, and IVC are exposed at raw surface of the residual liver. *IVC* Inferior vena cava, *MHV* middle hepatic vein, *HA* hepatic artery, *PV* portal vein

6.3 Postoperative Care

Common complications that can occur after central bisectionectomy include biliary tract leakage, pleural effusion, ascites, wound infection, abscess in the abdominal cavity, and liver failure (Fig. 6.1d). In the case of liver resection without reconstruction of the biliary tract, the possibility of biliary leakage which depends on the presence or absence of cirrhosis is reported to be about 4–12%. The possibility of bile leakage from small-sized bile duct cannot be predicted by intraoperative bile leakage tests. In the case of bile leakage, dead spaces after hepatic resection can lead to bacterial overgrowth, so proper following treatments are needed. Recently, nonsurgical drainage is performed with good results. Intraperitoneal infection is often an unavoidable complication and can even lead to sepsis if there is abscess in the abdominal cavity. For this reason, a close postoperative monitoring is needed during the entire admission period. In recent years, infection rate has decreased sharply, to less than 3%, which is attributed to several advances in the management of hepatic resection.

Recent trends in intraperitoneal drainage suggest that intrahepatic jejunal anastomosis is not needed during partial hepatic resection. In some cases, drainage is not performed, but in the case of central bisectionectomy, it is recommended to perform closed suction drainage to prevent retrograde infection. In my experience, abdomen CT is performed to evaluate liver regeneration and fluid retention in the abdominal cavity on 5 days after surgery. The drainage tube is removed when there is no bile collection or the signs of infection in the abdominal cavity. Conservative treatments such as enteral nutrition is considered with the improvement of patient's condition.

From January 1998 to April 2007, 27 cases of central bisectionectomy for liver cancer in the central region were performed at Yonsei University Severance Hospital [4]. The results show that the operation time ranged from 215 to 669 min (median value of 330 min), and the amount of bleeding ranged from 550 to 7000 mL (median value 1400 mL). Postoperative resection margins ranged from 0.1 to 4.0 cm (median value of 1.5 cm). Postsurgical complications occurred in 12 cases including 5 cases of biloma, 5 cases of pleural effusion, and 2 cases of ascites. Conservative treatment such as percutaneous bile drainage was required. There were eight cases of recurrence during the follow-up period (1.4–102.2 months, median value 19.1 months). Therefore, a careful follow-up is considered necessary.

6.4 Conclusion

Despite the chance of biliary tract complications, central bisectionectomy is one of the promising procedures that can be performed for the treatment of malignant tumors located in the middle part of the liver, while preserving the volume of the remaining liver.

References

1. Gallagher TK, Chan AC, Poon RT, Cheung TT, Chok KS, Chan SC, Lo CM. Outcomes of central bisectionectomy for hepatocellular carcinoma. HPB (Oxford). 2013;15(7):529–34.
2. Yoon YS, Han HS, Cho JY, Ahn KS. Totally laparoscopic central bisectionectomy for hepatocellular carcinoma. J Laparoendosc Adv Surg Tech A. 2009;19(5):653–6.
3. Yanaga K. Central bisectionectomy (bisegmentectomy) of the liver (with video). J Hepatobiliary Pancreat Sci. 2012;19(1):44–7.
4. Lee JG, Choi SB, Kim KS, Choi JS, Lee WJ, Kim BR. Central bisectionectomy for centrally located hepatocellular carcinoma. Br J Surg. 2008;95(8):990–5.

7 Left Lateral Sectionectomy

Tae-Jin Song

Abstract

The left lateral section, involving the second and third segments of the left lobe of the liver, is a frequent location of benign diseases such as intrahepatic cholelithiasis and malignant diseases such as primary hepatocellular carcinoma or metastatic cancer. Although it is considered to be an area that is relatively easy to access, severe peripheral adhesion due to repeated inflammation leads to deformation of the anatomical structure via association with the surrounding organs or after abdominal surgery, and is often difficult to access or resect.

The lateral sectionectomy method during liver resection depends on the surgical evaluation of the local lesion. Herein, anatomical resection of the second and third segments alone has been discussed, and excludes wedge resection and lesion-limited sub-segmental resection of segments 2 or 3, such as enucleation and atypical liver resection.

In recent years, due to the popularity of laparoscopic hepatectomy, left lateral sectionectomy is mostly performed via laparoscopy or robotic minimally invasive surgeries.

Keywords

Left lateral section · Left lateral sectionectomy · Atypical resection · Laparoscopic resection · Robotic resection

The left lateral section, involving the second and third segments of the left lobe of the liver, is a frequent location of benign diseases such as intrahepatic cholelithiasis, and malignant diseases such as primary hepatocellular carcinoma or metastatic cancer. It is the area that is considered relatively easy to access. However, severe peripheral adhesion due to repeated inflammation leads to deformation of the anatomical structure via association with the surrounding organs or after abdominal surgery, and is often difficult to access or resect. However, location in the lateral segments 2 or 3 may interfere with pre- and post-operative evaluation depending on the preference of each surgeon or different institution [1–3].

Supplementary Information The online version contains supplementary material available at https://doi.org/10.1007/978-981-16-1996-0_7.

T.-J. Song (✉)
Department of Surgery, Korea University College of Medicine, Korea University Ansan Hospital, Ansan-si, Gyeonggi-do, South Korea
e-mail: tjsong@korea.ac.kr

H. C. Yu (ed.), *Hepato-Biliary-Pancreatic Surgery and Liver Transplantation*,
https://doi.org/10.1007/978-981-16-1996-0_7

The method of lateral sectionectomy during liver resection depends on the surgical evaluation of the local lesion. However, anatomical resection of the second and third segments alone is discussed here, and excludes wedge resection and lesion-limited sub-segmental resection of segments 2 or 3, such as enucleation and atypical liver resection.

Initially, during the surgery, the patient assumes a position with the arms wide open or attached to the body depending on conditions in the supine position. Depending on the liver location, it may be convenient to tilt the operating table to raise the head (head-up position) or the patient's left-up position (left-up position), depending each operation.

The left hepatic exposure is generally adequate to open the epigastric midline, and in most cases, this degree of incision ensures sufficient observation and exposure around the lesion (Fig. 7.1). If necessary, visibility can be extended below the umbilical cord. Traction differs with each trachea, such as the Kent retractor, but it is good to perform traction to show the spleen outside the diaphragmatic adhesion site in the outer left lobe area from the left. To prevent spleen damage, the visual field is improved by placing 1–2 surgical cotton pads behind the spleen. The Pringle maneuver is usually unnecessary for two- to three-segment ablation, except in special circumstances [3].

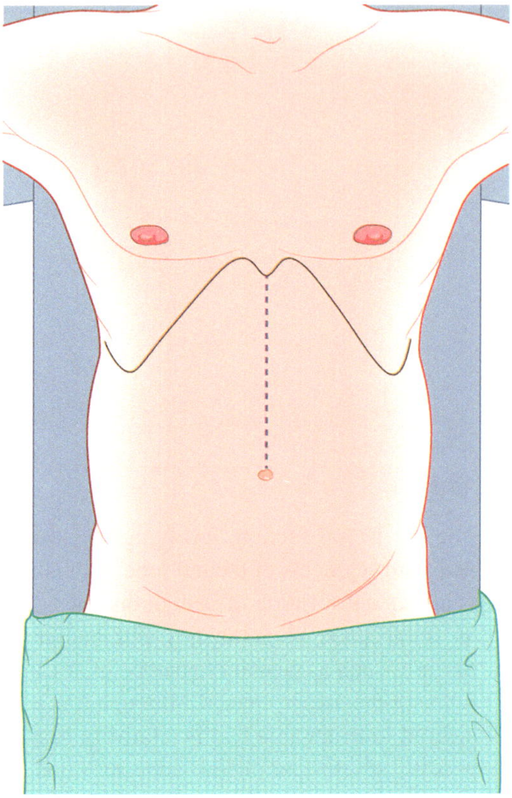

Fig. 7.1 Incision during resection of the lateral section of the liver

In the case of left lateral sectionectomy, the location of the operator and assistant on the right side of the patient is often adequate, and depending on the situation, it may be on the left side. When standing on the right, the first assistant is located on the upper left and the second assistant is located on the lower left. In some cases, the position of the operator and the first assistant can be changed, but differs depending on the situation. The liver is exposed first for the left lateral segment resection, to observe the lesion and the surroundings. As described above, the Pringle maneuver is usually unnecessary, so just in case the hepatic duodenal ligament is wrapped with a cotton tape sling and pulled, only a tourniquet is used for hemostasis. The umbilical ligament and the falciform ligament are cut during the laparotomy and double-ligated for traction. The left triangular ligament is used for traction by pulling the left abdominal wall, and both the sides are ligated and the liver is used for traction. If the falciform ligament contains a lot of fat and is enlarged, or if it is stretched like a curtain, it should be removed via partial resection [4].

Clearing and observation around the incision margin after securing the field of view can establish the lesion via surgical ultrasound and determine the incision margin in the left lateral area. The posterior side becomes the right left margin of the circular ligament. In most cases, the second and third segments of the Glissonian branch are separated, and the thread is slinged to prepare for ligation (Figs. 7.2, 7.3, 7.4 and 7.5). The parenchymal ablation of the liver can be started after appropriate towing and marking for electrosurgery. Before parenchymal resection, the Gleason branches 2 and 3 are ligated and sepa-

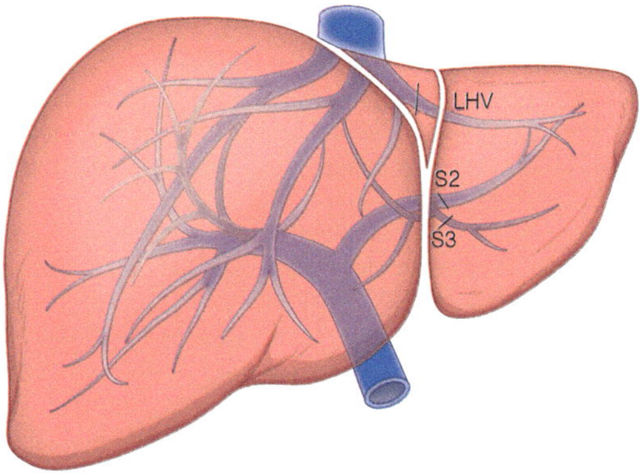

Fig. 7.2 The location of the hepatic vein branches and the second and third Glissonian pedicles in the actual liver

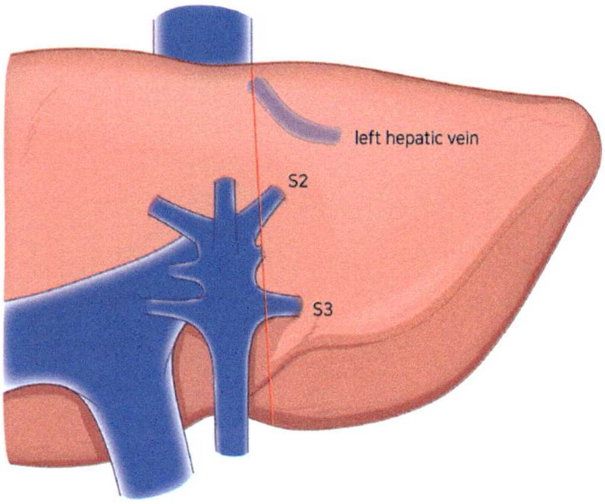

Fig. 7.3 Schematic diagram of the location of the hepatic vein tributary and the second and third Glissonian branches

rated (Figs. 7.4 and 7.5). Laparoscopic ultrasound scalpel (Harmonic scalpel®), which is used in laparoscopic surgery, facilitates the initial parenchymal resection. Monopolar or bipolar electrosurgery is preferred by surgeons.

During parenchymal resection for hemostasis of small blood vessels and bile ducts, if a branch of the left hepatic vein is encountered, it is ligated and cut with a sling (Figs. 7.2 and 7.3). During parenchymal transection, small blood vessels developed, which interfered with hemostasis, or additional hemostatic devices may be required if the patient has a history of anticoagulant use such as aspirin, but often it is not required for lesions associated with the second or third segment.

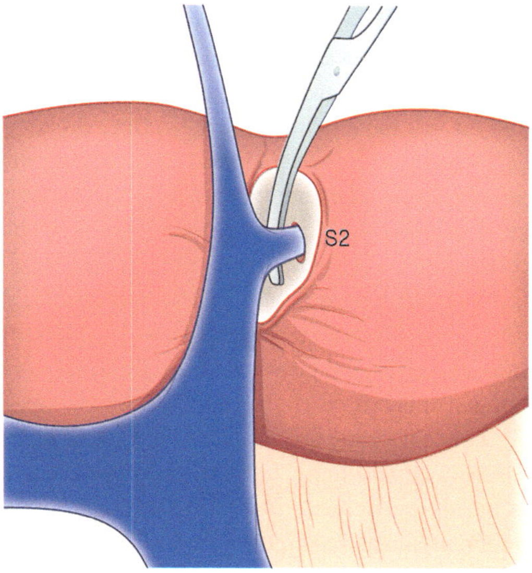

Fig. 7.4 Clamping technique for No. 2 Glissonian branch Sling

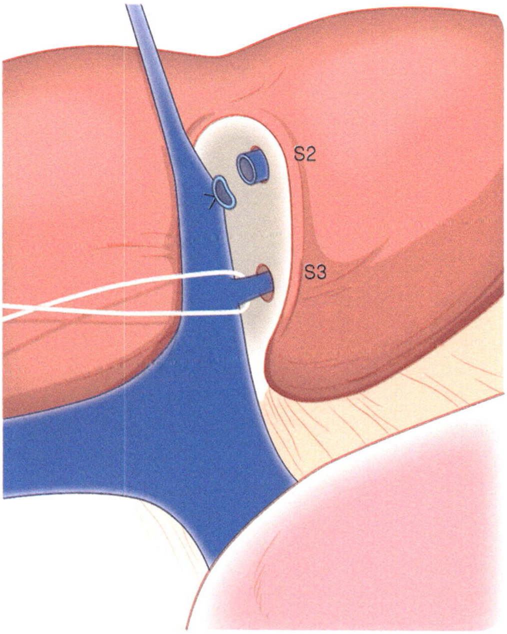

Fig. 7.5 No. 3 Glisson branch Sling

Other areas are the same, but even if the incision is small and not wide, special attention should be paid to bleeding. In some cases, closed suction drains, such as Jackson–Pratt drain may be required. Similar to general open surgery, the abdominal fascia is sutured, and the subcutaneous fat layer is closed. Even in open surgery, subcutaneous sutures are performed to cosmetically enhance the skin. Adhesive glue for skin closure and an automatic skin stapler or approximating suture tape can be selected according to the operator's convenience and preference. The left outer section of the liver is more accessible than the other places and can be relatively easy if it contains an appropriate margin. The philosophical differences between surgeons with different training at various institutions are minimal, and opinions may differ slightly [1–3].

In recent years, due to the popularity of laparoscopic hepatectomy, left lateral sectionectomy is mostly performed via laparoscopy or robotic minimally invasive surgeries [1, 2, 5].

References

1. Belli G, Fantini C, D'Agostino A, et al. Laparoscopic segment VI liver resection using a left lateral decubitus position: a personal modified technique. J Gastrointest Surg. 2008;12:2221–6.
2. Fong Y, Sun RL, Jarnagin W, et al. Analysis of 412 cases of hepatocellular carcinoma at a Western center. Ann Surg. 1999;229:790–9.
3. Song TJ, Ip EW, Fong Y. Hepatocellular carcinoma: current surgical management. Gastroenterology. 2004;127:S248–60.
4. Little SA, Fong Y. Hepatocellular carcinoma: current surgical management. Semin Oncol. 2001;28:474–86.
5. Buell JF, Cherqui D, Geller DA, et al. The international position on laparoscopic liver surgery: the Louisville statement, 2008. Ann Surg. 2009;250:825–30.

8 Right Anterior Sectionectomy

Koo Jeong Kang and Keun Soo Ahn

Abstract

The right anterior section consists of two segments, segment V and segment VIII. After clamp of the right anterior Glissonean pedicle or individual right anterior portal pedicle, ischemic margin of anterior section can be ensured. The hepatic parenchyma is transected right and left according to the demarcation line. Further hepatic transection is performed toward the root of right and mid-hepatic veins. Finally, the right anterior section is removed. In this chapter, the concept and technical details of both open and laparoscopic resections of right anterior sectionectomy are discussed.

Keywords

Hepatocellular carcinoma · Sectionectomy
Anterior section · Glissonean approach
Anatomical resection

8.1 Introduction

Anatomical resection of hepatocellular carcinoma require resection of the hepatic tumor including non-tumor areas. It can also ensure oncologic and surgical safety. The liver consists of eight segments according to the distribution of the portal and the hepatic venous systems. These segments are categorized into right anterior, right posterior, left medial, and left lateral sections (Fig. 8.1) The function of each segment or section is independent, with separate portal and hepatic veins and biliary drainage. Hepatocellular carcinoma spreads via retrograde flow of the portal venous system. Therefore, anatomical resection of each segment or section is safe in terms of hepatic function and oncologic safety. The right anterior section consists of two segments, V and VIII. In this chapter, the concept and technical details of both open and laparoscopic resections of right anterior sectionectomy are discussed.

Supplementary Information The online version contains supplementary material available at https://doi.org/10.1007/978-981-16-1996-0_8.

K. J. Kang (✉) · K. S. Ahn
Division of Hepatobiliary and Pancreatic Surgery, Department of Surgery, Keimyung University Dongsan Hospital, Daegu, South Korea
e-mail: kjkang@dsmc.or.kr

H. C. Yu (ed.), *Hepato-Biliary-Pancreatic Surgery and Liver Transplantation*,
https://doi.org/10.1007/978-981-16-1996-0_8

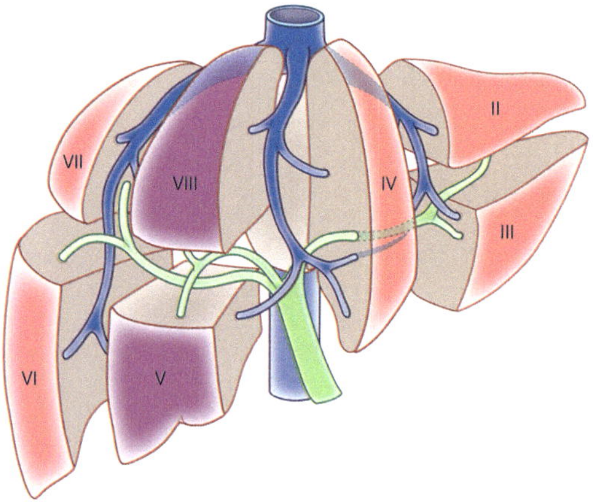

Fig. 8.1 Schematic diagram of the hepatic segments and sections. Right anterior sections include segments 5 and 8

8.2 Indications and Contraindications

Resection of tumors located in the right anterior section requires adequate function of the hepatic reservoir in terms of ICG R15 (<20%), prothrombin time (INR < 1.3), and bilirubin level (<2 mg/dL). Segmentectomy is feasible if the tumor is located in one segment (5 or 8). Tumor confined to the right anterior section with moderate degree of hepatic cirrhosis without extending beyond the right anterior section is a strong indication. If liver function is adequate, further resection including right hemihepatectomy is preferred for good surgical outcome based on convenience and oncologic safety. Otherwise, in case of large tumor or multiple metastatic tumors, the extent of resection should be increased similar to right hemihepatectomy [1].

8.3 Preoperative Evaluation

Preoperative evaluation includes complete blood count, coagulation profiles, and hepatic and renal function tests. Above all, liver function is essential for single section resection according to the resection criteria [2]. Functional assessment of the remaining liver and evaluation of the extent of cirrhosis should be conducted. A Child-Pugh-Turcotte score A is desirable, with a total bilirubin level <2 mg/dL and ICG R15 < 20%. Determination of the extent of hepatic resection and the relationship between vasculature and the volume of future liver remnant requires analysis of not only the cross-sectional images but also the coronary sections of the dynamic CT scan or contrast-enhanced magnetic resonance imaging (MRI) using gadoxetate disodium (Primovist™). In addition, 3D reconstruction images are very useful not only to increase the accuracy of resection margin and future liver remnant volume, but also to delineate anatomical structures (Fig. 8.2). The mass should be located between the right and the mid-hepatic vein, ensuring that the tumor is not in contact with the hepatic veins. Tumor invasion or portal vein thrombosis over the resection territory is not an indication for the right anterior sectionectomy [3].

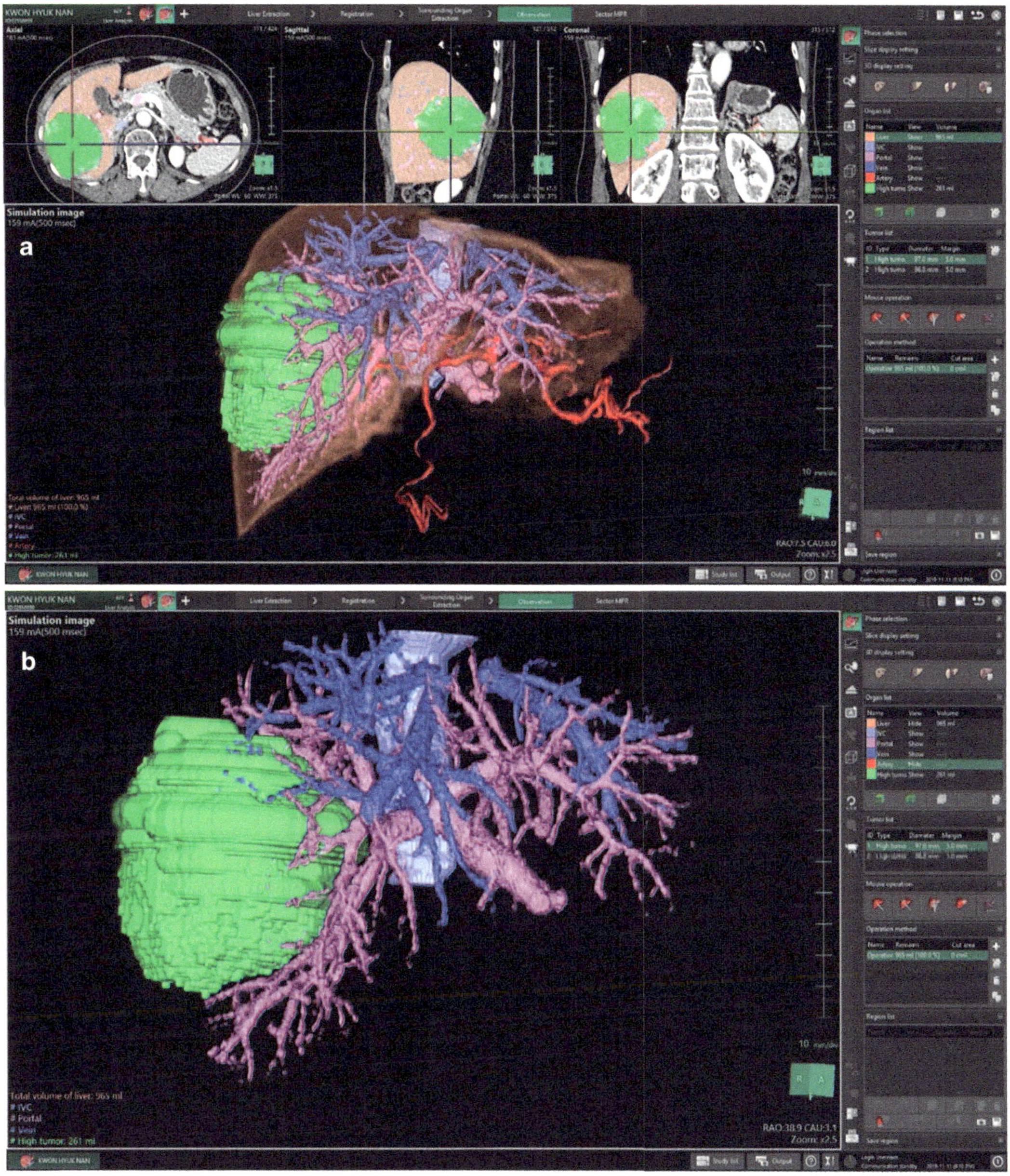

Fig. 8.2 Reconstruction image using Synapse 3D® system created by Fujifilm®. The green-colored mass is a huge hemangioma. (**a**) Relationship between tumor mass, portal veins, hepatic arteries, and hepatic veins. (**b**) Extracted tumor, portal vein, and hepatic vein from Fig. 8.2a

8.4 Surgical Technique

8.4.1 Open Surgery and Laparoscopy

(1) Positioning

For the open surgery, the patient is positioned supine with left arm on the table besides the trunk and right arm held away to maintain IV lines and monitor vital signs with an intra-arterial catheter by anesthesiologist. For laparoscopic surgery, lithotomy position is better for both the operator and assistants including photographer. A warm pad is used over the trunk except in the operation field. Deep vein thrombosis of the lower limbs is prevented via intermittent pneumatic compression.

(2) Incision

Depending on surgeon's preference, the liver may be exposed for mobilization via inverted "Y" shape (so-called Mercedes) incision, bilateral subcostal incision or an inverted "L" incision. Rarely, an upper midline incision is adopted, but it is inconvenient to adequately mobilize the right liver.

(3) Careful inspection and exploration of the abdominal cavity

Even though exploration is less important currently than in the era before dynamic CT or MRI, careful inspection and palpation of the entire intra-abdominal organs including pelvic cavity are used to identify extrahepatic metastasis, seeding or hidden tumor(s) before dissection around the liver.

(4) The hepatic suspensory ligaments including ligamentum teres hepatis are cut initially, followed by the falciform and coronary ligament and the bilateral triangular ligament. The right liver is mobilized by dissection of the right inferior hepatic peritoneal layer to enter the bare area to carefully divide the right adrenal gland attached to the liver. Next, proceeding along the retrohepatic IVC, the IVC ligament is encountered in the upward direction, and carefully divided without injury to the IVC. Upon completion of this procedure, the right liver is shifted to the anterior to ensure adequate exposure. After completing the mobilization of the right liver, the right hepatic vein is isolated and covered with an umbilical tape if possible.

(5) Intraoperative ultrasonography (IOUS) of the liver is used to delineate the vascular anatomy and the relationship between the tumor and hepatic portal veins, to validate the findings of dynamic CT and MRI preoperatively. Ultrasonogram can be used to identify the trunk of the right hepatic vein towards the periphery and the relationship with the tumor. The same procedure can be applied for the mid-hepatic vein (Fig. 8.3). The bifurcation of the main portal vein into right and left portal veins is then identified, and the right anterior and posterior branches are traced to determine the feeding portal vein territory for resection, and also identify possible tumor thrombus in the portal vein.

(6) Cholecystectomy and encircling of the right anterior Glissonean pedicle

Cholecystectomy is followed by isolation of the right main portal pedicle.

A. The Glissonean approach. To dissect the right main portal pedicle, an extra-Glissonean approach beginning at the upper border of the right main trunk is adopted without breaking the Glissonean sheath between right and left main portal pedicles. Next, a downward dissection toward the right caudate lobe of the liver is performed to break through the plane between portal pedicle and hepatic attachment (Fig. 8.4.) In this procedure, Yankauer suction tip enables dissection and suctioning of minor hemorrhage, and combination with periosteal elevator to expose the dissecting plane between portal pedicle and the liver (Fig. 8.5).

When the plane is tunneled, the right portal pedicle is covered with umbilical tape, followed by the same procedure to divide the right anterior and posterior pedicles and encircling with umbilical tapes individually. Test clamping of the

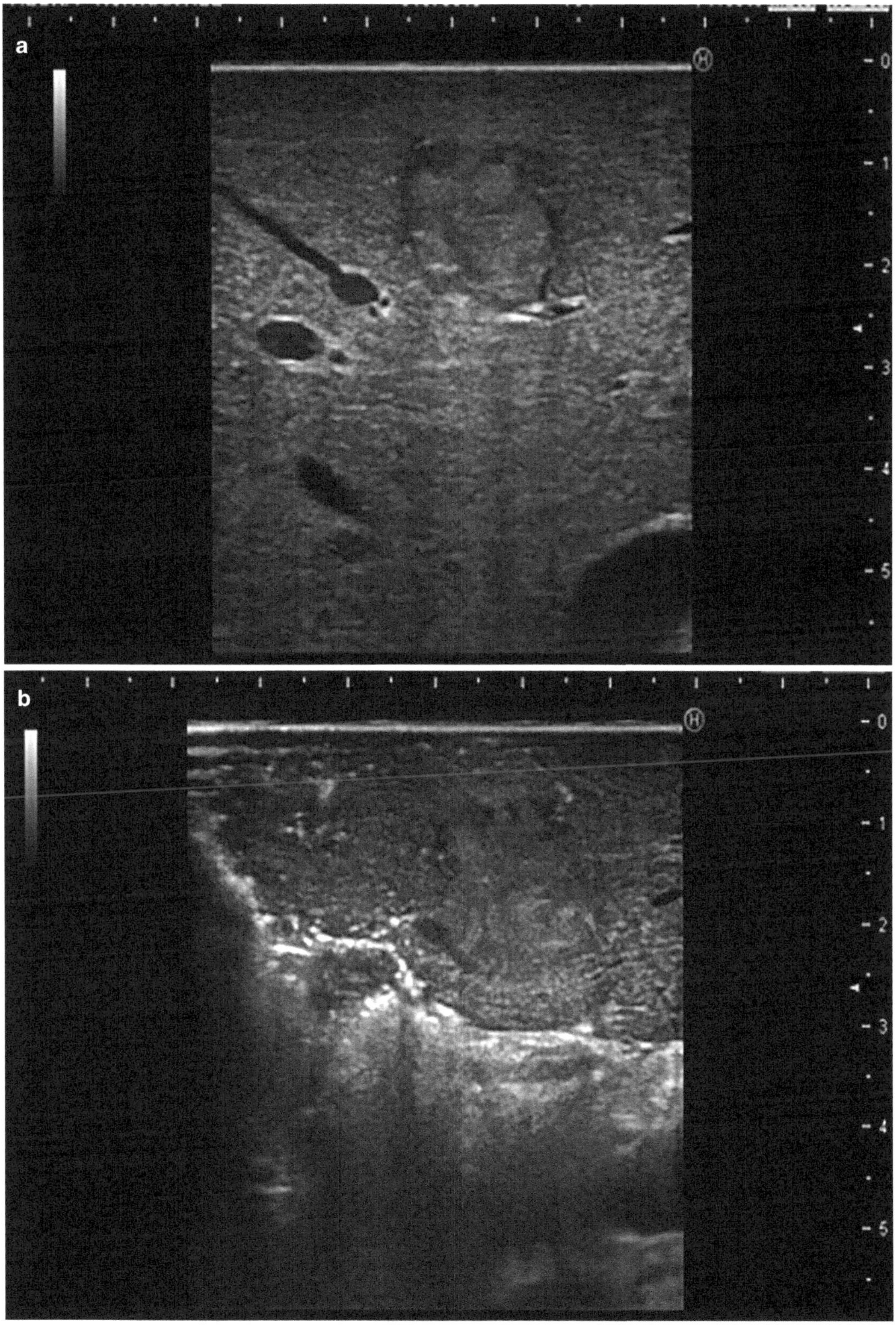

Fig. 8.3 Intraoperative ultrasonogram. (**a**) Tumor with portal and hepatic veins. (**b**) During hepatic transection, ultrasonogram reveals the relation between the tumor and transection plane to ensure adequate margin

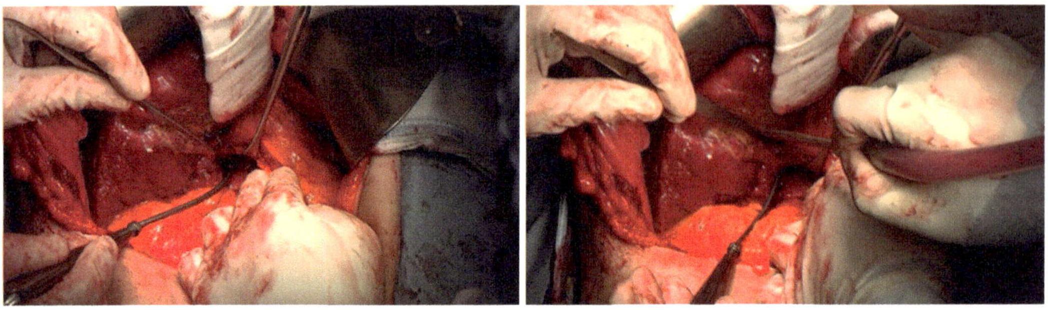

Fig. 8.4 The combination of Yankauer suction tip, periosteal elevator, and suction device facilitates the dissection of the extra Glissonean capsule to encircle the Glissonean pedicle

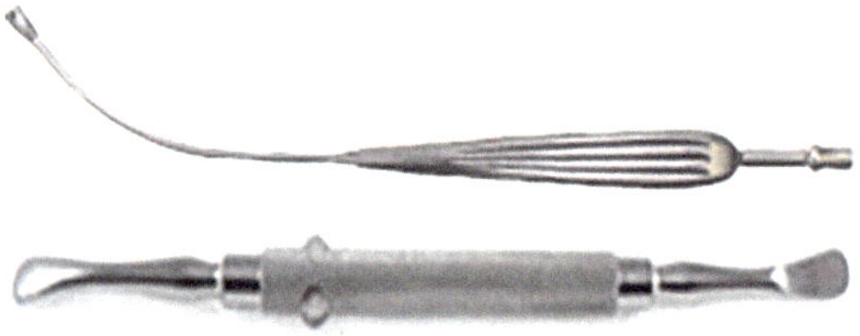

Fig. 8.5 The Yankauer suction tip with periosteal elevator

anterior portal pedicle with Bull-dog or small Satzinsky clamps ensures ischemic demarcation on the hepatic surface of the right anterior section, and marking of the ischemic margin via electrocautery (Fig. 8.6).

For laparoscopic approach, the laparoscopic Goldfinger retractor or Endo Mini-Retract™ is very useful (Fig. 8.7). After partial dissection of the Glissonean pedicle both superior and inferior border of the pedicle, the Goldfinger dissector or Endo Mini-Retract™ is inserted and encircled and hooked to the pedicle using an umbilical tape [4]. The next step is similar to the open surgery.

B. Individual Isolation of the Portal Vein

Alternatively, the portal vein can be isolated by separating the Glissonean sheath remaining in the bile duct and hepatic artery in the sheath, followed by test clamping of the portal pedicle after encircling the right anterior and posterior portal branches, for the demarcation of the intended sections. The demarcation may be weak in case of cirrhotic liver or variation and cross feeding portal vein branches. Therefore, the injection of indigo carmine dye into the isolated portal vein branch ensures discrete demarcation, which is one of the advantages of the individual isolation of the portal vein [5].

(7) Hepatic transection and division of the right anterior portal pedicle

The hepatic parenchyma is transected according to the demarcation line either right or left, depending on the anatomical location and tumor size. Generally, transection to the left of Cantlie line is preferable. The first transection is facilitated by hanging maneuver resulting in less bleeding. The upper end of hanging rope lies between the RHV and MHV, and the lower end between the right and the left Glissonean pedicles. Injury of the veins with intrahepatic portal pedicles can be prevented in the peripheral area via electrocautery or electric energy devices up to 2 cm in depth, and the CUSA® is useful for the deeper areas. When the transection reaches the Glissonean pedicle of both planes, the right anterior portal pedicle is divided as far distally as possible to avoid injury to the posterior or left portal pedicles using a vascular stapler TA™ (Fig. 8.8). Notably, when a rubber rope is used for hanging, the right posterior should not be pulled in the transection of the vascular TA. The right posterior bile duct is prone to injury during retraction of the right anterior

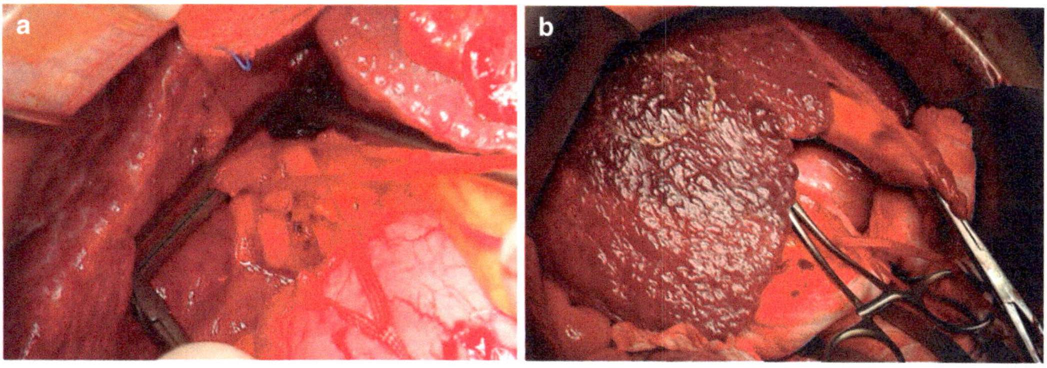

Fig. 8.6 Test clamping of the right anterior Glissonean pedicle with Satzinsky clamp (**a**) and ischemic demarcation of the right anterior section (**b**)

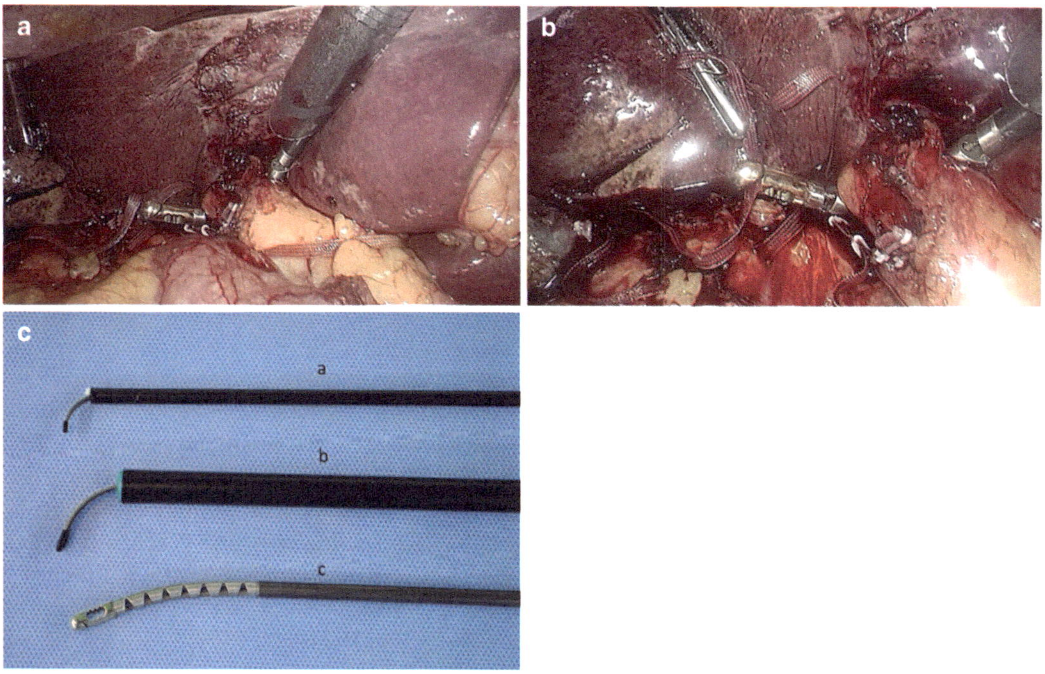

Fig. 8.7 Encircling the Glissonean pedicle for laparoscopy using Goldfinger retractor (**a**, **b**) and various instruments for dissecting and encircling the pedicle (**c**) (**a**) Endo Mini-Retract 5 mm (Covidien); (**b**) EndoRetract Maxi 10 mm; (**c**) Goldfinger dissector (Johnson and Johnson)

pedicle using a vascular stapler. Injury to the left duct is rare. Subsequent transections after the division of the right anterior pedicle are easy.

Further hepatic transection toward the root in addition to both right and mid-hepatic veins can be performed whether or not it is exposed on the transection plane. Bleeding from the side holes or large-bored fenestrations of the main hepatic veins can be stopped with 5-0 Prolene sutures or via light cauterization with bipolar cautery, especially during laparoscopy. Finally, the right anterior section is removed.

(8) Cut surface

The transected hepatic surface is inspected for bleeding and leakage of bile after hepatic resection. Hemostasis can be resolved using

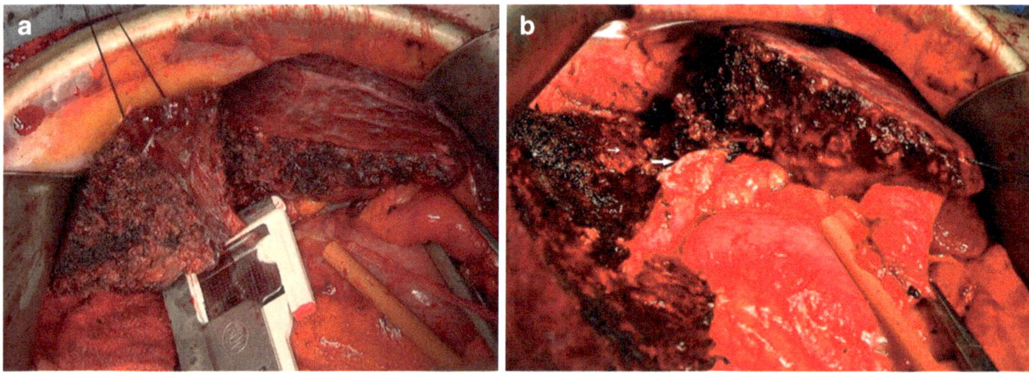

Fig. 8.8 Final step in anterior sectionectomy. (**a**) The right anterior pedicle is cut using vascular TA™. (**b**) The cut surface of the liver and the cut end of the right anterior portal pedicle

bipolar and monopolar electrosurgery and ligation of bleeding vessels with Prolene 5-0 sutures. Active topical hemostatic agents and sealants such as Tachosil™ or fibrin glue can be used for high-risk areas in subsequent bleeding or bile leakage. After lavage of the peritoneal cavity with normal saline solution, a drainage catheter is used to detect postoperative hemorrhage or bile leakage, and the abdominal wall layer is closed.

Tips

1. The Right anterior sectionectomy involves two methods: the Glissonean pedicle approach clamping the portal pedicle in the Glissonean sheath and individual isolation of the portal veins.
2. Discrete ischemic demarcation of the transection line using the Glissonean pedicle approach is facilitated by ensuring temporary clamping of both portal vein and hepatic artery together.
3. For the Glissonean pedicle approach, combination of Yankasuer's tonsil suction device and periosteal elevator is very useful in dissecting the Glissonean sheath in a bundle. Injury to the portal vein is prevented by preserving the Glissonean membrane of the sheath intact.
4. Goldfinger™ dissector is a good device for laparoscopic Glissonean pedicle approach.
5. During the transection down the right anterior portal pedicle close to the hilum, the anterior portal pedicle was cut using vascular TA™ as far peripheral as possible to avoid the right posterior or the left bile duct.

8.5 Complications

8.5.1 Bleeding

The cut surface is broader than in hemihepatectomy because of the two transection faces. The risk of hemorrhage or bile leakage during and after surgery can be reduced by maintaining the central venous pressure during hepatic transection as low as possible.

8.5.2 Bile Leakage

The risk of bile duct injury or bile leakage is higher in central hepatectomies, central bisectionectomy, or right anterior sectionectomy. Therefore, a careful dissection of the hilar plate is essential. Transection of the anterior portal pedicle should be as distal as possible to prevent injury to the left or right posterior branch of the bile duct. Intraoperative cholangiography should be performed to prevent unexpected bile duct injury, whenever biliary anatomy is unclear. Vascular TA is very useful to cut the pedicle.

8.5.3 Oncologic Safety

It is critical to ensure adequate tumor-free margins. The exposure of right and mid-hepatic veins is not absolutely necessary. However, in case of inadequate tumor-free margins, the procedure can be modified for further resection, including central bisectionectomy or right hemihepatectomy.

8.6 Conclusion

The right anterior sectionectomy is indicated for patients carrying tumors in the right anterior section and with insufficient hepatic reservoir function. Otherwise, the right hemihepatectomy is preferable due to oncologic safety, better anatomical incision and technical precision.

References

1. Chouillard E, Cherqui D, Tayar C, et al. Anatomical bi- and trisegmentectomies as alternatives to extensive liver resections. Ann Surg. 2003;238:29–34.
2. Makuuchi M, Kosuge T, Takayama T, Yamazaki S, Kakazu T, Miyagawa S, Kawasaki S. Surgery for small liver cancers. Semin Surg Oncol. 1993;9:298–304.
3. Lillemoe KD, Jarnagin WR. Hepatobiliary & Pancreatic Surgery. Philadelphia: Lippincott and Wilkins; 2013.
4. Honda G, Karata M, Okuda Y, Kobayashi S, Sakamoto K, Takahashi K. Totally laparoscopic anatomical hepatectomy exposing the major hepatic veins from the root side: a case of right anterior sectorectoy. J Gastrointest Surg. 2014;18:1379–80.
5. Ahn KS, Kang KJ, Park TJ, Kim YH, Lim TJ, Kwon JH. Benefit of systematic segmentectomy of the hepatocellular carcinoma; revisiting the dye injection method for various portal vein branches. Ann Surg. 2013;258:1014–21.

9 Right Posterior Sectionectomy

Yang-Seok Koh

Abstract

Right posterior sectionectomy entails division of the liver parenchyma following the right hepatic vein. Two traditional methods for inflow control including individual and the Glissonian approaches were adopted. The plane of dissection is wider than the other types of liver resection. The right hepatic vein is often resected to secure the safety margin.

Keywords

Right posterior sectionectomy · Right hepatic vein · Glissonian approach

Right posterior section includes the Couinaud segments 6 and 7 [1]. The right posterior hepatic artery and the right posterior portal vein supply blood, and the right posterior bile duct drains bile.

Supplementary Information The online version contains supplementary material available at https://doi.org/10.1007/978-981-16-1996-0_9.

Y.-S. Koh (✉)
Department of Surgery, Chonnam National University Medical School, Gwangju, South Korea
e-mail: yskoh@jnu.ac.kr

9.1 Indications

Tumors located in this section without invasion of the right hepatic vein and the right intrahepatic duct stone with or without intrahepatic duct strictures are indications for this procedure.

9.2 Technique

9.2.1 Incision

Reverse T incision, both subcostal incision, midline incision, right subcostal incision, and reverse L incision are used.

9.2.2 Cholecystectomy

The gallbladder and cystic plate should be removed to facilitate inflow control.

9.2.3 Hepatic Hilum for Inflow Control

Two types of inflow control are performed.

9.2.3.1 Individual Dissection

After cholecystectomy, the peritoneal incision of the right side of hepatoduodenal ligament with traction of the cystic duct stump to anterior and leftward

H. C. Yu (ed.), *Hepato-Biliary-Pancreatic Surgery and Liver Transplantation*,
https://doi.org/10.1007/978-981-16-1996-0_9

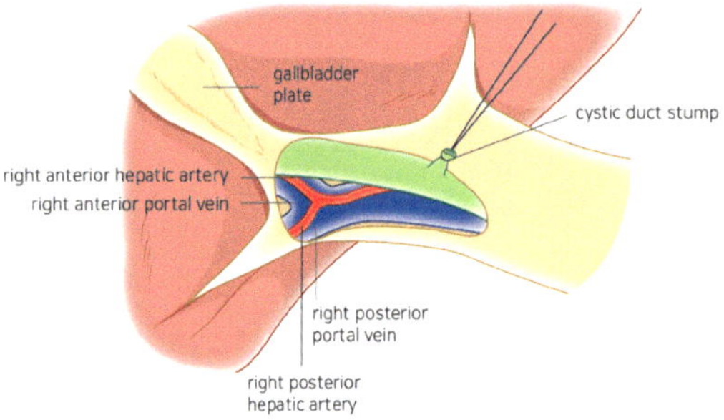

Fig. 9.1 Individual inflow control

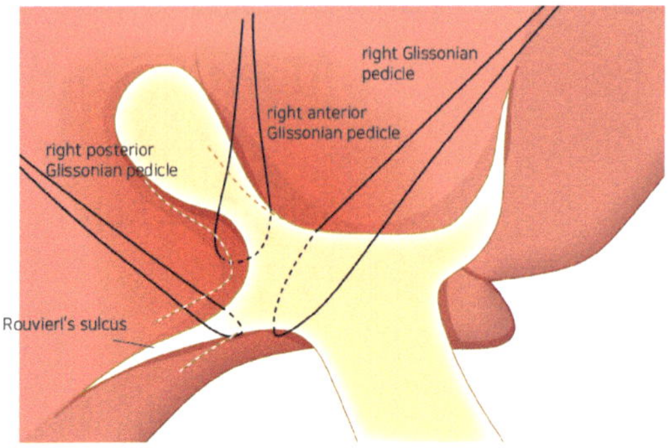

Fig. 9.2 Glissonian approach

is used to expose the right hepatic artery. Dissection until the bifurcation of the right anterior and posterior hepatic arteries is followed by the isolation of the right posterior hepatic artery (Fig. 9.1).

The right portal vein passes behind the right hepatic artery. Minor dissection up to the liver parenchyma exposes the right posterior portal vein aided by the ligation of small portal branches to the caudate lobe.

The right posterior hepatic duct is often ligated at the final stage of liver parenchyma division.

9.2.3.2 Glissonian Approach

It is a rapid and easy approach to inflow control. However, the risk of bleeding during the isolation and the relative distal control of the Glisson compared with the individual control should be borne in mind.

In most cases, the posterior Glisson lies in the Rouviere sulcus, whereas the anterior Glisson passes posterior to the cystic plate. The entry point is between the cystic plate and the Rouviere sulcus, and smooth circling around the Glisson using a right-angled clamp or similar instrument can be used to fully isolate the right posterior Glisson. Clamping leads to pale posterior section and visible demarcation line. Umbilical taping of the right posterior Glisson facilitates subsequent hanging (Fig. 9.2).

Minor bleeding from the hilar plate may be avoided using hemostatic materials such as Surgicell® or bipolar cauterization. When the Glisson capsule is thick and does not encircle in one motion, the Pringle maneuver is often performed to decrease the blood flow.

9.2.4 Liver Mobilization

The liver is retracted to the left by the assistant, and right triangular and coronary ligament are dissected until the right hepatic vein is exposed. The adrenal gland is easily exposed by upward traction of the liver anterior to the IVC, which in a few difficult cases prevent easy isolation, and minor portion of the liver covering the adrenal gland is removed. Short hepatic veins are serially divided from the caudal to the cephalad to fully expose the right hepatic vein. Vessel taping of the right hepatic vein may be a preventive measure to avoid bleeding. A Penrose drain insertion between the right and middle hepatic vein is often used for hanging of the liver to facilitate parenchymal division and reduce bleeding.

9.2.5 Parenchymal Division

The cutting is followed along the demarcation line. Sutures on both the sides of the line may facilitate tracts in opposite directions. CUSA and Kelly are two main instruments for the division of the liver. Tubular structures and vessels during dissection should be ligated meticulously to prevent subsequent bleeding or bile leak. The right hepatic vein is the land mark between the right anterior and posterior sections, and dissection should be continued to expose fully the point of intersection of the right hepatic vein and the IVC (Fig. 9.3).

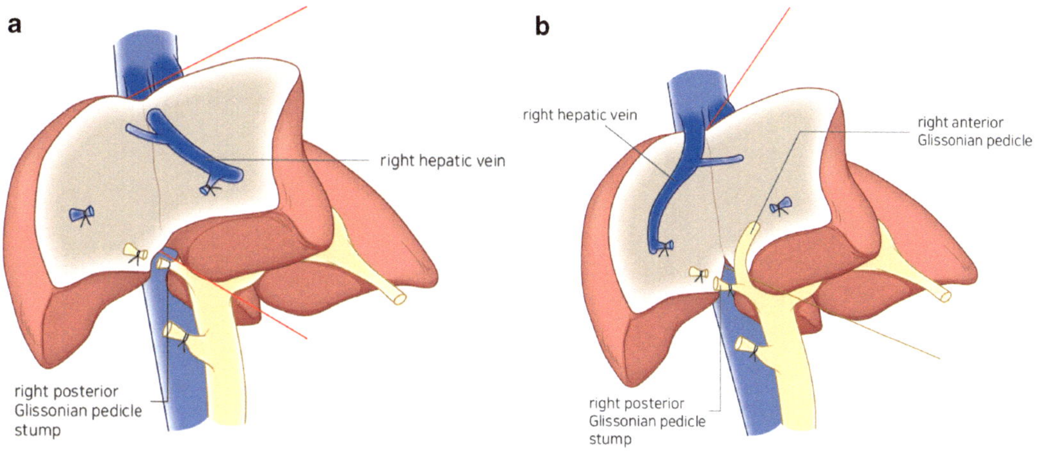

Fig. 9.3 RHV exposure during conventional right posterior sectionectomy (**a**) and during extended right posterior sectionectomy (**b**)

9.2.6 Cut Surface and Drain

When the specimen is extracted, the cut surface should be cautiously examined for possible bleeding and bile leakage. Hemostatic agents or materials are sprayed and placed on the cut surface to prevent bleeding from the right adrenal gland. One or two closed suction drains are placed.

Reference

1. Couinaud C. Liver anatomy: portal (and suprahepatic) or biliary segmentation. Dig Surg. 1999;16(6):459–67. https://doi.org/10.1159/000018770. PMID: 10805544.

S4 Segmentectomy With or Without Resection of Ventral Area of Right Anterior Section

10

Yang Won Nah

Abstract

In this manuscript and video, I will describe the liver resection procedure entailing resection of the ventral branches of the right anterior Glisson pedicle and the Glisson pedicles to segment 4. In this procedure, the left resection margin corresponds to the umbilical fissure and the right resection margin the right anterior Glisson pedicle. It is difficult to delineate the right resection margin, which is the core of this surgery. In the final step of the operation, the middle hepatic vein is divided at its junction with the left hepatic vein. This operation is based on the anatomical division of the portal basin of the right anterior section into ventral and dorsal areas, unlike the traditional Couinaud's segmental anatomy, which divides the basin of the right anterior portal vein into superior and inferior segments. In the absence of a specific term describing this procedure, I have arbitrarily designated it as central bisegmentectomy in this manuscript. Bisegments here mean segment 4 and ventral segment (area) of the right anterior section. Tumor adherent to the middle hepatic vein is a good indication for this parenchyma-sparing resection.

Keywords

Liver anatomy · Liver resection Segmentectomy · Parenchyma-sparing resection · Hepatocellular carcinoma · Right anterior section · Dorsal area · Ventral area Medial segmentectomy

Anatomical liver resections in which the left resection margin is in line with the falciform ligament include medial segmentectomy (segmentectomy 4), central bisectionectomy (segmentectomy 4, 5, 8), and right trisectionectomy (segmentectomy 4, 5, 6, 7, 8) (Table 10.1). The left resection margin is visible by connecting the falciform ligament and the umbilical fissure. In case of medial segmentectomy, the right resection margin on the Cantlie line is not discernible on the surface of the liver. However, ligation of Glisson pedicles to the medial segment leads to discoloration of the medial segment, which reveals the Cantlie line clearly (Fig. 10.1). Therefore, anatomical medial segmentectomy can be performed similar to other Glissonian approaches.

Anatomical hepatic resection is traditionally based on Couinaud's concept of liver anatomy

Supplementary Information The online version contains supplementary material available at https://doi.org/10.1007/978-981-16-1996-0_10.

Y. W. Nah (✉)
Department of Surgery, Ulsan University Hospital, University of Ulsan College of Medicine, Ulsan, South Korea
e-mail: nahyw@uuh.ulsan.kr

H. C. Yu (ed.), *Hepato-Biliary-Pancreatic Surgery and Liver Transplantation*,
https://doi.org/10.1007/978-981-16-1996-0_10

Table 10.1 Anatomical liver resections where the left resection margin is aligned with the falciform ligament and umbilical fissure

Surgical procedure	Important structure along the right resection margin	Major hepatic vein(s) being divided
According to Couinaud's anatomy		
Left medial segmentectomy (left medial sectionectomy)	MHV	None
Central bisectionectomy	RHV	MHV
Right trisectionectomy	None	MHV, RHV
According to Hjortsjo's anatomy		
Central bisegmentectomy[a]	Right anterior Glisson pedicle	MHV

MHV middle hepatic vein, *RHV* right hepatic vein

[a] Resection of segment 4 and ventral area (segment) of right anterior section

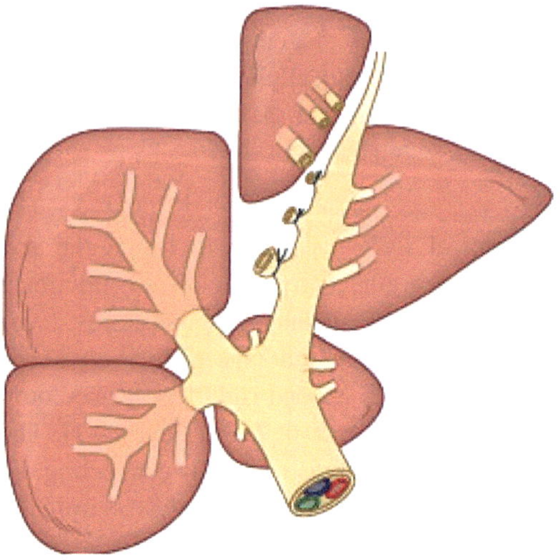

Fig. 10.1 Left medial segmentectomy. The right resection margin is visible by dividing the respective Glisson cords. It is compatible with the Cantlie line (modified from reference [3, 7])

grounded in portal vein ramification (Table 10.1) [1]. According to Couinaud's classification, the right anterior portal vein is divided craniocaudally into superior (segment 8) and inferior (segment 5) portal branches. Recently, other patterns of right anterior portal ramification including ventro-dorsal bifurcation or trifurcation have been reported [2–6].

In this manuscript and video, I will describe the resection procedure in which the territory supplied by the Glisson pedicles to segment 4 and the ventral branches of the right anterior Glisson pedicle are resected. In this procedure, the left resection margin corresponds to the umbilical fissure, and the right resection margin represents the right anterior Glisson pedicle (Fig. 10.2). In the final step of the operation, middle hepatic vein was divided at its junction with the left hepatic vein. This operation is based on the anatomical division of the portal basin of the right anterior section into ventral and dorsal areas, unlike the traditional Couinaud's segmental anatomy, which divides the basin of the right anterior portal vein into superior and inferior segments.

In the absence of a specific term defining this procedure, I have arbitrarily designated it as central bisegmentectomy involving segment 4 and ventral segment (area) of right anterior section. The procedure is completely different from the central bisectionectomy, because the trunk and dorsal branches of the right anterior Glisson pedicle are preserved in this central bisegmentectomy procedure. Particularly, it is difficult to understand and identify the right resection margin and is the core of this surgery. In this proce-

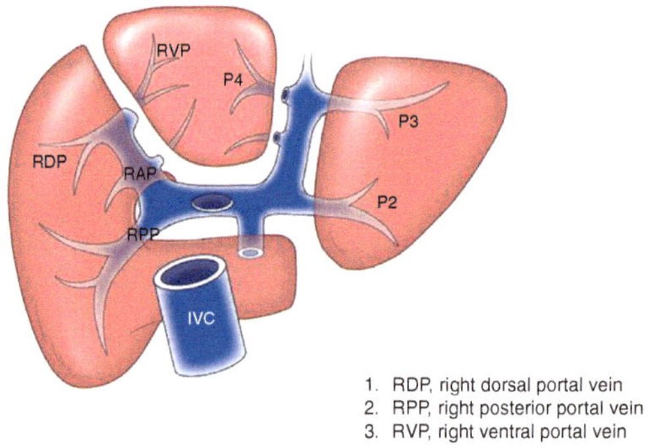

Fig. 10.2 Central bisegmentectomy (resection of segment IV and ventral area of the right anterior section). The right resection margin is compatible with the right anterior Glisson pedicle. Its ventral branches are divided (modified from reference [3])

dure, the left and right hepatic veins are preserved, and the middle hepatic vein is amputated as mentioned before (Table 10.1). Tumor adherent to the middle hepatic vein is a good indication for this parenchyma-sparing resection. In this study, the focus is on surgical techniques alone.

10.1 Surgical Procedures

10.1.1 Patient Position, Incision and Peritoneal Exploration

Abdominal incision is based on the general principles of open surgery based on adequate room for maneuver surgically. An inverted L-shaped incision is preferred. Upper midline incision from the xiphoid process to just above the navel was made and extended transversely to the right at the bottom of the incision, to avoid left abdominal incision and thereby reduce pain in the left abdomen, and thus reduce pulmonary complications.

10.1.2 Mobilization of the Liver

The falciform ligament is separated from the abdominal wall, and the round ligament is ligated, cut, and held with Kelly forceps for traction. The major hepatic veins are exposed at the area of contact between the falciform ligament and the diaphragm. The root of middle hepatic vein is localized. Usually, the left coronary and triangular ligaments are not incised. However, the right coronary and triangular ligaments are cut so that the right liver can be easily grasped. Most often, detachment of the liver from the inferior vena cava is not necessary during medial segmentectomy or central bisegmentectomy.

10.1.3 Localization of the Tumor

Adequate mobilization of the liver facilitates tumor localization. When a small tumor is located deep inside the liver parenchyma, it is difficult to palpate manually. In this case, the location of the tumor is detected via ultrasonography during surgery. Therefore, it is desirable to acquire ultrasound images before surgery when the tumor is located deep inside the liver. If the tumor location is consistent with the results of preoperative imaging, the location is marked by tattooing at the liver surface with electrocautery.

10.1.4 Cholecystectomy

Cholecystectomy is essential for the left medial segmentectomy or central bisegmentectomy. Once the gallbladder is removed, the base of the right anterior Glisson pedicle can be exposed from the hilar plate after dividing the cystic plate.

10.1.5 Hepatectomy

Generally, liver transection is initiated from the left resection margin, which facilitates the identification of landmarks for resection, including the falciform ligament along the superior liver surface and umbilical fissure along the inferior liver surface. The junction between the middle and left hepatic vein is rather superficial and easy to expose.

Ligation of Glisson pedicles to medial segment is performed along the right border of the umbilical fissure. The liver parenchyma was transected mainly using the Kelly clamp crushing method. The Cavitron Ultrasonic Surgical Aspirator (CUSA) is often used to separate large Glisson cords or hepatic veins from the parenchyma.

10.1.5.1 Left Resection Margin

The line connecting the falciform ligament and the umbilical fissure, which can be seen with the naked eye from the outside, becomes the left resection margin. A couple of small superficial Glisson cords that run from the tip of umbilical portion to the S4b can be easily isolated after dividing the superficial liver tissue partially between S3 and S4. The Glisson cords were ligated and divided aided by traction of the round ligament aids (Fig. 10.3).

Usually, one to two large portal branches to segment 4b run from the upper area of the umbili-

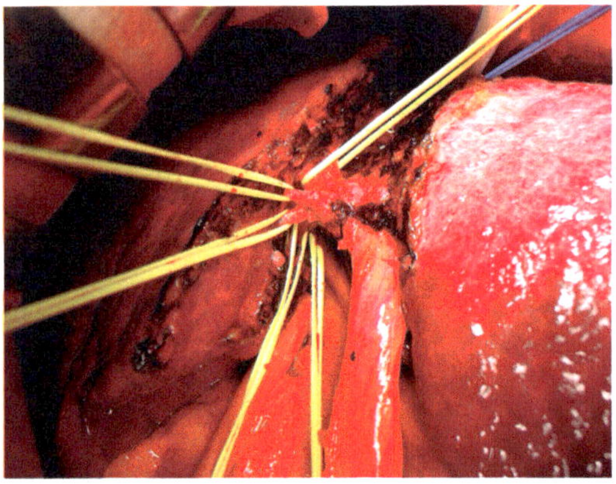

Fig. 10.3 Intraoperative view of the Glisson pedicles to segment IV. There are several Glisson pedicles to the segment IV (yellow taped)

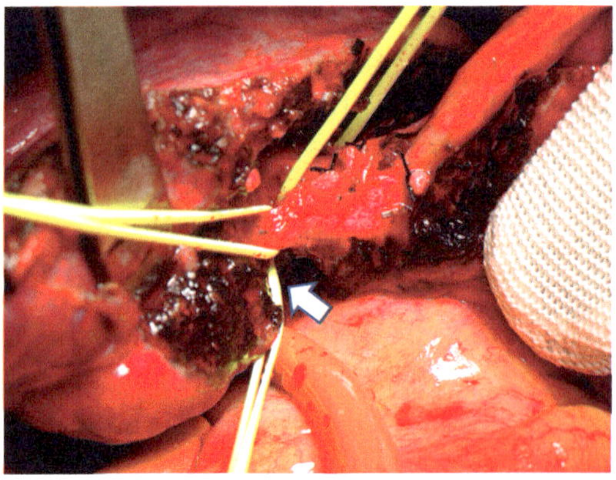

Fig. 10.4 Intraoperative view of the Glisson pedicles to segment IV. Three large Glisson pedicles supply the segment IV (yellow taped) after division of three superficial small branches. The lowest one (arrow) is the branch to segment IVa

cal portion in the left portal vein, and a branch to segment 4a originates from the lower area of umbilical portion. These portal branches are grouped with arteries and bile ducts to form the Glisson cord and batch-ligated and divided (Fig. 10.4). The parenchyma is further transected toward the direction of the middle hepatic vein. The middle hepatic vein is exposed in the last course of the left resection, and if possible, a tape is hung over the middle hepatic vein after full exposure.

10.1.5.2 Right Resection Margin

Medial Segmentectomy

Segment 4 will be demarcated clearly by dividing the respective Glisson cords. Resection of segment 4 is completed by dissecting the liver parenchyma along the discolored line, which is compatible with the Cantlie line and preserving the middle hepatic vein. During transection of the liver parenchyma along the direction of the middle hepatic vein, several branches of the hepatic vein running from the medial segment to the middle hepatic vein are divided.

Central Bisegmentectomy

In the case of central bisegmentectomy (resection of medial segment and ventral area of right anterior section), the identification of the right anterior Glisson pedicle is the first step for accurate anatomical resection. It can be performed by continuing the peeling of the hilar plate off the liver parenchyma in the direction from G4a to the right. A large right anterior Glisson pedicle is encountered at the right end of the transverse portion. Further dissection exposes the origin of right anterior Glisson pedicle by 180° (Fig. 10.5). The direction of dissection is altered by following the anterior Glisson pedicle. Thus, the direction of liver transection is from the bottom to the top, at the inferior surface of the liver.

Projecting an imaginary line toward the liver edge following the direction of the exposed right anterior Glisson pedicle leads to the origin of the right resection at the liver surface, which is located in Couinaud's segment 5. The extension line from this point to the right edge of the middle hepatic vein represents the right resection margin, which is marked with electrocautery on the liver surface.

Subsequently, the liver parenchyma is transected along the electrocautery mark from the superior surface of the liver toward the right anterior Glisson pedicle until the pedicle is exposed 180°. Branches from the right anterior Glisson pedicle to the ventral or leftward direction are ligated and cut in turn (Fig. 10.6). Usually, 2–3 large branches are ligated, and these are the ventral branches of right anterior Glisson pedicle.

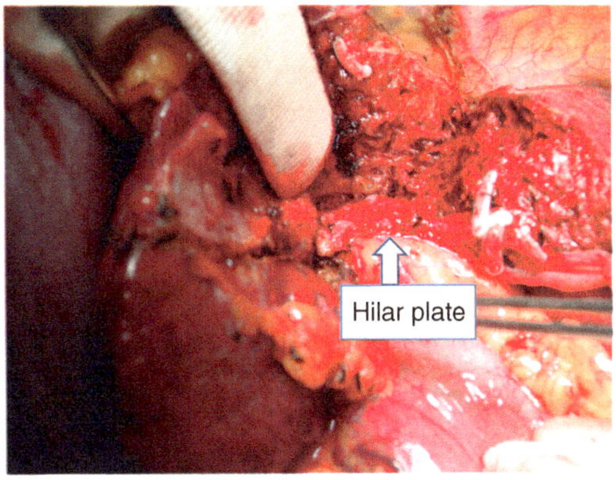

Fig. 10.5 The right anterior Glisson pedicle can be identified via rightward dissection at the liver hilum along the right Glisson pedicle

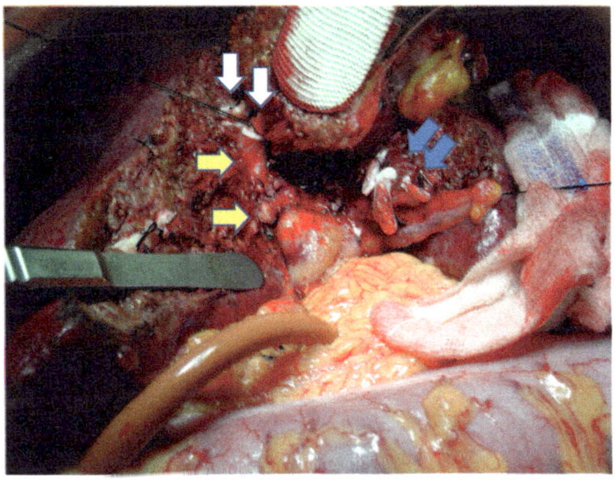

Fig. 10.6 Ventral branches (white arrows) from the anterior Glisson pedicle (yellow arrows) are being ligated. Glisson pedicles to segment IV (blue arrows) are already clipped and divided

The hepatic vein branch from Couinaud segment 8 to the middle hepatic vein emerges along the parenchymal transection cephalad. It may be preserved and followed to the middle hepatic vein, or ligated and divided according to the relationship with the tumor. Upon completion of the parenchymal transection, only the middle hepatic vein remains, which is clamped and divided. The specimen is removed. The middle hepatic vein stump is closed manually with a 4/0 Prolene suture (Fig. 10.7). The middle hepatic vein can be managed with a vascular stapler.

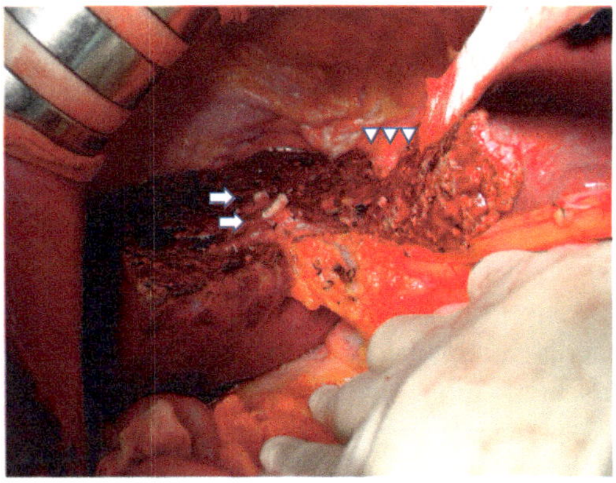

Fig. 10.7 View after central bisegmentectomy (resection of segment IV and ventral area of right anterior section). Note the ventral branches of the anterior Glisson pedicle (arrows, Hem-O-Locked) and suture-closed stump of middle hepatic vein (arrowheads)

10.1.6 Hemostasis, Drainage, and Closure

The principles of general liver resection should be followed. A meticulous hemostasis cannot be overemphasized. I use two negative pressure drain tubes: one drain tube is placed in the right sub-diaphragmatic space and the other in the Morrison pouch.

10.2 Precautions for Surgery

10.2.1 Bleeding

Blood loss is one of the most important factors influencing morbidity after liver resection. Blocking inflow of blood by the Pringle maneuver is an effective way to reduce bleeding during liver transection. In addition, since the massive hemorrhage during liver resection usually originates in the hepatic vein, it is important to maintain the central venous pressure low, usually below 5 mmHg. Bleeding from the hepatic vein branch can be stopped, at least temporarily, simply using finger pressure. Therefore, in case of invisible bleeding, direct suture of the bleeding vessel in a pool of blood must be avoided, and instead, light finger pressure should be used at the bleeding point for 1–3 min until the origin of bleeding is visible and easily controlled.

Intra-hepatic anatomy is also important in reducing bleeding during liver resection. For example, if the location of the hepatic veins can be predicted during parenchymal transection, the bleeding can be managed effectively. A thorough preoperative imaging analysis is essential along with considerable surgical experience.

10.2.2 Tips for Liver Parenchymal Transection

Excessive pulling of the liver bilaterally during surgery can tear the blood vessels. If the Kelly clamp crushing method is used, it is better to reduce the traction strength during crushing. It is necessary to adjust the power of crushing according to the degree of liver fibrosis in order to reduce bleeding and shorten the transection time of the liver. Substantial liver fibrosis can result in tearing of blood vessels upon soft crushing because the fibrotic tissue is stronger than the vessel wall. Instead, bold crushing may be a strategy to reduce the transection time in this case rather than soft crushing, especially for cirrhotic liver. The degree of bold crushing should be guided by experience. A precaution: do not crush the liver until the end but leave behind residual liver tissue at the end of crushing.

Acknowledgments I appreciate Drs. Park Hyung-woo and Yoon Jong-hee of Ulsan University Hospital for organizing and editing this manuscript and video.

References

1. Strasberg SM. Nomenclature of hepatic anatomy and resections: a review of the Brisbane 2000 system. J Hepato-Biliary-Pancreat Surg. 2005;12(5):351–5.
2. Kogure K, Kuwano H, Fujimaki N, et al. Reproposal for Hjortsjo's segmental anatomy on the anterior segment in human liver. Arch Surg. 2002;137(10):1118–24.
3. Cho A, Okazumi S, Miyazawa Y, et al. Proposal for a reclassification of liver based on portal ramifications. Am J Surg. 2005;189(2):195–9.
4. Fasel JH, Schenk A. Concepts for liver segment classification: neither old ones nor new ones, but a comprehensive one. J Clin Imaging Sci. 2013;3:48–54.
5. Fujimoto J, Hai S, Hirano T, et al. Anatomic liver resection of right paramedian sector: ventral and dorsal resection. J Hepatobiliary Pancreat Sci. 2015;22(7):538–45.
6. Cazauran JB, Pâris L, Rousset P, et al. Anatomy of the right anterior sector of the liver and its clinical implications in surgery. J Gastrointest Surg. 2018;22(10):1819–31.
7. Yamamoto M, Katagiri S, Ariizumi S, et al. Tips for anatomical hepatectomy for hepatocellular carcinoma by the Glissonean pedicle approach. J Hepatobiliary Pancreat Sci. 2014;21:E53–E56.

S5 & S6 Segmentectomy

11

Soon-Chan Hong and Chi-Young Jeong

Abstract

With respect to bisegmentectomy (s4 and s5), performing accurate anatomical hepatic resection seems to be rare, and more importantly, it seems necessary to pay more attention to ensuring a sufficient resection margin for the tumor and selecting the liver resection range that minimizes venous congestion or an ischemic injury after surgery. Recently, laparoscopic bisegmentectomy (s4 and s5) has been performed frequently due to the development of techniques and instruments for laparoscopic liver resection. This chapter describes laparoscopic liver resection.

Keywords

Anatomical segmentectomy · Bisegmentectomy · Laparoscopy · Segment 5 · Segment 6

11.1 Method

After cholecystectomy is performed, liver mobilization is conducted up to the right hepatic vein. Then, with laparoscopic ultrasound, the middle hepatic vein, which borders segment IV, is checked, and the right boundary line is marked with electrocautery. Alternatively, a right-side Glissonean approach is used to temporarily ligate the right Glisson to check the boundary between segments IV and V along the ischemic line (Fig. 11.1).

In the case of open surgery, the boundary between segments V and VI can be confirmed based on counterstaining identification of P8 and ultrasonically guided puncture and injection of the dye into P6. However, in cases of laparoscopic surgery, which is based on the virtual line of the horizontal plane of the left and right branches of the portal vein, it is reasonable to select the resection line considering the position of the tumor. After confirming the tumor with laparoscopic ultrasound, the resection line is secured and marked with electrocautery. For counter traction, stay suturing can be performed. For the pringle maneuver, U-tape is placed in the hepatoduodenal ligament, and the laparoscopic endo-bulldog can be used to save the trocar port

Supplementary Information The online version contains supplementary material available at https://doi.org/10.1007/978-981-16-1996-0_11.

S.-C. Hong · C.-Y. Jeong (✉)
Department of Surgery, Gyeongsang National University School of Medicine, Jinju, South Korea
e-mail: hongsc@gnu.ac.kr

H. C. Yu (ed.), *Hepato-Biliary-Pancreatic Surgery and Liver Transplantation*,
https://doi.org/10.1007/978-981-16-1996-0_11

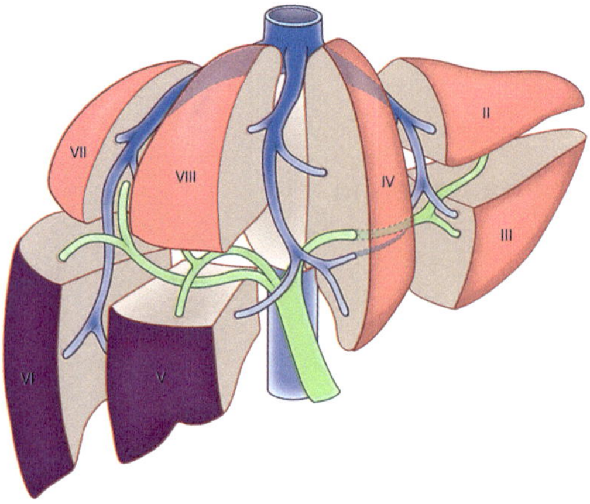

Fig. 11.1 Couinaud's liver segments 5 and 6

for clamping. At this time, it is safer and more effective to clamp the hepatoduodenal ligament on the patient's left side. Liver resection starts at the boundary with segment IV, and the operator stands between the legs of the patient. A liver resection of 1 cm from the surface is performed with a harmonic scalpel at the border between segments IV and V, followed by liver resection with a laparoscopic cavitron ultrasonic surgical aspirator (CUSA®). Here, if counter traction is not properly performed, it becomes difficult to use CUSA®; therefore, the patient's position is tilted toward the left side to use gravity, and counter traction is performed using stay sutures. During liver resection, even if the vessel is small, careful ligation is advantageous to maintain a clean field of view and a good resection surface. At this point, if the middle hepatic vein is encountered, it is dissected with CUSA® suctioning and then ligated. In the case of liver cirrhosis, CUSA® becomes less effective; therefore, liver resection can be performed with the crush clamping technique using LigaSure®. When using a LigaSure®, activating it by opening and closing the jaw using the foot switch and not completely closing it can ligate thick blood vessels and bile ducts, while complete closure of the jaw can stop bleeding. In case of an increase in the amount of bleeding or difficulties in continuing with CUSA®, it can be a useful technique to try. After resection between segments IV and V, the operator moves to the left side of the patient and performs resection between segments VI and VII. At this time, if a branch of the thick middle hepatic vein drains segment VI alone, it is ligated and excised. When the resection between segments VI and VII proceeds, traction and hanging are performed as the U-tube is hung by the groove of the resected liver parenchyma (sling suspension technique), and the lateral posterior parenchyma of segment VI is brought close to the eye. After completion of liver resection, bleeding or bile leakage in the liver resection margin is checked and fibrin glue is applied.

S7 & S8 Segmentectomy

12

Hee Jung Wang and Sung Yeon Hong

Abstract

Resection of liver tumors located in Couinaud segments 7 and 8 is challenging due to their intricate location and difficulty of identifying feeding Glissonean pedicles. Various surgical approaches can be employed case by case according to individual segmental anatomy of the patient. In this chapter, the role of preoperative 3D imaging and the technique of anatomical liver resection for tumors located in segments 7 and 8 are discussed.

Keywords

Hepatocellular carcinoma · Sectionectomy
Anterior section · Glissonean approach
Anatomical resection · Segmentectomy 7 and 8

12.1 Introduction

In segmental anatomy, liver segments 7 and 8 are located at the superior aspect of the liver with no noticeable surface structure to outline their borders. Moreover, their segmental portal branches are deeply situated thereby rendering difficulties in ligation before parenchymal transection. Segment 7, alongside segment 6, forms the posterior-right lateral portion of the liver stretching up to the right border of the spinal body and medially neighboring the inferior vena cava. Internally, segment 7 is located at the right posterior aspect of the right hepatic vein or right portal fissure. The borderline between segments 7 and 6 is usually a coronal plane. However, it is possible to identify it by ischemic demarcation after the ligation of the segment 7 branch or by intraoperative ultrasound during surgery. The boundaries of segment 8 are at the main portal fissure toward the left side and the right portal fissure toward the right side. The posterior border of segment 8 is the superior leaf of the right coronary ligament, and the anterior border is roughly at the coronal plane of the porta hepatis. Internally, segment 8 is located at the anterior-superior aspect of right and middle hepatic veins (RHV and MHV), and the inferior vena cava (IVC) is not found at the border. However, IVC can be exposed at the superior part of the posterior border where a confluence of RHV and MHV is seen (Fig. 12.1).

Supplementary Information The online version contains supplementary material available at https://doi.org/10.1007/978-981-16-1996-0_12.

H. J. Wang (✉)
Department of Surgery, Inje University Haeundae Paik Hospital, Busan, Korea
e-mail: wanghj@ajou.ac.kr

S. Y. Hong
Division of Hepatobiliary Surgery and Liver Transplantation, Department of Surgery, Ajou University School of Medicine, Suwon, Korea

H. C. Yu (ed.), *Hepato-Biliary-Pancreatic Surgery and Liver Transplantation*,
https://doi.org/10.1007/978-981-16-1996-0_12

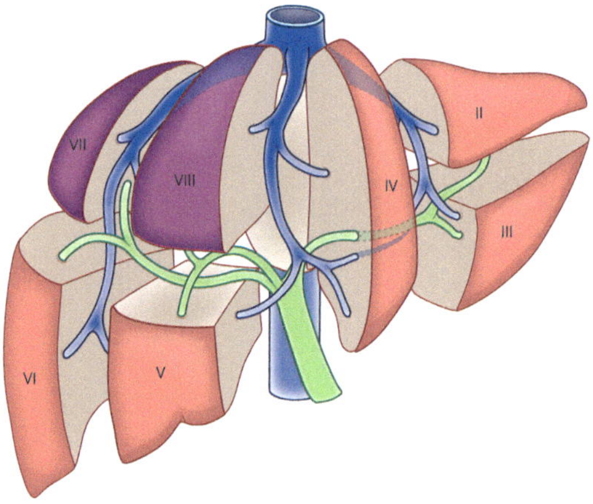

Fig. 12.1 Schema of Couinaud 8 segments of the liver

12.2 Indications and Contraindications

Segmentectomy 7 and 8 can be performed in selected patients with liver tumors located at the superior aspect (dome) of the liver and with compromised liver function to permit a larger extent of hepatic resection. For successful surgery, the tumor must be confined to the corresponding liver segment, and the segmental anatomy must not have such anatomical variations as severe sliding of origin of the Glissonean pedicles. Gross tumor thrombosis in the portal vein or hepatic vein is a contraindication to the surgery.

12.3 Preoperative Assessment and Designing the Liver Resection

Patients with hepatocellular carcinoma confined to the corresponding liver segments with preserved liver function (i.e., no ascites, serum bilirubin less than 1.0 mg/dl, and ICG-R15% less than 20–25%) and no severe systemic disease are indicated for this type of liver segmentectomy. Abdominal CT scans and MRIs are used to assess the anatomical structure and its relation to tumors. Recently, three-dimensional depiction of the liver segmental anatomy has become possible, and a more delicate approach in the form of navigation, according to individual liver anatomy has been practised.

12.4 Comprehending 3D Image and its Necessity in Planning the Surgery

Couinaud's eight-segment scheme, despite its usefulness and simplicity, can serve as a dogma that divides the liver in a man-made fashion. In general, the liver has constant first and second-order inflow branches that divide the organ into two hemilivers and three sections which have a watershed plane where the hepatic veins are located. However, this schema of anatomical description renders or even precludes inflow-oriented anatomical liver resection as it neglects the variation of inflow vessels in terms of number and sliding of their origins. In the next section, the variation in inflow in the right hemiliver by the present author's experience in cadaveric liver dissection and 3D image analysis will be discussed.

Our institution adopted Synapse 3D (Fuji film) in 2016, and we analyzed the variation in third-order inflow branches to the right anterior and posterior sections (RAS and RPS) in 96 liver donors from 2017 to 2018. The result showed that the portal pedicles to the RAS have four different branching types; A-D. A cranio-caudal type or type A is when the third-order branch structure corresponds to the Couinaud's segments 5 and 8 anatomies and comprised 45.8% (44) of the cases. Ventral-dorsal type or type B (13, 13.5%) is responsible for the segments 5 and 8 of which are supplied by two or more fourth-order branches from a different third-order branch. A radial type or type C (33, 34.4%) is when there are multiple or usually more than four third-order branches present. In this case, segments 5 and 8 cannot be distinguished. In the slidden type or type D (6, 6.3%), the third- or fourth-order branches of the RAS and RPS traverse to other territories (Fig. 12.2).

The RPS, likewise, has four distinct anatomical entities. Type A is whereby the right posterior portal pedicle has a common trunk (a second-order branch) and further gives its branches (two) to each segment 6 and 7, and comprised 34.4% (33) of the cases. In type B, similarly, the right posterior section pedicles branch to each segment but in the absence of a common trunk (14, 14.6%). The right posterior portal pedicle in type

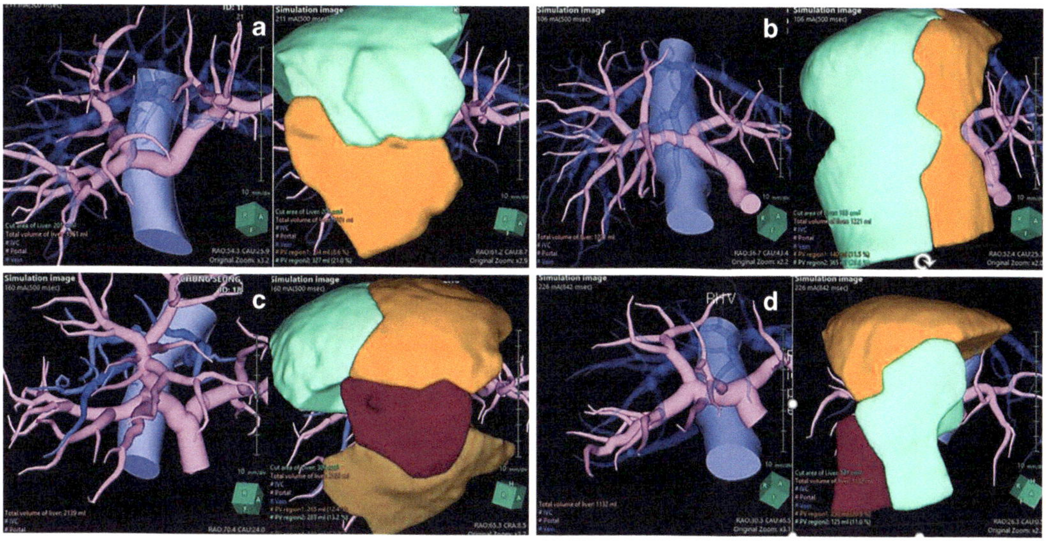

Fig. 12.2 (**a**) Classic cranio-caudal type (**b**) ventral-dorsal type variation (**c**) radial type variation (**d**) variation with third or fourth-order branches of RAS and RPS traversing to other territories

C runs through the liver parenchyma toward segment 7 and gives multiple branches to segment 6 (43 cases, 44.8%). Lastly, type D is likewise of type D of RAS variation.

In conclusion, a strictly controlled anatomical resection of segments 7 and 8 can be performed in only 48.0% (A type of RPS variant) and 45.8% (A type of RAS variant) of all the cases, respectively. However, given that 3D CT image reconstruction is available, a higher success rate of anatomical resection can be achieved by designing the resection plane according to the individual anatomy. Otherwise, a larger extent of liver resection or nonanatomical wedge resection must be selected in patients with variant anatomy.

12.5 Operative Technique

12.5.1 Laparotomy and Liver Mobilization

A right subcostal incision followed by a midline incision or a Hockey-stick incision is generally preferred. Falciform ligament and coronary ligament are dissected up to the IVC. Cholecystectomy is performed subsequently and a nelaton catheter is encircled around the hepaticoduodenal ligament for Pringle maneuver.

12.5.2 The Procedure of Anatomical Resection of Segments 7 and 8

12.5.2.1 Segmentectomy 8

1. Type A Branching Pattern of RAS on Preoperative 3D Image Analysis

   In type A RAS portal pedicle anatomy, two approaches can be undertaken. The first approach is known as Makuuchi's method [1], whereby ultrasound-guided indocyanine green dye injection to a single P8 is performed for liver surface staining of segment 8 (Fig. 12.3). Cantlie's line and a transverse liver transection along the demarcation line are the first steps to find a single P8. Subsequently, P8 is ligated and liver parenchymal transection is continued thereby exposing the ventral portion of the RHV. A specimen containing segment 8 can thus be taken out after completion of liver dissection to the IVC at the superior border. When P8 puncture is unpliant, a second method known as Takasaki's approach can be attempted. In this procedure, the main right portal pedicle is temporarily clamped to induce ischemic demarcation to the right hemiliver. The demarcation line or interlobar plane is dissected and a superior-ventral portion of the

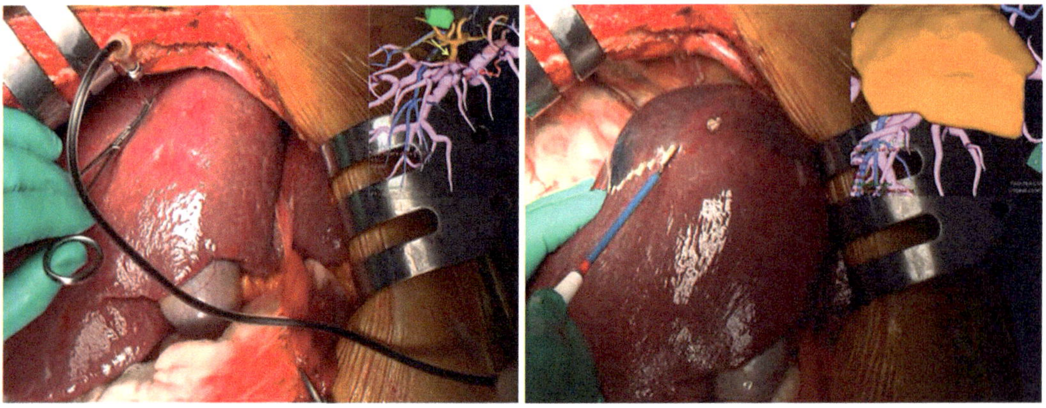

Fig. 12.3 Delineation of segment 8 by US-guided ICG dye injection. (Makuuchi's method)

main portal fissure is found. Then, the P8 is ligated at its root. Ischemic demarcation of segment 8 can be seen and the process afterward is identical to Makuuchi's method. The difference between the two procedures is that the operator can see the anterior and right border of segment 8 before liver parenchymal transection in Makuuchi's method, whereas in Takasaki's method, only the left border can be noticed before commencing the liver transection. If 3D images are available and if there is only one P8, the two methods are considered as equally simple and feasible.

2. Type B or C Branching Type of RAS on Preoperative 3D Image Analysis.

   In type B RAS branching pattern, the third-order branches of the right anterior portal vein spread in the ventral-dorsal direction. The P8s consist of two or more fourth-order branches arising from the ventral and dorsal third-order branches. In such cases, the success rate of Makuuchi's approach is low. Hence, Takasaki's approach is preferred. The right portal pedicle is temporarily clamped and the superior-ventral portion of the main portal fissure is dissected along the ischemic demarcation line. The ventral branches of segment 8 are subsequently ligated and the liver parenchymal transection is continued posteriorly to find the dorsal branches. After ligation of the dorsal branches, segment 8 is demarcated and the operator can complete segmentectomy 8. However, it remains controversial whether performing a segmentectomy by ligating multiple fourth-order branches can be called anatomical resection. If the ventral cone unit of RAS encompasses the tumor, resecting the territory of the corresponding third-order branch can be a more ideal approach as an anatomical resection.

   In the case of irregular branching (more than 4) of the third-order branches or type C branching pattern of RAS, segmentectomy 8 can be a challenging task. In such a case, Makuuchi's approach is not recommended. Likewise, liver parenchymal transection can be carried out by finding and ligating multiple P8s in the ventral to the dorsal direction. Since it is not likely to be able to ligate all P8s at their roots, the success rate of anatomical resection is low. If the operator is determined to perform an anatomical resection, the trans-fissural approach can be used as an alternative. As a first step, the hilar plate is lowered by blunt dissection, and the right Glissonean pedicle is encircled with a nelaton tube. The ischemic demarcation of the right hemiliver can be observed by temporary clamping. The demarcation line is the main portal fissure. Subsequently, transection of the liver parenchyma through the main portal fissure using CUSA or a Kelly clamp crushing is carried out until the dissection reaches the hilar plate. Afterward, the dissection plane is tilted toward the right side following the right anterior portal pedicle to find P5 and P8 within 2 cm from the hilar plate. Temporary clamping of P8 allows visualizing the segment 8 territory at the liver surface. The ischemic demarcation of segment 8 is marked at the surface using bovie. Parenchymal transection is continued toward the right side until RHV is exposed. Following the RHV, the dissection proceeds to suprahepatic IVC. Meanwhile, dissection of the connective tissue to the right-hand side of the anterior surface of the IVC allows visualization of the RHV trunk. An additional parenchymal dissection parallel to the RHV separates segment 8 from the liver. After extraction of the specimen, the cut-surface of the liver is coagulated with an argon beam laser or a bipolar coagulator. Finally, the surgeon finishes the procedure by reassuring hemostasis with a tachocomb seal or fibrin glue spray (Fig. 12.4).

3. Type D Branching Type of RAS on Preoperative 3D Image Analysis.

   Anatomical resection is rarely achievable in type D variant anatomy of the RAS. A wedge resection is rather convenient. However, Takasaki's procedure or main portal fissure approach can be applied in the case of the anterior section dominant type. On the contrary, in the case of posterior section dominant type, wedge resection is preferred unless small contracted segment 8 can confine a small tumor.

4. Preoperative 3D Image is Not Available.

   Using a 2-dimensional study only limits the success rate of Makuuchi's procedure when conducting anatomical resection. Also, unawareness about P8's anatomical variation may consume an excess amount of parenchymal dissection to find the root of P8 when attempting Takasaki's procedure. A considerable amount of hemorrhage can result since hemostasis becomes difficult. Even so, the success rate of anatomical resection remains low. At the time when the 3D image was not available in our institution, I managed to perform segmentectomy 8 by transfissural approach with a success rate of 80%. This approach allows the visualization of P8 root in most of the cases, but it is an invasive procedure. The detailed procedure is described in section ②.

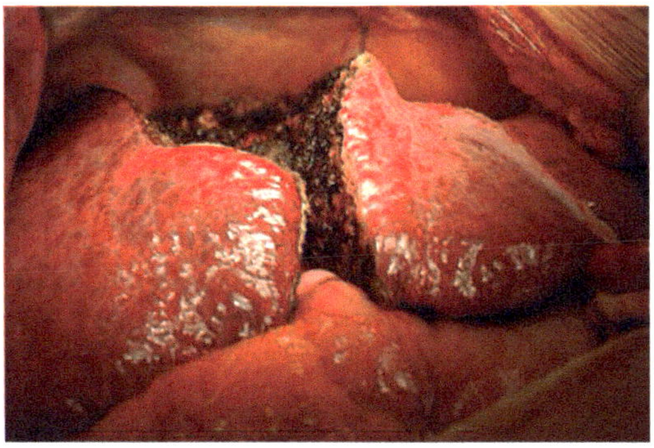

Fig. 12.4 The operative field after monosegmentectomy of segment 8 using transfissural approach

12.5.2.2 Segmentectomy 7

Anatomical resection of segment 7 is the least successful procedure of all the segmentectomies, although the definition of the anatomical resection may vary. Two approaches are used in our institution. The first approach is Takasaki's approach [2] where the Glisson sheath is lowered from the hilar plate and the right posterior pedicle is separated. Temporary clamping of the right posterior pedicle induces ischemic demarcation of the RPS thereby revealing the right portal fissure. The superior aspect of the right portal fissure is dissected and the surgeon finds the P7. Ligation of P7 follows and further dissection along the RHV completes segmentectomy 7 (Fig. 12.5). The second approach is the

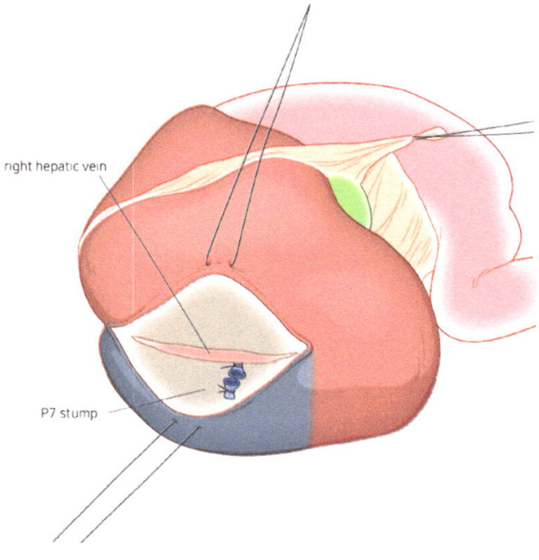

Fig. 12.5 Takasaki approach. Delineation of segment 7 by detecting and clamping the root of S7 pedicle through the parenchymal dissection on the dorsal 2/3 of the right portal fissure

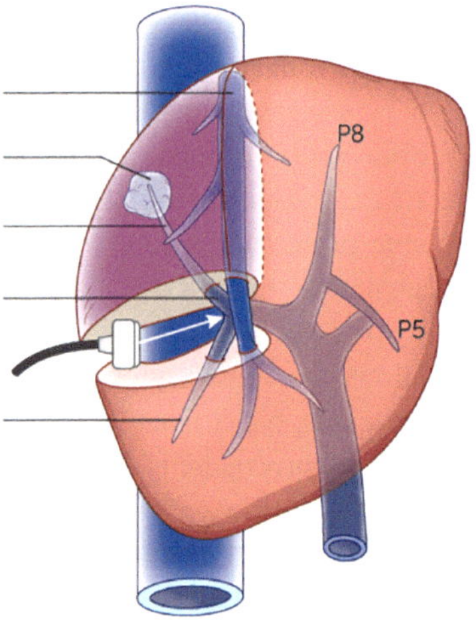

Fig. 12.6 Lateral approach. Delineation of segment 7 by identifying and clamping the root of S7 pedicle through the parenchymal dissection from right lateral to medical direction of the coronary plane. We can decide this plane by detecting the confluence of S6 and S7 Glisson pedicles using intraoperative ultrasonography

ultrasound-guided method. It is used when finding P7 by the above-mentioned approach is unpliant or in case of severe liver fibrosis. An ultrasound probe is applied to half the area of the right portal fissure in search of the bifurcation point of P6 and P7. Parenchymal transection is performed along the plane perpendicular to the right portal fissure. After ligation of P7, the dissection line follows RHV. Despite the satisfactory surgery, the second approach can be criticized for not following the strict rule of anatomical resection (Fig. 12.6).

References

1. Makuuchi M, Hasegawa H, Yamazaki S. Ultrasonically guided subsegmentectomy. Surg Gynecol Obstet. 1985;161:346–50.
2. Takasaki K. Glissonean pedicle transaction method for hepatic resection. 1st ed. Japan: Springer; 2007.

Laparoscopic Left Hemihepatectomy

13

Ki-Hun Kim and Hwui-Dong Cho

Abstract

Left hemihepatectomy refers to the resection of segments II, III, and IV of the liver according to the Couinaud classification. If the tumor is not too close to the liver hilum or major vessels such as IVC and middle hepatic vein, the indication of laparoscopic left hemihepatectomy is the same as that of the open procedure. With proper patient selection and laparoscopy surgical technique, the left hemihepatectomy can be performed safely.

Keywords

Laparoscopic liver resection · Laparoscopic left hemihepatectomy · Pure laparoscopy Surgical procedure · Surgical technique

13.1 Definition

Left hemihepatectomy refers to the resection of segments II, III, and IV of the liver without the middle vein according to the Couinaud classification, and resection with the middle vein is called extended left hemihepatectomy. In the pure laparoscopic procedure, the entire resection of the liver is completed through laparoscopic ports; hand-assist devices or working incisions are not used, although a small incision may be made for specimen extraction. Hand-assisted laparoscopy is defined by the elective placement of a hand port for facilitating the procedure. And, the hybrid technique is defined as a procedure, which is started as a pure laparoscopic, or a hand-assisted procedure but the resection is performed through a mini-laparotomy incision [1]. The contents to be described below are pure laparoscopy-oriented explanations.

13.2 Indications

Laparoscopic left hemihepatectomy is performed if the liver tumor is in segment IV or left lateral segments (segment II/III) when it is expected that

Supplementary Information The online version contains supplementary material available at https://doi.org/10.1007/978-981-16-1996-0_13.

K.-H. Kim (✉) · H.-D. Cho
Division of Hepatobiliary Surgery and Liver Transplantation, Department of Surgery, Asan Medical Center, University of Ulsan College of Medicine, Seoul, South Korea
e-mail: khkim620@amc.seoul.kr

H. C. Yu (ed.), *Hepato-Biliary-Pancreatic Surgery and Liver Transplantation*,
https://doi.org/10.1007/978-981-16-1996-0_13

sufficient resection margin would not be obtained as left lateral sectionectomy. However, to perform safe laparoscopic surgery, the tumor must not be attached to the liver hilum and major vessels such as IVC and middle hepatic vein. It can also be performed when symptomatic intrahepatic stones are in the left lobe, and there is stenosis of the left biliary tract that causes suspicion of malignancy.

13.3 Preoperative Examination

The preoperative examination should be done to ensure that the liver function is enough for resection and to recognize the patient's anatomy. The general blood test is the same as the open procedure. It is recommended to perform a three-dimensional CT or MRI that reconstructs the hepatic arteries, portal vein, and biliary tract of the liver. The anatomy of the liver has a lot of variations; it is necessary to recognize the patients' liver anatomy and make a plan before surgery. In particular, the right posterior hepatic duct drains to the left hepatic duct in about 30% of the cases, and determining the left bile duct resection site is very important to prevent damage to the right posterior bile duct (Fig. 13.1) [2].

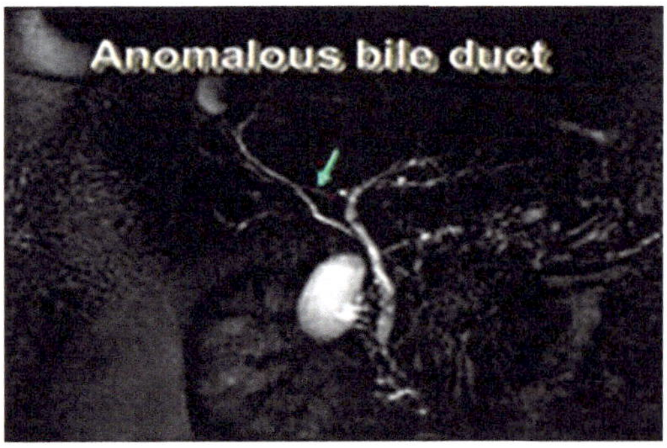

Fig. 13.1 The right posterior bile duct has an anomalous drainage to the left bile duct

13.4 Patient Position

The patient lies in the lithotomy position under general anesthesia. At this time, the operator stands between the two legs of the patient (French position); the first assistant stands at the upper left side of the patient and the second assistant stands with the camera at the lower left side. Occasionally, the operator would stand on the right side of the patient, but in experience, standing between the legs of the patient is optimal for laparoscopic liver resection.

13.5 Trocars Site

Generally, a total of five trocars are used. The procedure is feasible with four trocars, but adding a 5 mm trocar can provide a much more convenient resection. The pneumoperitoneum is made by the open or closed method, and the trocar for the camera is located just above the umbilicus or slightly upper left side. The operator utilizes two trocars. The main working trocar for hepatectomy is 12 mm in size and is inserted at the point where the right rib meets the midclavicular line under visualization of the camera. The second trocar measuring the same size is inserted directly below the rib cage along the right anterior axillary line. At this trocar site, an atraumatic grasper is often used to pull the liver, or an automatic anastomosis device can be inserted depending on the angle of the left hepatic vein.

Two trocars are used by the first assistant. A 12 mm trocar is placed directly below the xiphoid process, whose main functions are suction and irrigation. The other 5 mm trocar is inserted at the point where the left rib meets along the left middle clavicle line. The first assistant uses an atraumatic grasper to pull the liver through this trocar during resection (Fig. 13.2) [3, 4].

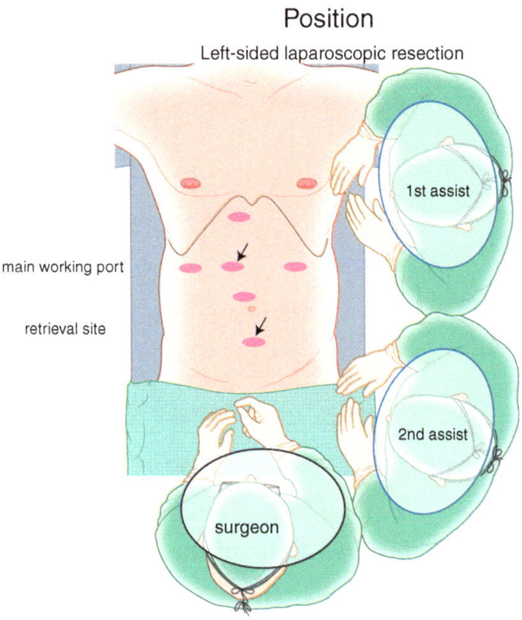

Fig. 13.2 The patient was placed in the lithotomy position in the 30° reverse Trendelenburg position, with the surgeon standing between the donor's legs. The 1st assistant and the 2nd assistant were located on the left side of the patient

13.6 Pneumoperitoneum

In general, abdominal pressure is maintained below 12 mmHg. It has been reported that raising the abdominal pressure during bleeding may help stop the bleeding, but raising the abdominal pressure for a long time is considered a high risk for air embolism; therefore, special care should be taken.

13.7 Bleeding Control

Usually, laparoscopic liver resection causes less bleeding than conventional open liver resection due to several reasons. The pneumoperitoneum itself can lead to less bleeding and a magnified view by the camera can lead to a more meticulous surgery. Careful parenchymal resection of the liver and Pringle maneuver are performed to minimize bleeding unless there is a contraindication (15 min of occlusion and 5 min of reperfusion). In the case of bleeding from small vessels with a stump, the dissector is used to hold the tip of the stump and apply a clip underneath. If a hole is formed in the main hepatic vein, hemostasis can be done with a bipolar device or with a suture using prolene 6-0. Under conditions of nonfeasibility, the hole should be with hemostatic agents or gauze and the procedure should be delayed until the bleeding stops. In most cases, this will lead to hemostasis. If you carefully dissect around the parenchyma of the bleeding focus while pressing that area, you can eventually find the exact bleeding focus and stop bleeding. However, if you fail to control bleeding with these measures, you must boldly switch to an open conversion. The transition to open surgery is never a problem and is necessary for the patient's safety.

13.8 Surgical Technique

13.8.1 Round Ligament Division

The round ligament is first excised for the mobilization of the liver. In the case of right hemihepatectomy, the falciform ligament should be adequately left for fixation of the remnant left liver, but in the case of left hemihepatectomy, it is not necessary.

13.8.2 Cholecystectomy

In the case of a left hemihepatectomy, cholecystectomy is not performed routinely unless there is a problem with the gallbladder. When resecting the liver, it is convenient to perform surgery while holding the gallbladder with an atraumatic grasper with the surgeon's left hand and pulling it outwards.

13.8.3 Left Hilar Dissection and ICG (Indocyanine Green) Technique

There are two methods of the left hilar dissection. The first is the Glissonean pedicle approach [5] and the second is the individual isolation approach. Since biliary malformations can be present in 30% of cases [2], a thorough review of the preoperative imaging studies is mandatory and, if necessary, intraoperative cholangiography should be performed before and after biliary division, to ensure that the division has been safely performed.

In the method of the Glissonean pedicle approach, after confirming the hepatic hilum, the liver parenchyma around the left Glissonean pedicle is dissected to make space. When the Glissonean pedicle is clamped with a Bulldog clamp, the ischemic boundary for resection of the lobe can be seen.

In the individual isolation method, the first assistant lifts the left lobe for the operator, and the operator dissects the left hepatic artery using the dissector, clips the Hem-o-lok® clip twice on the remnant side, and seals the artery stump of the specimen side using an energy device (Fig. 13.3). The left hepatic portal vein may be divided after isolation, but if there is a risk of bleeding during the left portal vein isolation due to the small portal branches around it, it may be ligated with a small clip and divided with the left hepatic duct with Endo-GIA™ after parenchymal transection of the liver (Fig. 13.4).

Regarding the ICG injection, 2.5 mg of ICG is injected intravenously after isolation and clamping of the Glisson of the liver to be resected. Then, ICG is administrated into the entire remnant liver segment, excluding the clamped side (Video 13.1).

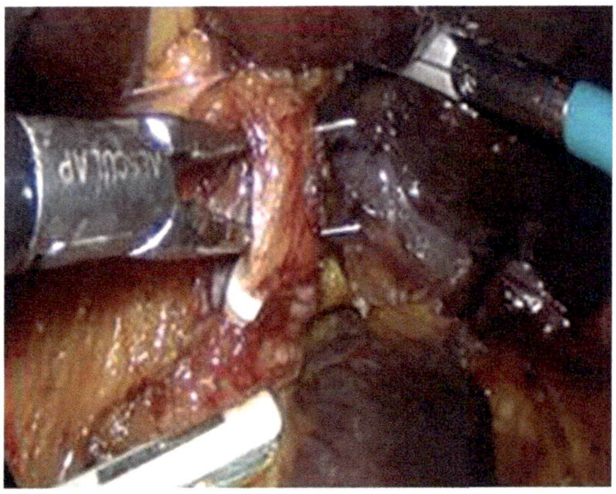

Fig. 13.3 The Left hepatic artery was applied with Hem-o-lok® clip

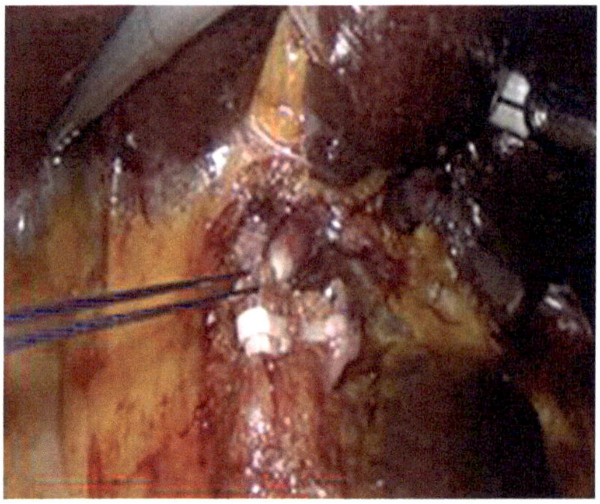

Fig. 13.4 The left portal vein was tied off

13.8.4 Liver Mobilization

For benign diseases, liver mobilization may be performed first, but in the case of malignant tumors, it is recommended to first block the blood inflow to avoid the chance of tumor spread. After removing the left coronary ligament and the left triangular ligament using the energy device, the lateral side of the left hepatic vein is exposed. If the lateral side of the liver is large, it is convenient to separate the ligament after placing the gauze between the spleen, omentum, and liver.

When dividing the hepatogastric ligament, there may be blood vessels going to the liver in the ligament, which can be ligated using a Hem-o-lok® clip on the remaining side and divided using an energy device.

13.8.5 Liver Parenchymal Transection

The surface of the liver is transected using an energy device along the ischemic boundary, and the deep part of the liver is transected with an ultrasonic aspirator equipped with a long tip for laparoscopy. An ultrasonic aspirator has to move widely to the left and right and shallow to the top and bottom to reduce the Glissonean pedicle injury and for safe parenchymal transection. As in the left hemihepatectomy, full exposure of the middle hepatic vein is important during parenchymal transection for the anatomical resection. Occasionally, a small branch of the middle vein may be damaged and bleed, but in most cases, it is stopped by transient pressing with a gauze-type hemostatic agent.

13.8.6 Left Hilar Division

The left Glissonean pedicle exposed after parenchymal transection is divided using the Endo-GIA™. If the bile duct has an anatomical variation such that the right-side bile duct drains to the left bile duct, using the Endo-GIA™ in the distal part to the maximum extent possible to prevent biliary damage is preferred (Fig. 13.5).

13.8.7 Left Hepatic Vein Division

After the division of the left Glissonean pedicle, the left hepatic vein is exposed easily when the remaining parenchyma is removed and divided using the Endo-GIA™ (Fig. 13.6).

13.8.8 Specimen Extraction

The resected left lobe is placed in an Endo-bag and removed from Pfannenstiel incision, the transverse incision just above the pubic symphysis. The length of the incision is determined according to the volume of the resected liver.

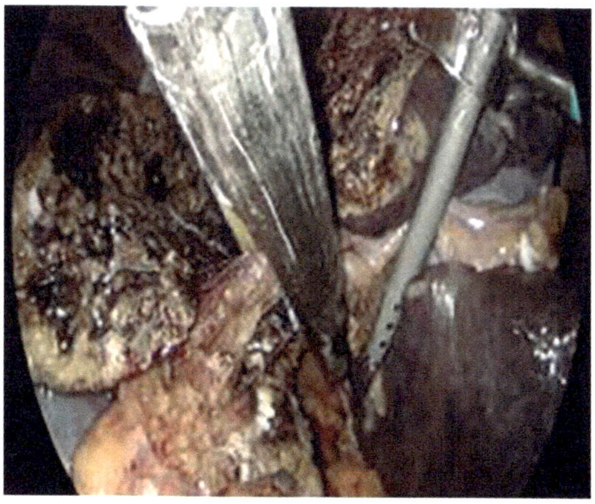

Fig. 13.5 The left bile duct was divided using Endo-GIA™

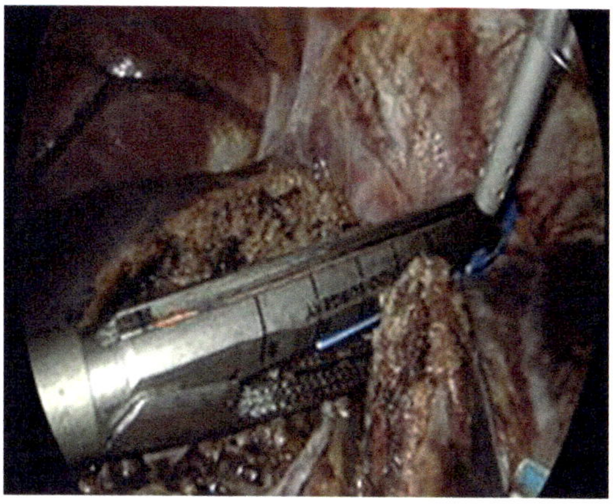

Fig. 13.6 The left hepatic vein was divided using Endo-GIA™

13.8.9 Check Resection Margin and Drain Tube Insertion

Occasionally, there may be bleeding at the resection margin when using the Endo-GIA™, so it is better to clip using small clips at the resection site. After bleeding control, a hemostatic agent should be applied to the resection margin and the drain tube should be placed on the resection margin.

13.9 Summary

Laparoscopic left hemihepatectomy can be performed with surgical indications such as the open left hemihepatectomy. With the proper patient selection and surgical technique for laparoscopy, the left hemihepatectomy can be performed safely.

References

1. Buell JF, Cherqui D, Geller DA, O'Rourke N, Iannitti D, Dagher I, et al. The international position on laparoscopic liver surgery: the Louisville statement, 2008. Ann Surg. 2009;250(5):825–30.
2. Choi JW, Kim TK, Kim KW, Kim AY, Kim PN, Ha HK, et al. Anatomic variation in intrahepatic bile ducts: an analysis of intraoperative cholangiograms in 300 consecutive donors for living donor liver transplantation. Korean J Radiol. 2003;4(2):85–90.

3. Cho HD, Kim KH, Hwang S, Ahn CS, Moon DB, Ha TY, et al. Comparison of pure laparoscopic versus open left hemihepatectomy by multivariate analysis: a retrospective cohort study. Surg Endosc. 2018;32(2):643–50.
4. Namgoong JM, Kim KH, Park GC, Jung DH, Song GW, Ha TY, et al. Comparison of laparoscopic versus open left hemihepatectomy for left-sided hepatolithiasis. Int J Med Sci. 2014;11(2):127–33.
5. Takasaki K. Glissonean pedicle transection method for hepatic resection: a new concept of liver segmentation. J Hepato-Biliary-Pancreat Surg. 1998;5(3):286–91.

14 Laparoscopic Left Lateral Sectionectomy

In Seok Choi and Ju Ik Moon

Abstract

Laparoscopic left lateral sectionectomy can be applied easily among several laparoscopic hepatic segmental resection procedures. This chapter discusses the technical aspects of laparoscopic left lateral sectionectomy, including instrument and patient position, location of trocars, liver traction, and surgical procedures steps. Also, the authors provide useful tips for laparoscopic left lateral sectionectomy.

Keywords

Laparoscopy · Left lateral sectionectomy
Laparoscopic liver resection · Glisson

Supplementary Information The online version contains supplementary material available at https://doi.org/10.1007/978-981-16-1996-0_14.

I. S. Choi (✉) · J. I. Moon
Department of Surgery, Konyang University Hospital, Konyang University School of Medicine, Daejeon, South Korea
e-mail: choiins@kyuh.ac.kr

14.1 Indication

- Malignant tumors located on the left side of the falciform ligament (hepatocellular carcinoma, metastatic liver cancer, and intrahepatic liver cancer).
- Benign tumors (cystic adenoma, hemangioma, and other cystic tumors).
- Intrahepatic stones (when intrahepatic stones without stenosis in the main left bile duct are localized in the left lateral section).

14.2 The Patient's Posture and the Position of the Operators

- Operate in a supine state with elevated head position (Reverse Trendelenburg).
- Depending on the preference of the operator or the patient's body mass, you can choose French posture with both legs spread apart.
- The surgeon is on the right side of the patient, and the assistant and scopist are on the left side. Depending on the preference of the operator, the operator can be positioned between both legs to perform surgery (Fig. 14.1).

H. C. Yu (ed.), *Hepato-Biliary-Pancreatic Surgery and Liver Transplantation*,
https://doi.org/10.1007/978-981-16-1996-0_14

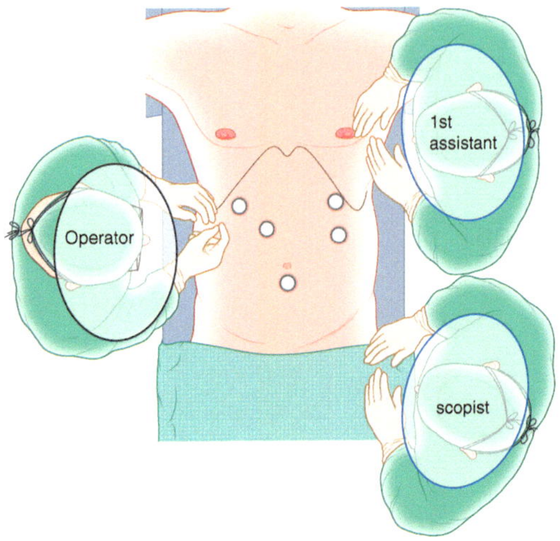

Fig. 14.1 Position of the operator and trocar

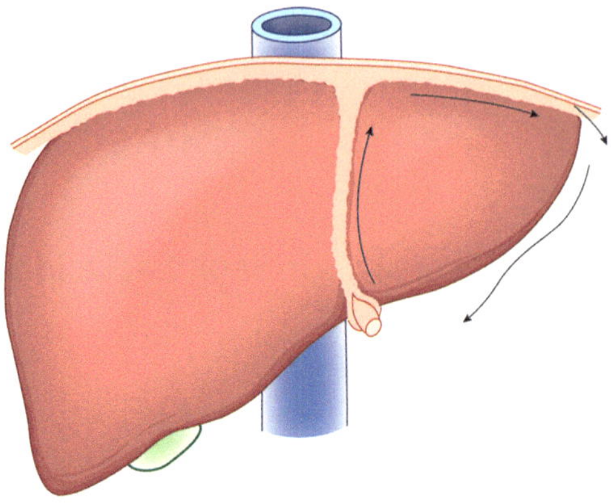

Fig. 14.2 Liver mobilization

14.3 Locations of Trocars

- For the first trocar (A), after making an incision of 1 cm in size at the bottom of the umbilicus, an 11–12 mm trocar is inserted following the Hasson method to create pneumoperitoneum and then a camera is inserted.
- In the case of the second trocar (B), a 12 mm trocar is inserted in the right part of the midline into the patient's right upper abdomen and used as the primary (main) port for the operator.
- In the case of the third trocar (C), a 5 mm trocar is inserted 2–3 cm below the rib cage of the clavicle midline in the patient's right upper abdomen and is used by the operator's left hand.
- In the case of the fourth trocar (D), a 5 mm trocar is inserted in the patient's upper left abdomen 5–7 cm below the costal margin of the clavicle midline and used by the assistant surgeon.
- Tip: Depending on the level of the assistant's skills or the progress of the surgery, a 5 mm trocar may be added to the upper left abdomen if necessary.

14.4 Steps of Surgery

14.4.1 Mobilization of the Liver (Fig. 14.2)

- Using an ultrasonic energy device, the falciform ligament is dissected upward close to the parenchyma, approaching the diaphragm, and exfoliated to the area where the inferior vena cava and the left hepatic vein meet.
- Dissect the left coronary ligament while pulling down the left lateral lobe of the liver. At this time, to avoid injuring the diaphragm, the ligament is peeled off by contacting the parenchyma, and when the left triangular ligament is exposed, it is ligated with a clip or hemlock.
- After the left triangular ligament is cut, the left lateral segment is lifted to expose the hepatogastric ligament. To easily expose the left hepatic vein, the ligament may be exfoliated, and depending on the operator, exfoliation may not be performed.
- Ligamentum teres is used for traction after cutting according to the taste of many other surgeons. In the case of this author, it is used for traction without cutting.

14.4.2 Liver Traction (Fig. 14.3)

- For laparoscopic liver resection, retraction of the liver is an essential process, and in the case of the author's experience, a 2-0 prolene straight needle is used to insert the straight needle from the outer side of the right upper abdomen, tied to the ligamentum teres, and then pulled out to the needle to the right-side traction. Left-side traction is performed by stay suture to the parenchyma of the left lateral lobe using a 2-0 prolene straight needle and a rubber band and then pulled out toward the left lateral abdominal wall.

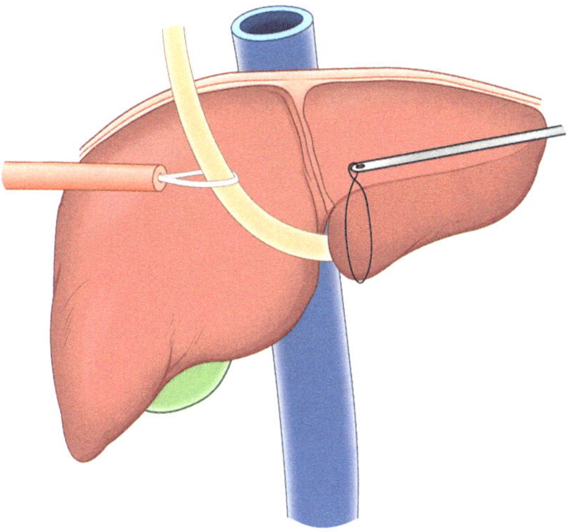

Fig. 14.3 Liver traction method

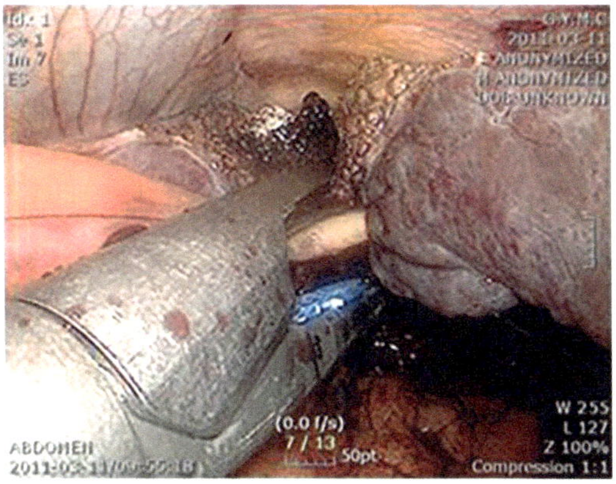

Fig. 14.4 Glisson's approach with the endoscopic automatic anastomosis device

- For the beginners, the right-side traction can be done by pulling the ligament teres with the left hand of the operator, and the left-side traction using the liver retractors (snake retractor or fan retractor) can easily expose the cut surface of the liver.

14.4.3 Liver Resection by Glissonean Approach

- By traction of the left and right lobes of the liver toward the left and right sides, the parenchyma on the left side of the falciform ligament gets well exposed. First, the cutting line is marked on the left side of the falciform ligament using an electric cauterizer, and the parenchyma is cut 1–2 cm from the liver surface using an ultrasonic energy device or a vessel sealing device. For deeper parenchymal dissection or blood vessel exposure, CUSA is used to dissect the hepatic parenchyma.
- Dissect the parenchyma to expose the Glisson branches. After that, secure enough space for the endoscopic anastomosis. Glisson branch is processed in batch using an endoscope automatic anastomosis machine measuring 60 mm in size (Blue, Gold cartilage) (Fig. 14.4).
- Tip: Depending on the preference of the operator or the thickness of the Glisson, an automatic endoscopic anastomosis device of appropriate thickness should be used, and multiple cartilages may be used as needed.
- Tip: Endoscopic automatic anastomosis device is inserted into the hepatic parenchyma in the horizontal direction with the falciform ligament to the maximum extent possible.
- Tip: Individual Glisson method for 2 and 3 segments: Along the left side of the umbilical portion, the soft tissue around the area suspected to be the Glisson area in segment 3 is removed, and the Glisson branch and the hepatic parenchyma are carefully dissected with a suction tip. With the suction tip and right-angle device, the upper and lower parts of the branch are continuously peeled off, and when the upper and lower parts of the branch are penetrated, the proximal and distal parts of the detached segment 3 Glisson branch are ligated and cut with a hemolock. After cutting the Glisson branch in segment 3, if the hepatic parenchyma is slightly dissected, the Glisson branch in segment 2 is exposed and cut in the same way. Subsequently, the hepatic parenchyma is peeled to expose the hepatic vein.
- Tip: Liver resection by an individual approach is practically not used much recently because the umbilical portion has a difficult anatomical structure, and it is difficult to individually cut and treat the hepatic portal vein and hepatic artery.

After the Glisson branch is cut using the endoscopic automatic anastomosis device, the remaining hepatic parenchyma is separated using ultrasonic energy devices, vessel sealing devices, or CUSA to expose the left hepatic vein, and the hepatic vein is cut using the endoscopic automatic anastomosis device measuring 60 mm in size (white cartilage) (Fig. 14.5).

- Tip: In patients with intrahepatic duct stones, residual stones need to be checked if the Glisson branches draining to the left lateral segment are thickened by inflammation and it is difficult to separate the Glisson branches or if the intrahepatic duct stone is in the intrahepatic duct proximal to the umbilicus. The intrahepatic bile duct on the resected surface should be exposed. First, the liver portal vein and the hepatic artery are individually separated, and then the lateral bile ducts are partially exposed after cutting the vessels. After exposing as much of the bile duct as possible to the upper parenchyma of the bile duct using CUSA and the ultrasonic energy device, cut the bile duct using the device. After removing intrahepatic stones through an open bile duct, the bile duct is sutured and closed.

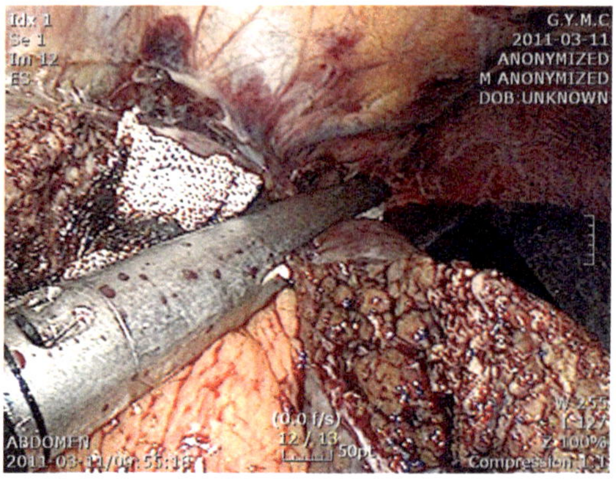

Fig. 14.5 Ligation of left hepatic vein

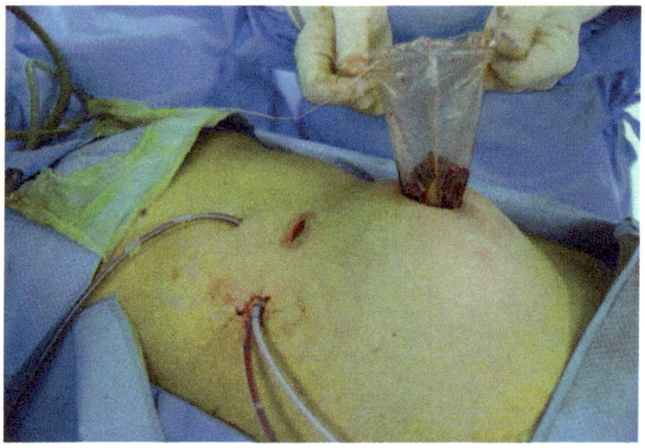

Fig. 14.6 Hepatic specimen removal using an umbilical port

14.4.4 Drain Insertion and Extraction of the Surgical Specimen

- After applying fibrin glue to the liver resection surfaces, place the drainage tube around it.
- The excised left lateral section is placed in an endoscopic plastic bag and removed through an incision extending toward the 12 mm trocar region of the umbilicus or the Pfannenstiel incision (Fig. 14.6).

15 Laparoscopic Right Hemihepatectomy

Ho-Seong Han and Jai Young Cho

Abstract

As the potential applications for LLR have expanded considerably, laparoscopic left lateral sectionectomy is now regarded as a standard treatment option (Guro H, Cho JY, Han HS, Yoon YS, Choi Y, Periyasamy M. Clin Mol Hepatol. 22:212–218, 2016). However, laparoscopic major liver resection including laparoscopic right hepatectomy is still considered a difficult operation. Recently, laparoscopic right hemihepatectomy has been increasingly performed in patients with hepatocellular carcinoma or metastatic liver tumors by the accumulation of experiences and development of instruments (Guro H, Cho JY, Han HS, Yoon YS, Choi Y, Kim S, Kim K, Hyun IG. Surg Oncol. 27:31–35, 2018; Han HS, Yoon YS, Cho JY, Ahn KS. Ann Surg Oncol. 17:2090–2091, 2010). Successful laparoscopic donor right hepatectomy has also been reported (Han HS, Cho JY, Yoon YS, Hwang DW, Kim YK, Shin HK, Lee W, Surg Endosc. 29:184, 2015). This manuscript describes details of standard surgical techniques, instruments, and precautions in a stepwise manner.

Keywords

Laparoscopy · Right · Major · Donor

15.1 Indication

1. Hepatocellular carcinoma occupying the right hemiliver, metastatic tumor with no evidence of extrahepatic disease, and intrahepatic cholangiocarcinoma confined to the right lobe of the liver.
2. Benign liver tumors with the presence of symptoms, the danger of rupture, and uncertainty of diagnosis.
3. Hepatolithiasis associated with duct stricture, atrophy of the diseased liver parenchyma, or both.
4. The living donor with favorable anatomy for adult-to-adult living donor liver transplantation.

Supplementary Information The online version contains supplementary material available at https://doi.org/10.1007/978-981-16-1996-0_15.

H.-S. Han (✉) · J. Y. Cho
Department of Surgery, Seoul National University Bundang Hospital, Bundang-gu, South Korea
e-mail: hanhs@snubh.org

H. C. Yu (ed.), *Hepato-Biliary-Pancreatic Surgery and Liver Transplantation*,
https://doi.org/10.1007/978-981-16-1996-0_15

15.2 Patient Position and Trocar Placement

1. The patient is always placed in a supine position with split legs. The table is usually kept in reverse Trendelenburg's position with the right side up.
2. Five trocars are usually used (Fig. 15.1). The diameter of the trocar depends on the instrument used, so 12 mm trocar for the scope, CUSA, stapler, fan retractor, and the rest is 5 mm. The 12 mm trocar placement for the main working port (Port C in Fig. 15.1) is adjusted according to the size of the patient's body and abdominal cavity and location of the tumor.
3. The operator usually stands between the patient's legs. Occasionally, the operator moves to the right side of the patient during the operation.

15.3 Operative Technique

1. After insertion of the first trocar, pneumoperitoneum is established and maintained at 10–12 mmHg. A flexible laparoscope is used. After exploration of the peritoneal cavity for signs of unresectable disease, intraoperative ultrasound is performed to define the location and extent of the lesion.
2. Complete mobilization of the right lobe of the liver by dissection of triangular and coronary ligaments and diaphragmatic attachments is performed. Separation of the falciform ligament from the anterior abdominal wall is done using ultrasonic shears till full exposure of inferior vena cava is achieved. A few short hepatic veins are ligated using clips (Fig. 15.2).
3. Inflow control can be done by the Glisson approach or by individual ligation. When the Glissonean approach is adopted for right-

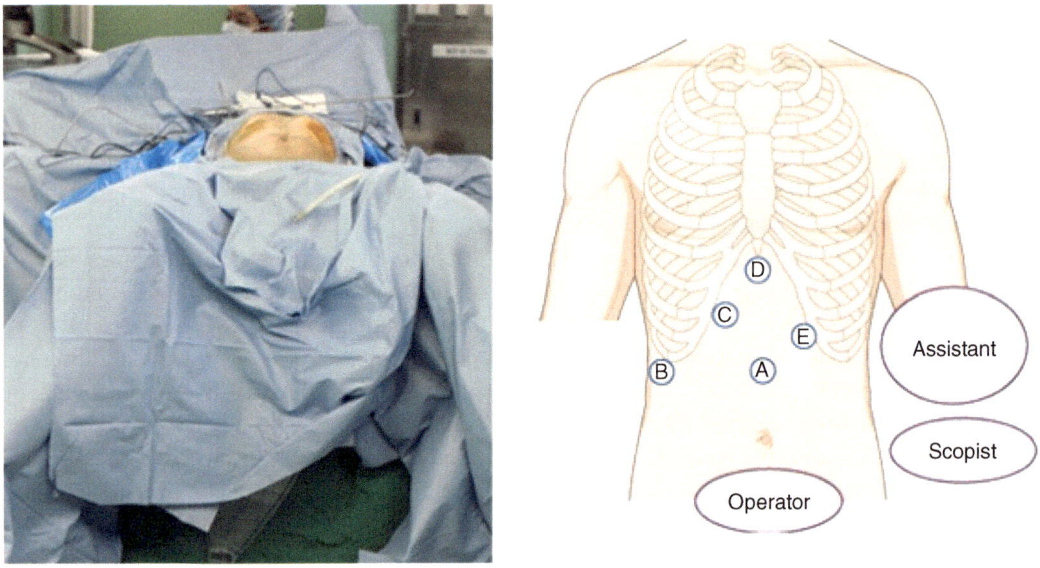

Fig. 15.1 Trocar placement and position of the surgeons

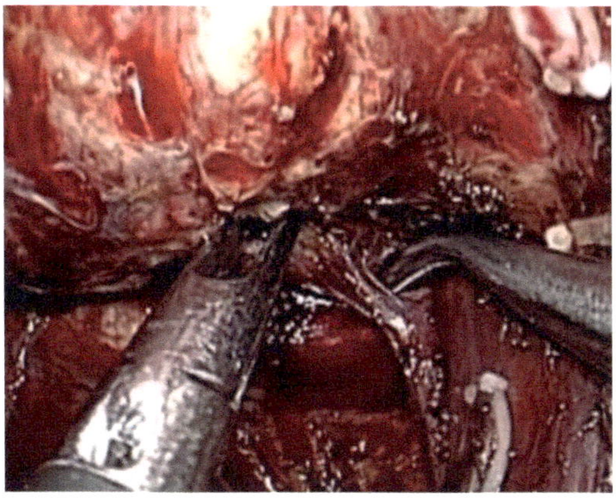

Fig. 15.2 Dissection of the inferior vena cava

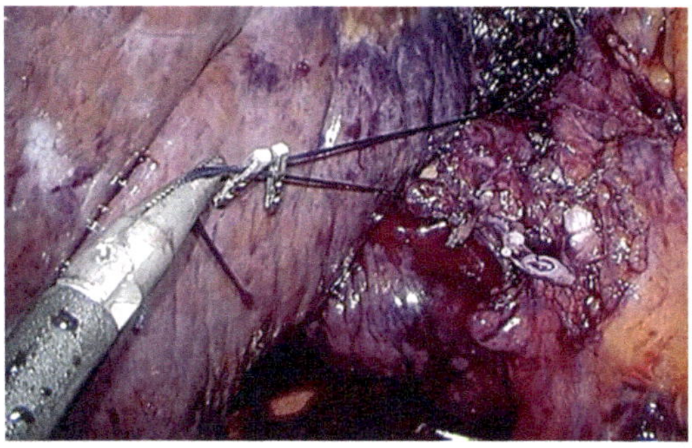

Fig. 15.3 Isolation of right Glisson pedicle

sided resection, hilar dissection is performed to isolate the right Glisson's pedicles at the inferior surface of the quadrate lobe. To isolate and tape the right pedicle, a long right-angle type clamp or curved dissector is considered as valuable. After taping the right pedicle, the whole pedicle can be ligated en masse by an Endo stapler (Fig. 15.3).

4. For living donors or patients with hepatolithiasis, individual ligation is preferred (Fig. 15.4). After right hepatic artery isolation with meticulous dissection, the right portal vein could be isolated with blunt atraumatic forceps. The demarcation line is made after temporary clamping of the artery and portal vein.
5. For parenchymal dissection for superficial liver tissue, ultrasonic shear is very useful and considered a fast energy device (Fig. 15.5). If the donor has significantly large V5 and/or V8 branch, those should be widely and safely dissected for future reconstruction. Then CUSA is used to dissect the deep part of parenchyma with bipolar diathermy. The hanging maneuver is beneficial to facilitate parenchymal dissection (Fig. 15.6).

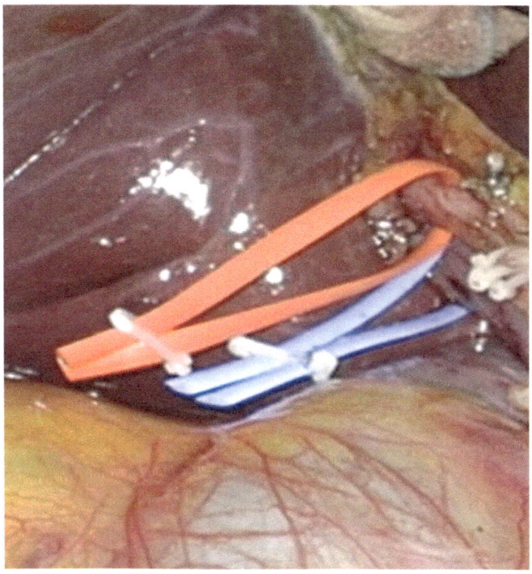

Fig. 15.4 The right hepatic artery and portal vein are isolated and taped

6. The final step is ligation of the right hepatic vein at the origin of the vein root using a stapler (Fig. 15.7). After retrieval of graft or right liver through the suprapubic incision, hemostasis and drain insertion are done.

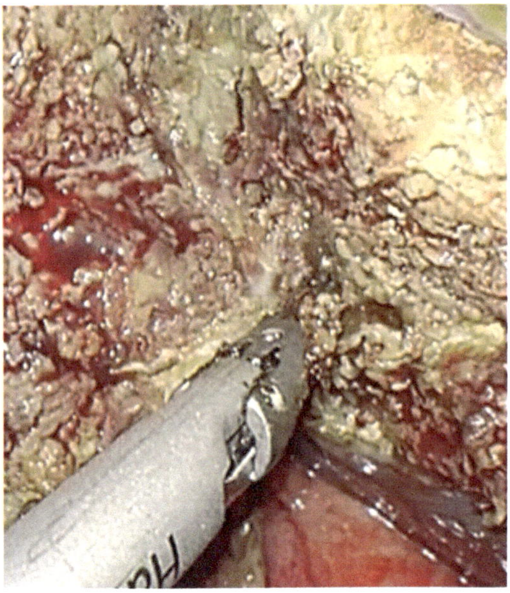

Fig. 15.5 Superficial parenchymal dissection using ultrasonic shears

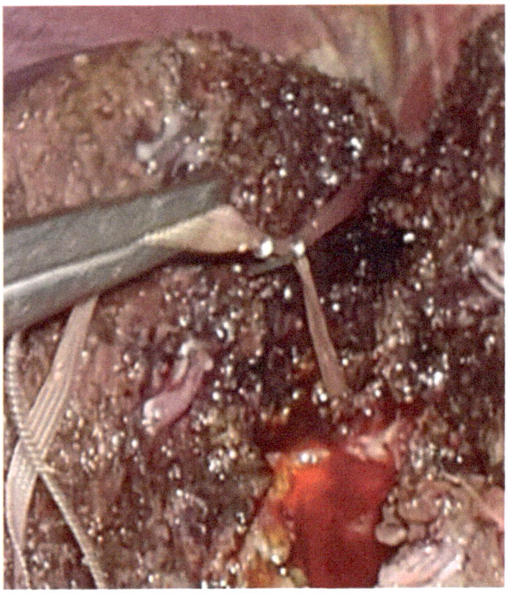

Fig. 15.6 Hanging maneuver during laparoscopic right hepatectomy

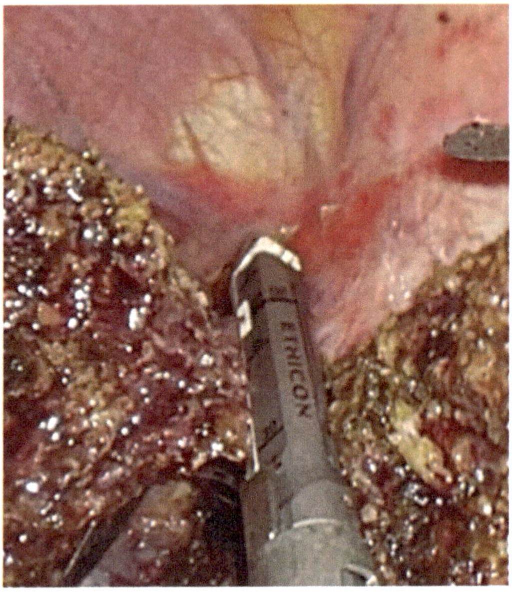

Fig. 15.7 The right hepatic vein is ligated using a stapler

Further Reading

Guro H, Cho JY, Han HS, Yoon YS, Choi Y, Periyasamy M. Current status of laparoscopic liver resection for hepatocellular carcinoma. Clin Mol Hepatol. 2016;22:212–8.

Guro H, Cho JY, Han HS, Yoon YS, Choi Y, Kim S, Kim K, Hyun IG. Outcomes of major laparoscopic liver resection for hepatocellular carcinoma. Surg Oncol. 2018;27:31–5.

Han HS, Yoon YS, Cho JY, Ahn KS. Laparoscopic right hemihepatectomy for hepatocellular carcinoma. Ann Surg Oncol. 2010;17:2090–1.

Han HS, Cho JY, Yoon YS, Hwang DW, Kim YK, Shin HK, Lee W. Total laparoscopic living donor right hepatectomy. Surg Endosc. 2015;29:184.

Part II

Deceased Donor Liver Transplantation

16 Liver Procurement in a Deceased Donor

Hee Chul Yu and Jae Do Yang

Abstract

The goal of donor management and selection is maximizing the number of organs procured and transplanted for each deceased donor while maintaining optimal function of those organs [1]. The concept of multiple abdominal organ procurement techniques was outlined by Starzl [2–4].

For the deceased donors, wide exposure to the abdominal and thoracic organs is required, as well as access to the aorta and the provision of sufficient venous venting [5–8]. The basic concepts of liver procurement include less warm dissection, good perfusion, and rapid cooling [9].

These concepts must be integrated into simple and systematic procedures in order to promote a stable operation [10, 11].

Keywords

Deceased donor · Liver procurement · Warm dissection · Perfusion

Supplementary Information The online version contains supplementary material available at https://doi.org/10.1007/978-981-16-1996-0_16.

H. C. Yu (✉) · J. D. Yang
Department of Surgery, Jeonbuk National University Medical School, Jeonju, South Korea
e-mail: hcyu@jbnu.ac.kr

16.1 Procedures

A skin incision is made via the xiphoid process to the point just above the symphysis pubis and is transversely extended up both flanks at the level of the umbilicus (Fig. 16.1a, b).

If thoracotomy is needed for the donor, the incision line is extended toward the suprasternal notch, followed by opening the chest using a sternal saw and a Finochietto sternal retractor (Fig. 16.1c).

In order to provide sufficient exposure of the liver, the round and the falciform ligament of the liver is divided and tied (Fig. 16.2a, b). Examination of the intra-abdominal organs is carried out to exclude the presence of potential malignant disease. The quality of the liver is usually assessed at this stage, and a liver biopsy is recommended to evaluate the percentage of microsteatosis. Next, the left lateral section of the liver is separated from its ligamentous attachments by the division of the left coronary and triangular ligaments (Fig. 16.2a, c).

Careful exposure of the hepatogastric ligament must be performed. Inspection and palpation of the arterial supply of the liver can be performed at this time by paying close attention to anatomical variants, such as accessory or replace the right hepatic artery from the superior mesenteric artery (SMA) and accessory or replace the left hepatic artery from the left gastric artery (Fig. 16.3a, b).

H. C. Yu (ed.), *Hepato-Biliary-Pancreatic Surgery and Liver Transplantation*,
https://doi.org/10.1007/978-981-16-1996-0_16

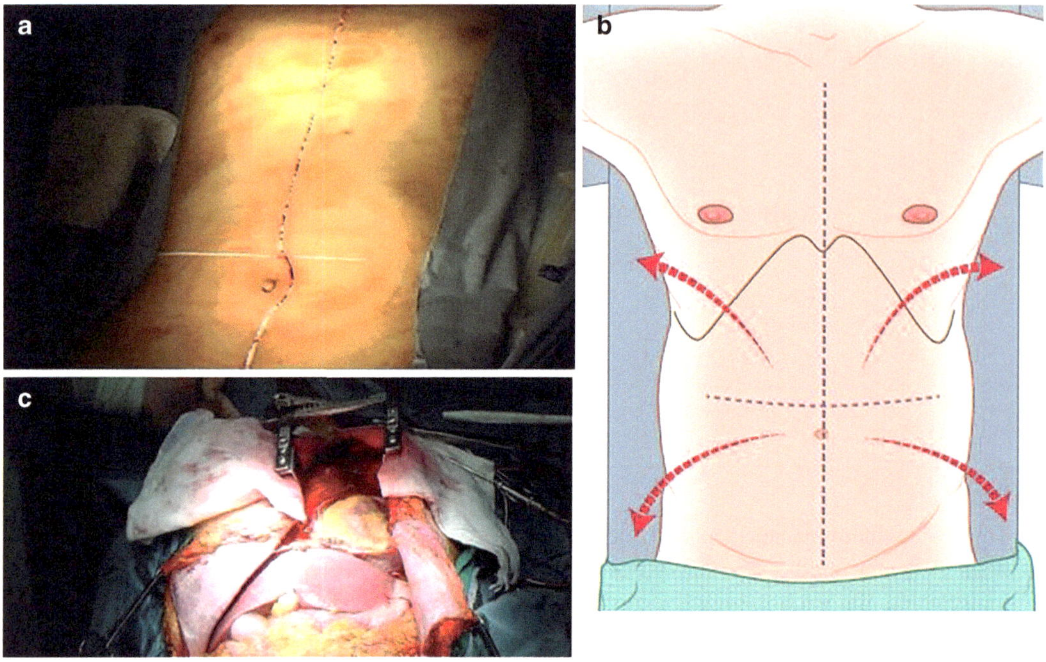

Fig. 16.1 (**a**) A skin incision. (**b**) A schematic view of midline and vertical incisions. (**c**) The towel clip fixed to the abdominal wall, and the chest is opened using the Finochietto retractor

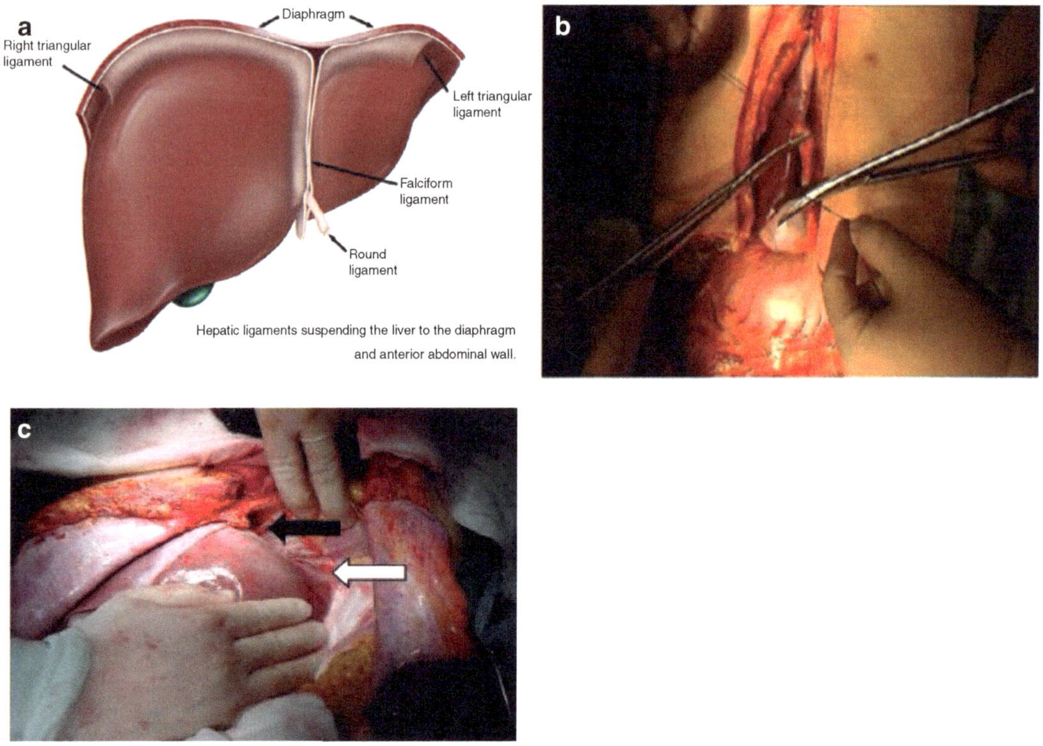

Fig. 16.2 (**a**) The peri hepatic ligaments. (**b**) Resection of the round and falciform ligament. (**c**) Left coronary (black arrow) and triangular ligament (white arrow)

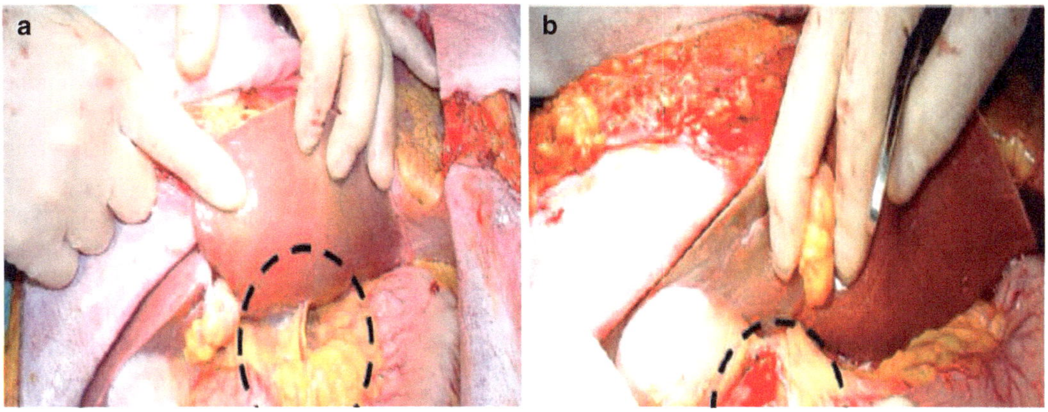

Fig. 16.3 Identification of anatomical variations of the hepatic artery. (**a**) Inspection of the gastrohepatic ligament for the left hepatic artery. (**b**) Inspection of the foramen of Winslow for the right hepatic artery

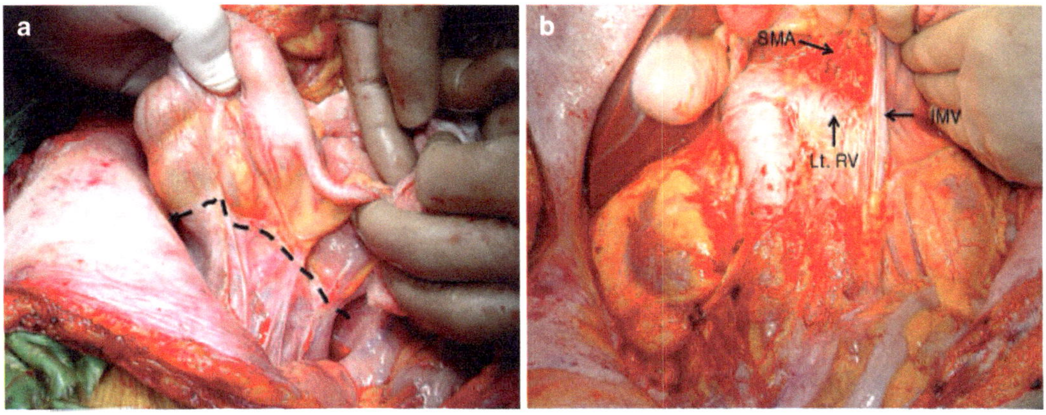

Fig. 16.4 Mobilization of the intestinal and retroperitoneal vessels. (**a**) Dissection of the ascending colon along the white line of Toldt. (**b**) Division of the Lt RV, SMA, and IMA after Kocherization

Preparation of aortic cannulation. The right colon and the terminal small intestine are moved cephalad and retracted to the left side (Fig. 16.4a) The Kocher maneuver is performed to mobilize the duodenum. Peritoneal reflections between the duodenum and retroperitoneal areas are dissected and incised, thereby exposing entire retroperitoneal structures like the aorta, inferior vena cava (IVC), renal vein (RV), SMA, inferior mesenteric artery (IMA), and the inferior mesenteric vein (IMV) (Fig. 16.4b).

IMV (or SMV in case of without pancreas procurement) is looped with a 3–0 black silk for portal cannulation. Arterial perfusion is usually performed by cannulating at the infrarenal aorta. The aorta is encircled above the iliac artery bifurcation using umbilical tape (Fig. 16.5).

At this time, careful dissection is needed to avoid damaging the vertebral artery that posteriorly branches out from the aorta.

The abdominal or thoracic aorta is used to cross-clamp based on the circumstances.

If the chest is not opened, the cross-clamp at the abdomen is applied over the supraceliac aorta.

Umbilical tape is used to encircle the aorta after dissection of the diaphragmatic crus in addition to a retracted left lateral section to the right side and esophagus to the left side (Fig. 16.6a, b).

If the chest is opened, the intrathoracic descending aorta is cross-clamped by opening the left side of the chest (Fig. 16.6c).

Histidine-Tryptophan-Ketoglutarate (HTK) solution and a cannula (aorta 18–22 fr, portal 10-12Fr) are connected, and crushed ice is prepared. At least 3 minutes before infusion of the preserving solution, a dose of 300 U/kg of heparin should be given intravenously. The gallbladder is incised and irrigated using saline to reduce autolysis of the bile duct membrane (Fig. 16.7).

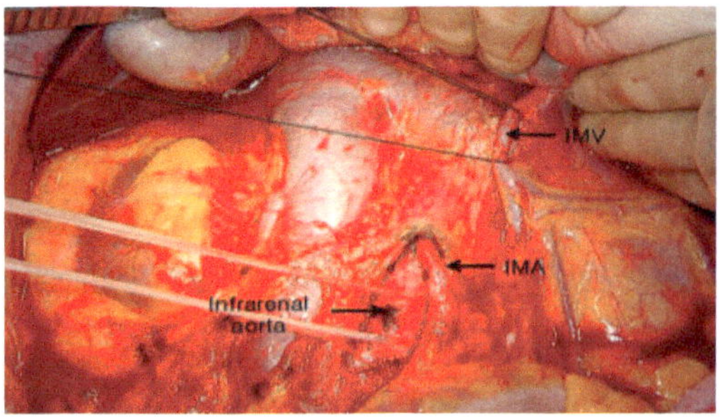

Fig. 16.5 Exposure of the IMV for portal cannulation (3-0 black silk tapping) and infrarenal aorta for aortic cannulation (umbilical tapping)

The abdominal aorta is ligated distally using the umbilical tape above the bifurcation of the iliac artery and is proximally incised up to about one-third toward the interior while holding using the thumb and index finger.

After lumen examination, place the tube so that its end is located below the renal artery and ligated (Fig. 16.8a, b). The IMA or SMV is cannulated at the portal perfusion (Fig. 16.8b).

Immediately before the infusion of the preserving solution, the aorta (abdominal or thoracic) should be clamped and must be infused with cold preserving solution under 150 mmHg pressure measured using a pneumatic cuff. The

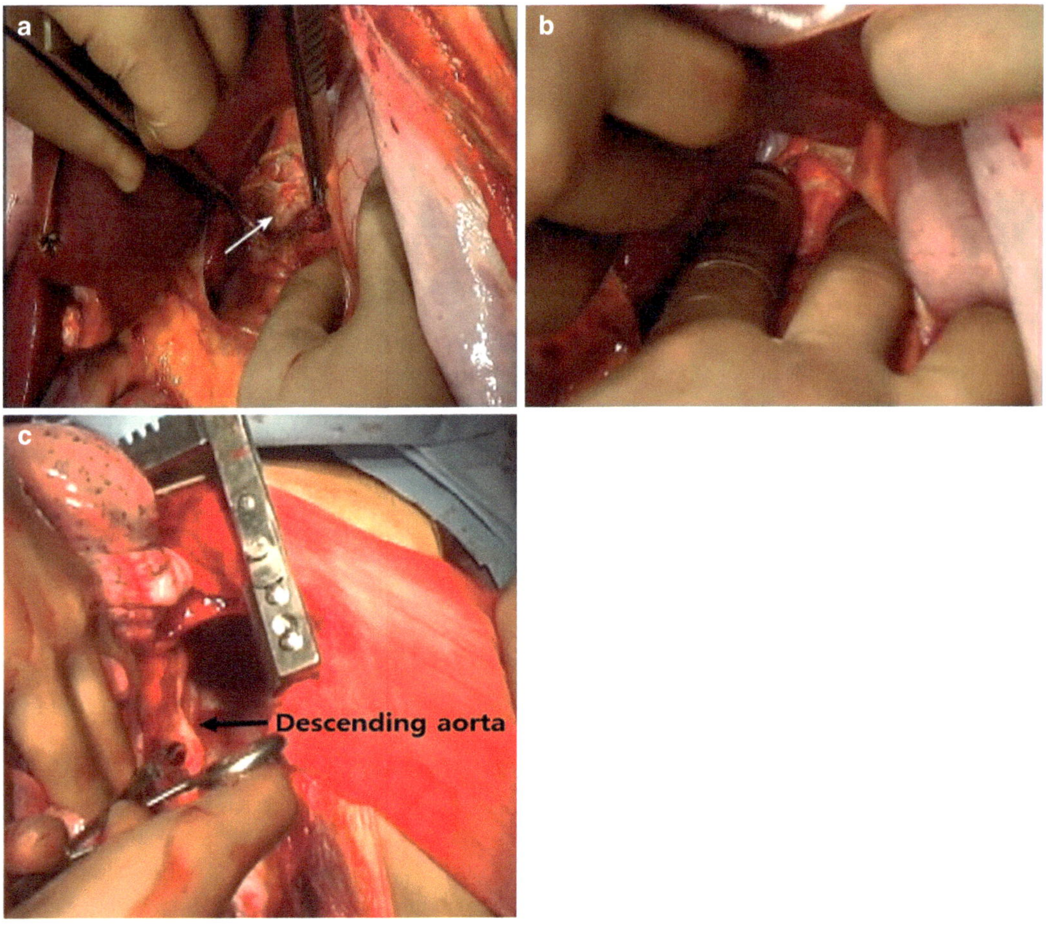

Fig. 16.6 (**a**) Dissection of the diaphragmatic crus (white arrow). (**b**) Exposure of the abdominal aorta. (**c**) Dissection of the descending (thoracic) aorta

suprahepatic IVC (or caval-atrial junction, infrarenal IVC) should be transected to allow exsanguinations of the abdominal organ (Fig. 16.9a–d). Five liters of HTK solution should be run through the aortic perfusion. The aortic (30–60 ml/kg) and IMV/SMV (1–2 L) cannulae are flushed in both the perfusions. The liver, kidney, and pancreas are completely covered with ice to facilitate rapid cooling of the abdominal viscera.

Liver procurement involves the common bile duct, gastroduodenal artery (GDA), portal vein (PV), splenic artery (SA), SMA, infrahepatic IVC, and perihepatic ligaments. After perfusion, the caval-atrial junction at the venting site is completely divided (Fig. 16.10a). In the case of a thoracic cross-clamp, the lower part of the clamping site is divided and dissected to the abdominal aorta (Fig. 16.10b). The gastrohepatic ligament is divided into the gastroesophageal junction along the lesser curvature of the stomach (Fig. 16.10c).

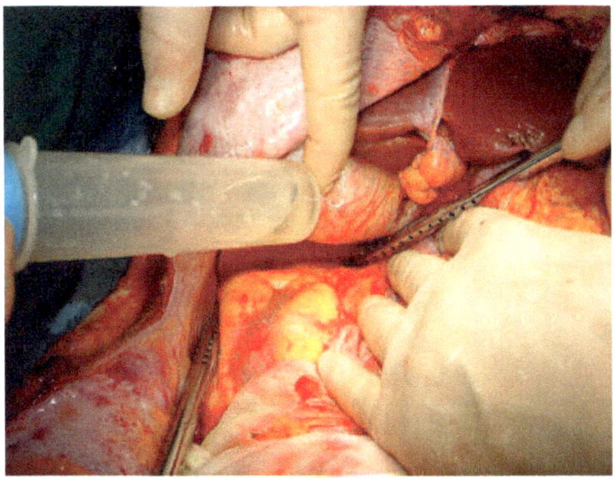

Fig. 16.7 The gallbladder is incised and irrigated using saline fluid

The duodenum and antrum of the stomach are retracted inferiorly (Fig. 16.11a). CBD resects the duodenal upper border without causing any vascular injury (Fig. 16.11b). GDA is dissected at the left part of the CBD (Fig. 16.11c).

PV is identified by dividing the fibrous tissue at the superior margin of the pancreas. If the pancreas is not procured, the head of the pancreas is divided (Fig. 16.12a). SMV/splenic vein (SV) (distal part) is identified, cut, and moved proximally along with the PV (Fig. 16.12b).

The common hepatic artery (CHA) is identified and cut after dissection of the CA up to the SA along the superior margin of the pancreas (Fig. 16.13a, b). If the pancreas is procured, PV and SA should be divided from the superior border and the proximal part of the pancreas in order to avoid vessel injury.

At the inferior part of the pancreas, the origin of the SMA at the aorta is dissected. If the pancreas is not procured, a midline incision (2–3 cm) at this point is performed, while preventing injury to the accessory or aberrant hepatic arteries. After the SMA is divided and the right renal artery or accessory vessel is identified, the aorta is cut and mobilized (Fig. 16.14a, b).

To identify both the renal veins in the lumen, a partial incision of the infrahepatic IVC is performed at the superior part of the left renal vein (Fig. 16.15a). After cutting the IVC (Fig. 16.15b), the hepatorenal ligament is carefully divided,

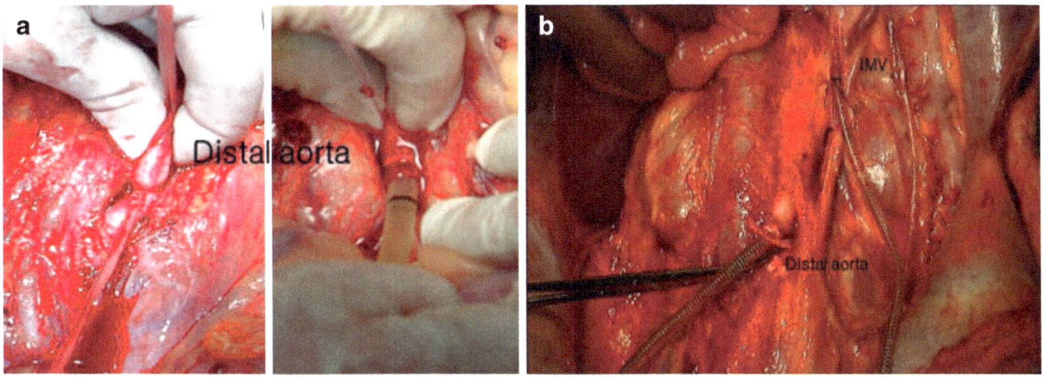

Fig. 16.8 (**a**) Cannulation and ligation of the distal aorta. (**b**) Cannulation of the distal aorta and IMV for perfusion

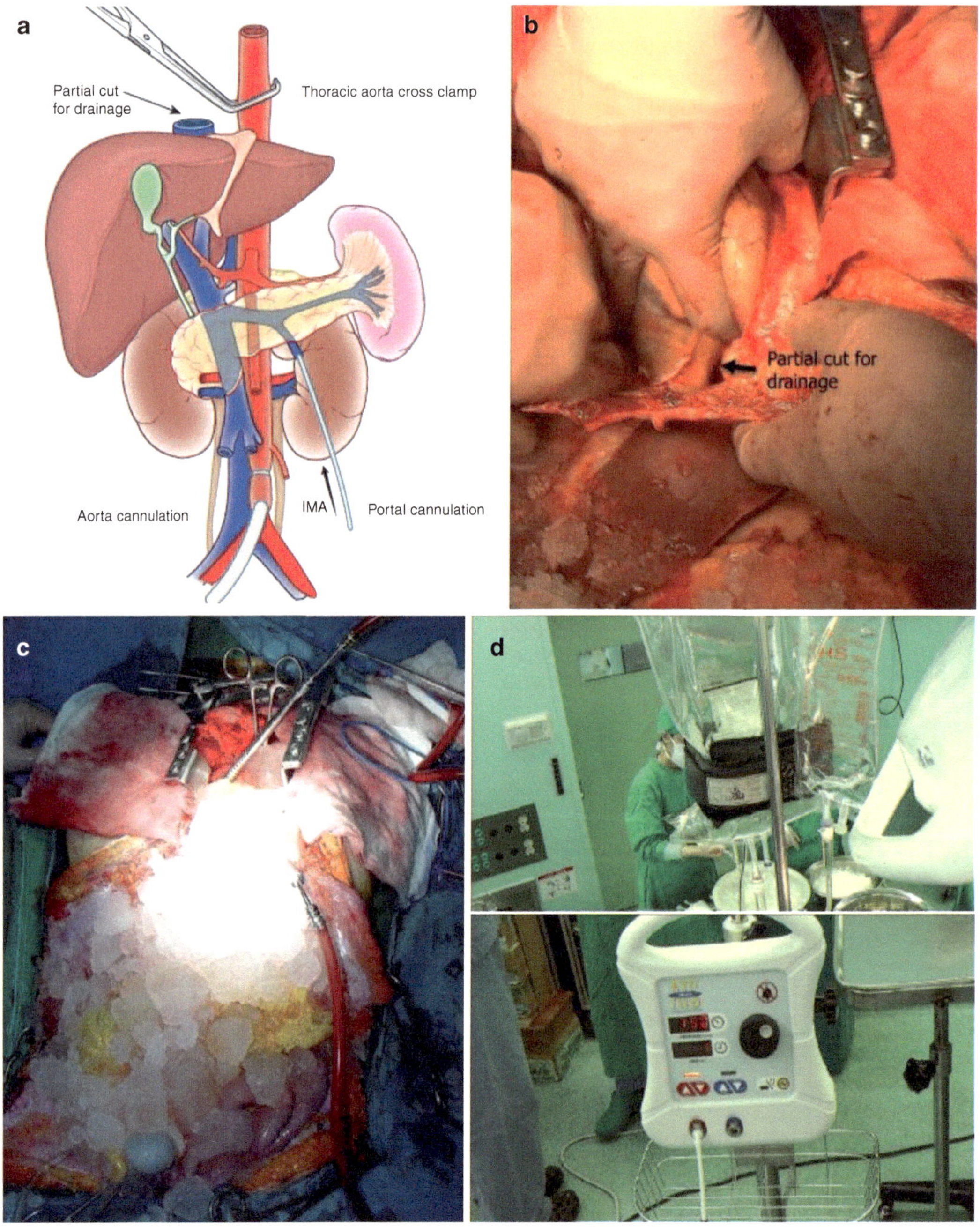

Fig. 16.9 (**a**) Perfusion of HTK solution after clamping of the thoracic aorta. (**b**) Suprahepatic IVC and partial incision of the caval-atrial junction for venting. (**c**) Rapid cooling of visceral organs using ice. (**d**) Preserving solution infused under 150 mmHg of pressure using a pneumatic cuff

while the right kidney is retracted inferiorly to protect from injury (Fig. 16.15c).

A finger is inserted into the lumen of the suprahepatic IVC in order to avoid injury, the areas of the diaphragm surrounding the liver are divided (Fig. 16.16a). After identification of the CBD, GDA, and SA, the liver, along with the aorta, SMA, and CA is divided (Fig. 16.16b). Finally, the liver is procured.

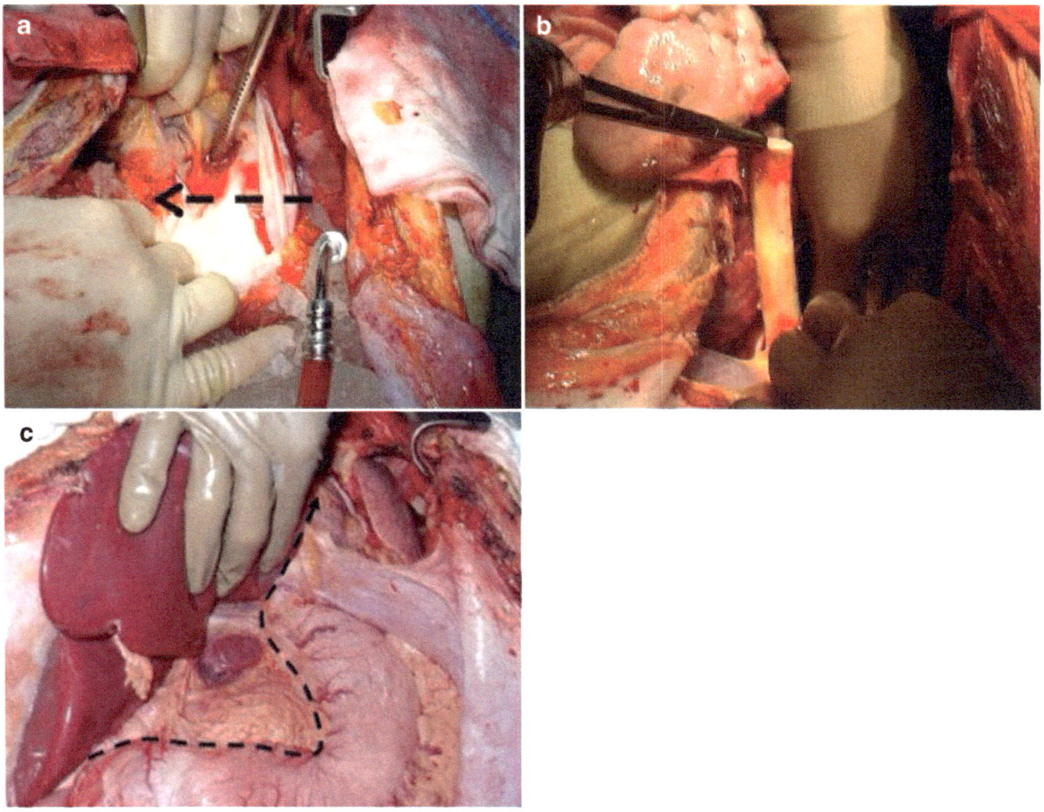

Fig. 16.10 (**a**) Division of the suprahepatic IVC-atrial junction. (**b**) Abdominal aorta dissection after cutting of the thoracic aorta. (**c**) Gastrohepatic ligament dissection at the gastroesophageal junction

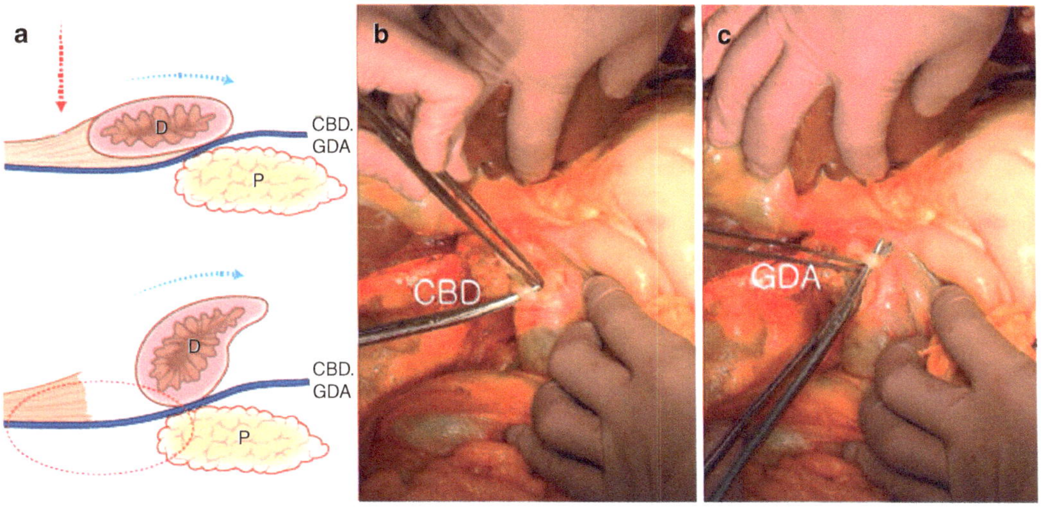

Fig. 16.11 (**a**) Schematic view after inferior traction of the first portion of the duodenum. (**b**) Dissection of the CBD on the superior margin of the duodenum. (**c**) GDA dissection on the left side of the CBD

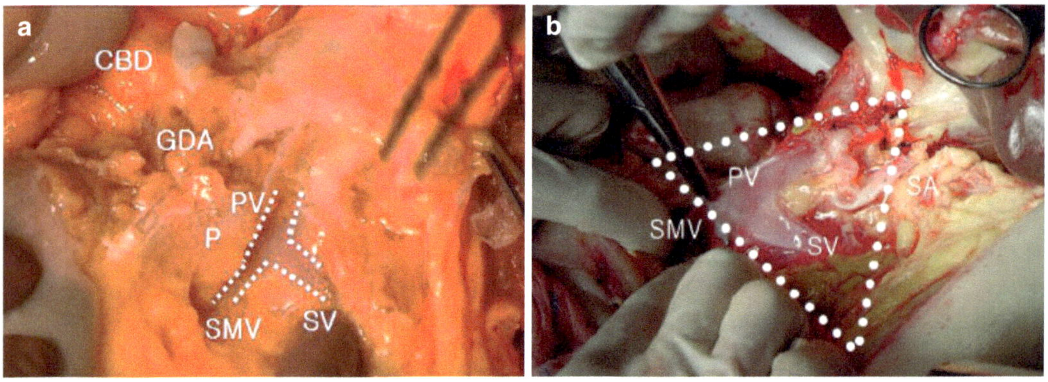

Fig. 16.12 (**a**) Exposure of PV/SV and SMV after incision of the pancreatic head. (**b**) Division of PV after dissection of the SMV and SV

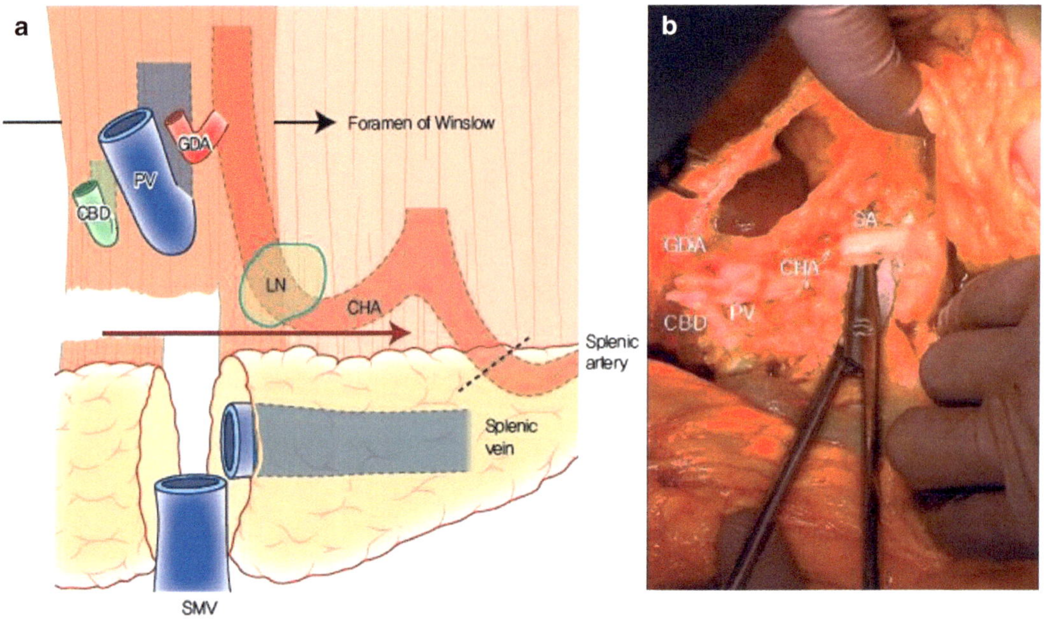

Fig. 16.13 (**a**) Schematic view of resection parts including the CBD, PV, and the common hepatic artery (CHA). (**b**) SA is resected after dissection along the superior border of the pancreas

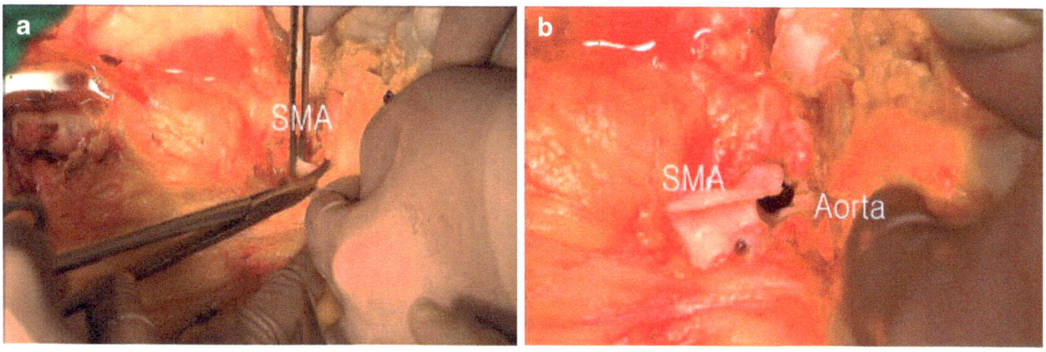

Fig. 16.14 (**a**) SMA resection at the abdominal aorta. (**b**) Identification of the right renal artery and accessory renal vessels after partial incision of the SMA

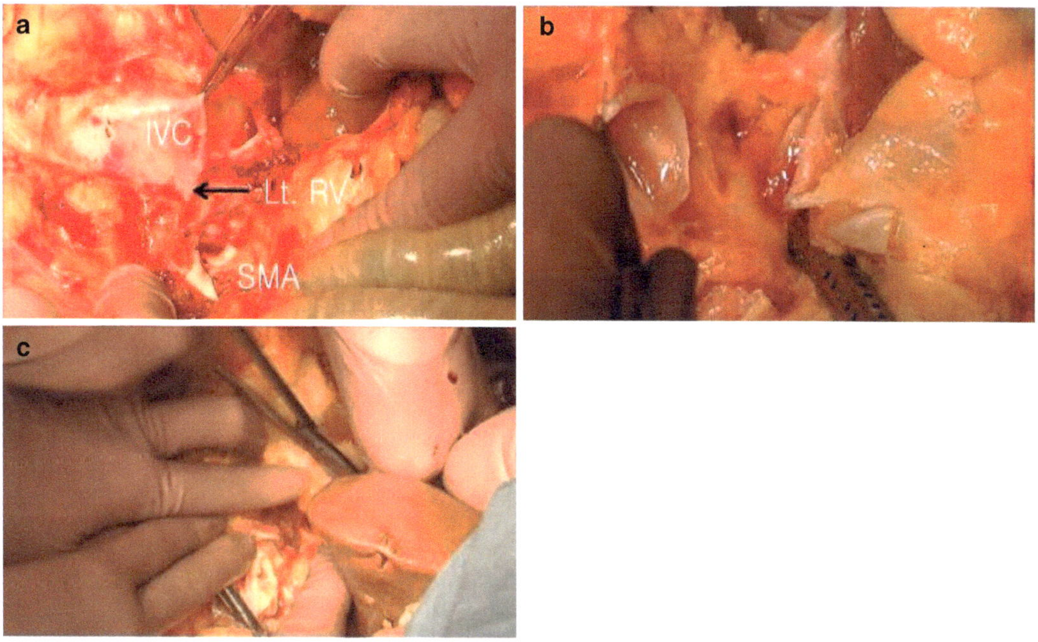

Fig. 16.15 (**a**) Partial incision of the infrahepatic IVC above the left renal vein. (**b**) Complete resection of the infrahepatic IVC. (**c**) Resection of the hepatorenal ligament for the division of the liver (lower part)

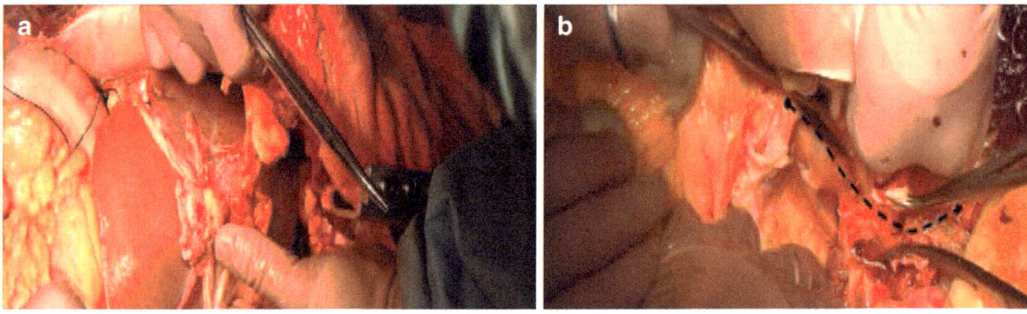

Fig. 16.16 (**a**) Insertion of a finger into the lumen of the suprahepatic IVC to prevent injury and aid in the dissection of the diaphragm around the liver. (**b**) Dissection of the inferior part of the liver after hand traction of perihilar structures for protection

References

1. Abu-Elmagd K, Fung J, Bueno J, Martin D, Madariaga JR, Mazariegos G, Bond G, Molmenti E, Corry RJ, Starzl TE, Reyes J. Logistics and technique for procurement of intestinal, pancreatic, and hepatic grafts from the same donor. Ann Surg. 2000;232:680–7.
2. Casavilla A, Selby R, Abu-Elmagd K, Tzakis A, Todo S, Reyes J, Fung J, Starzl TE. Logistics and technique for combined hepatic-intestinal retrieval. Ann Surg. 1992;216:605–9.
3. Starzl TE, Hakala TR, Shaw BW Jr, Hardesty RL, Rosenthal TJ, Griffith BP, Iwatsuki S, Bahnson HT. A flexible procedure form multiple cadaveric organ procurement. Surg Gynecol Obstet. 1984;158:223–30.
4. Starzl TE, Miller C, Broznick B, Makowka L. An improved technique for multiple organ harvesting. Surg Gynecol Obstet. 1987;165:343–8.
5. Imagawa DK, Olthoff KM, Yersiz H, Shackleton CR, Colquhoun SD, Shaked A, Busuttil RW. Rapid en bloc technique for pancreas-liver procurement. Improved early liver function. Transplantation. 1996;61:1605–9.
6. Marroquim CE, Kuo PC. Adult cadaveric liver transplantation. In: Kuo PC, Davis RD, editors. Comprehensive atlas of transplantation. Philadelphia: Lippincott W & W; 2005. p. 99–114.
7. Renz JR, Yersiz H. The donor operation. In: Busttil RW, Klintmalm GM, editors. Transplantation of liver. Philadelphia: WB Saunders; (2005):545–559.
8. Sturdevant ML, Humar A. Multiorgan procurement from the deceased donor. In: Humar A, Matas AJ, Payne WD, editors. Atlas of organ transplantation. London: Springer-Verlag; (2006):1–14.
9. Yu HC, Cho BH. How to do I make an organ procurement in deceased donor? Korean Soc Transplant. 2006;20:14–24.
10. Van Buren CT, Barakat O. Organ donation and retrieval. Surg Clin North Am. 1994;74:1055–81.
11. Vikraman D, Marroquim CE. Surgical techniques: Liver procurement and transplantation. In: Blazer III DG, Kuo PC, Pappas T, Clary BM, editors. Contemporary surgical Management of Liver, biliary tract, and pancreatic disease. Danvers: World Scientific Publishing Co. Pte. Ltd.; (2014):237–244.

Recipient Hepatectomy Without Venovenous Bypass

17

Jin Sub Choi

Abstract

The recipient hepatectomy with preservation of the vena cava blood flow is technically difficult than traditional recipient hepatectomy including vena cava. However, this procedure provides an advantage of hemodynamic stability and no venous bypass-related complications to the recipient.

Keywords

Recipient hepatectomy · Vena cava Preservation · Venous bypass

The traditional recipient hepatectomy for deceased liver donor liver transplantation involves removal of the entire diseased liver including retro hepatic IVC (inferior vena cava). The ends of supra and infra hepatic IVC are anastomosed with the upper and lower ends of graft IVC as end-to-end type (Fig. 17.1). However, the anastomosis of IVC is very difficult, or sometimes anastomotic stenosis may result in a patient with a deep surgical field or large liver graft. The massive bleeding or air embolism may occur if the supra hepatic IVC slips out of the vascular clamp.

Recipient hepatectomy with vena cava preservation has been proposed as an alternate procedure for the traditional liver transplantation. This procedure is sometimes technically difficult than traditional recipient hepatectomy and offers advantages of maintaining the caval blood flow during the anhepatic stage and avoidance of complications of the veno-venous bypass (Fig. 17.2).

Supplementary Information The online version contains supplementary material available at https://doi.org/10.1007/978-981-16-1996-0_17.

J. S. Choi (✉)
Division of Hepatopancreaticobiliary Surgery, Department of Surgery, Yonsei University College of Medicine, Seoul, South Korea
e-mail: choi5491@yuhs.ac

H. C. Yu (ed.), *Hepato-Biliary-Pancreatic Surgery and Liver Transplantation*,
https://doi.org/10.1007/978-981-16-1996-0_17

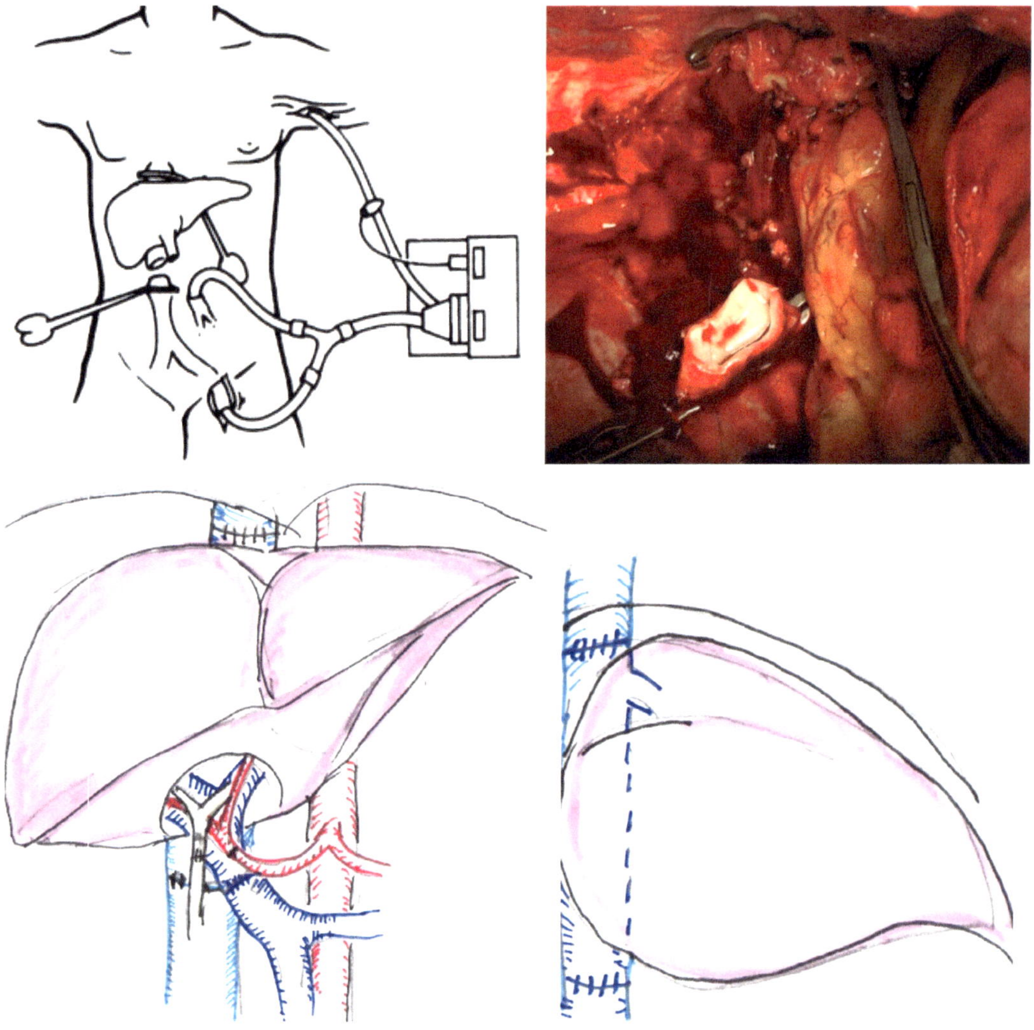

Fig. 17.1 Recipient hepatectomy with venous bypass and traditional liver transplantation

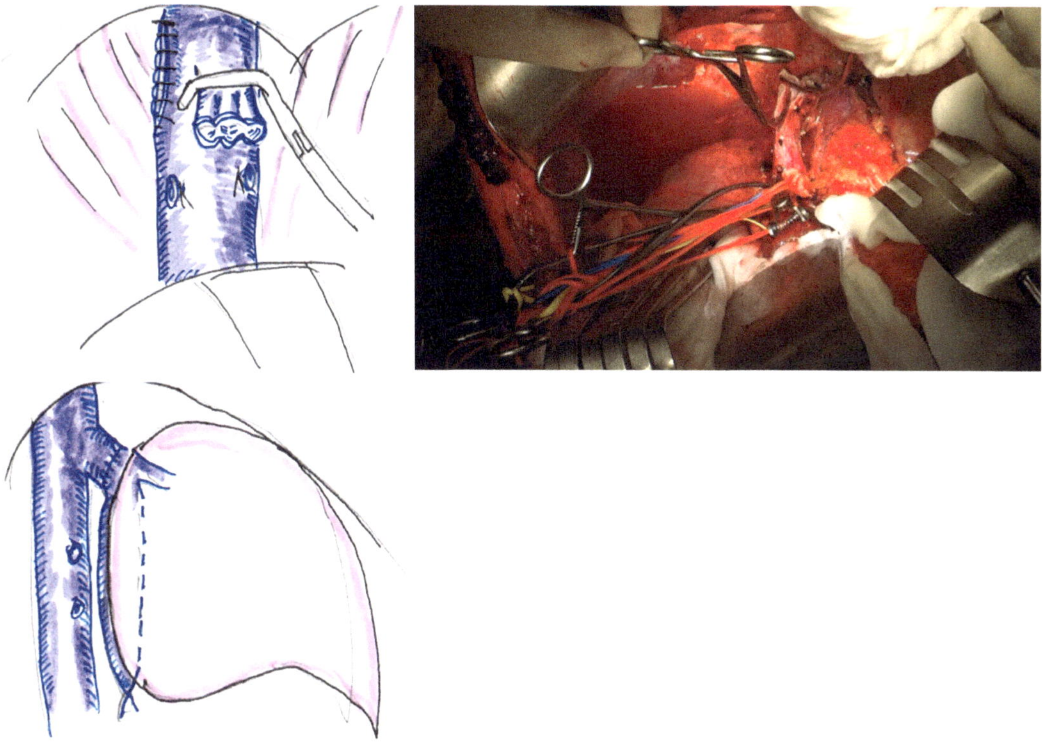

Fig. 17.2 Recipient vena cava preserving hepatectomy and piggyback anastomosis

17.1 Liver Mobilization

The bilateral subcostal incision with vertical midline extension is the most commonly used abdominal incision for the adult liver transplantation that is extended from the right mid axillary line to the left mid clavicular line. This wide incision exposes an entire liver and guarantees easy access to the subdiaphragmatic area, retroperitoneum, and IVC.

The umbilical ligament containing the dilated umbilical vein must be ligated and divided. The falciform ligament is dissected upwards and the supra hepatic IVC is exposed within the loose connective tissue. There are some collateral veins in the falciform ligament that can be easily controlled by electrocautery.

The hilar dissection begins by the incision of the anterior peritoneum of the hepatoduodenal ligament along the hepatic margin. Branches of the hepatic artery are ligated and divided. The right gastric or pyloric artery is ligated and divided during the proper hepatic artery dissection. The gastroduodenal artery is dissected about 1–1.5 cm distal area to use as a Carrell patch of artery anastomosis. The common hepatic artery is dissected to a 2 cm proximal area from the bifurcation of the gastroduodenal artery. The perivascular adventitia tissue of the artery must be preserved. The common bile duct is dissected with arterial dissection. The main portal vein trunk is freed from surrounding lymphatic soft tissue and dissection proceeds distal as far as to the right and left portal veins.

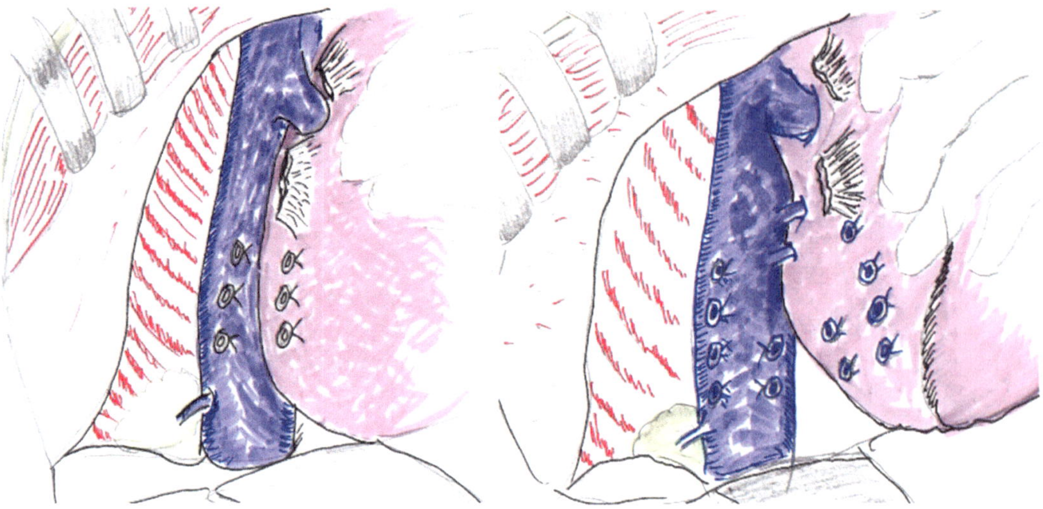

Fig. 17.3 IVC dissection on the right side

After all the components of the hepatoduodenal ligament are skeletonized, the right triangular ligament is divided to initiate liver mobilization. The liver is raised to the anterior and left side. The right posterior and inferior aspect of the liver is detached carefully from the diaphragm, renal capsule, and adrenal gland. After dividing the dorsal ligament of IVC, the lateral wall of IVC and the right adrenal vein are exposed. The right adrenal vein may be ligated and divided or preserved. The anterior aspect of retro hepatic IVC is gradually detached from the liver by progressive division and ligation of several accessories or short hepatic veins along the caudocranial direction as far as the main hepatic veins. The left edge of the caudate lobe and IVC ligament are separated from IVC to free the right hepatic vein (Fig. 17.3).

The left side dissection begins by the division of the left coronary ligament and the left triangular ligament. The lesser omentum is divided after raising the left liver. The accessory or aberrant left hepatic artery in the lesser omentum is ligated and divided. The peritoneum attached to the caudate lobe is divided. The left side of the caudate lobe is raised to expose the IVC and some short hepatic veins are ligated. The common or individual trunk of the middle and left hepatic vein is (are) isolated and encircled (Fig. 17.4).

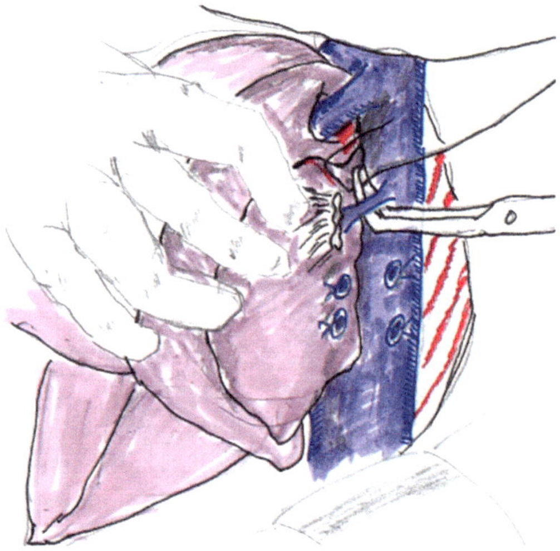

Fig. 17.4 IVC dissection on left side

After the anterior aspect of IVC is freed, the liver is hanged between the hepatoduodenal ligament and the trunk of three major hepatic veins.

17.2 Liver Removal

Before clamping the trunk of the right hepatic vein, the right portal vein is ligated to prevent hepatic congestion. The trunk of the right hepatic vein is clamped with an angled vascular clamp on

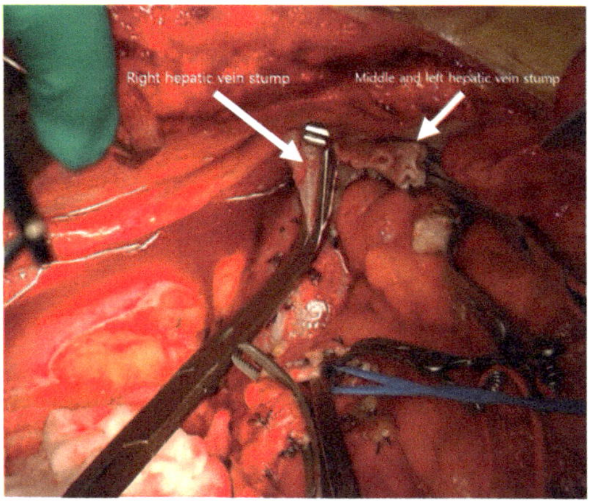

Fig. 17.5 Cava preserving recipient hepatectomy

the caval side, sutured on the liver side, and divided. The caval stump of the right hepatic vein is closed with monofilament 5-0 suture. The portal trunk is clamped with a curved vascular clamp. The common trunk of the middle and left hepatic vein is clamped with an angled vascular clamp laterally from the left side and the liver is removed. The septum of the hepatic vein is divided to make a wide common orifice of the hepatic vein. Sometimes the incision can be extended to the anterior wall of IVC to make a wide opening for hepatic vein anastomosis after lateral IVC clamping (Fig. 17.5).

To prevent the splanchnic congestion during the anhepatic stage, the end-to-side porto-caval shunt between the right portal vein stump and IVC can be made and this temporary porto-caval shunt can be closed just before portal venous anastomosis.

17.3 Anastomosis

The graft is placed in the operating field at a proper position and covered with cold saline-soaked surgical tapes to keep the graft in cold condition. The upper caval anastomosis of graft is carried out first with monofilament 3-0 stitches with the evaginated method. The liver graft should be flushed during the caval anastomosis and the lower stump of graft IVC is closed with a vascular stapler or monofilament 3-0 stitch. The liver graft is revascularized after the portal venous anastomosis. The hepatic artery and the bile duct are reconstructed following a traditional transplantation method.

With a severe size mismatch between the recipient hepatic vein and the graft IVC, the piggyback caval anastomosis is often not easy and results in severe anastomosis stenosis. The alternative to piggyback anastomosis is the side-to-side anastomosis between the recipient IVC and the graft IVC which is made along the longitudinal axis of IVC. The upper and lower stumps of the graft vena cava should be closed during the graft flushing and the side-to-side IVC anastomosis should be completed. After the portal vein is anastomosed and graft revascularization, hepatic artery, and biliary anastomoses are followed.

Recipient Hepatectomy with Venovenous Bypass

18

Gi-Won Song

Abstract

To avoid unnecessary intraoperative bleeding, total hepatectomy must be carried out along the precise surgical plane under good visualization. Although postoperative bleeding can occur at any site of dissection around the liver, special attention should be paid to the right adrenal gland, subphrenic area, and hepatic hilum for secure hemostasis. To acquire healthy vascular inflows with sufficient length, we must perform the fine dissection around the hepatic artery, portal vein, and bile duct with sufficient information about the vascular anatomy of the hepatic hilum. In the case of total occlusion of inferior vena cava during the implantation, the veno-venous bypass can provide hemodynamic stability and decompression of mesenteric blood pressure. But, the risk of complications such as venous thrombosis, air embolism, lymphocele, etc. should be considered.

Keywords

Deceased donor liver transplantation · Total hepatectomy · Veno-venous bypass

G.-W. Song (✉)
Division of Hepatobiliary Surgery and Liver Transplantation, Department of Surgery, Asan Medical Center, University of Ulsan College of Medicine, Seoul, South Korea

18.1 Mobilization of the Recipient's Liver

18.1.1 Patient Position and Incision

The patient is placed in the supine position with the right arm abducted at 90° and the left arm close to the body.

Expose left inguinal region with left thigh placed abducted and externally rotated and positioned with a prop under the left knee. Inverted T incision is made with meticulous bleeding control and ligation of collaterals on the abdominal wall. To provide excellent exposure to the operation field, xyphoid process is resected followed by fastidious hemostasis. In patients with a large number of ascites which were not drained preoperatively, ascites should be drained through a slit on incision before full laparotomy to prevent contamination and mess of the operation field. Round ligament (ligamentum teres) is ligated and divided from the abdominal wall during laparotomy, followed by division of falciform ligament to dissect anterior surface of the liver from the abdominal wall. Retractors are set up for full exposure of the right upper quadrant and its contents.

H. C. Yu (ed.), *Hepato-Biliary-Pancreatic Surgery and Liver Transplantation*,
https://doi.org/10.1007/978-981-16-1996-0_18

18.1.2 Division and Mobilization of the Recipient's Liver

Falciform ligament and coronary ligaments are divided with electrocautery cephalad to expose three major hepatic veins entering the IVC. Then, the right coronary ligament and triangular ligament are divided to mobilize the right liver lobe from the diaphragm, followed by traction of the right liver ventrally to mobilize the right liver lobe from the retroperitoneum. While traction of the right liver to the left side, right adrenal is met during dissection toward IVC, which should be divided carefully with ligation when it is adherent to the liver. The adrenal gland is one of the most common sites of postoperative bleeding, so careful hemostasis is necessary after the division of the adrenal from the liver. After the division of the right adrenal is completed, IVC is exposed and mobilized further from the retroperitoneum to pass through the left space on the posterior side of IVC. Different from LDLT, IVC is removed during the recipient hepatectomy in DDLT with cavo-caval end-to-end anastomosis. The short hepatic veins posterior to the caudate lobe are recommended to be resected in order to provide additional exposure to IVC with the secure length for anastomosis. Following the division of short hepatic veins with sufficient length of IVC for cavo-caval anastomosis, a vessel loop is applied to the infrahepatic IVC. After dissection of the right side is completed, the left coronary ligament and triangular ligament are divided and the left liver lobe is mobilized from the diaphragm. Several collaterals also exist in this area so vigilance is needed during dissection. During division on the triangular ligament, ligation before each division is necessary to prevent bleeding. During traction of the left liver to the right side, the gastrohepatic ligament is divided up to the hepatic vein. Thereafter, dissection around the left side of IVC from retroperitoneum is performed so that IVC is fully mobilized and freed on the posterior side.

18.1.3 Division of the Hepatic Hilum

After both sides of the liver are fully mobilized, division around the hepatic hilum is followed. First of all, cholecystectomy is started with cautious attention in dividing around the cystic duct and cystic artery for collaterals around the gallbladder. Occasionally, the cystic artery and cystic duct are ligated and divided with the gallbladder still attached to the liver to avoid profuse bleeding from the gallbladder fossa. After cholecystectomy, dissection of the hepatic hilum is started from the left side and proceeded to the right side. The left side of the hepatoduodenal ligament is dissected first to expose the left hepatic artery and a vessel loop is applied. Different from LDLT, hepatic artery anastomosis in DDLT is mostly performed at bifurcation level of right and left hepatic artery or bifurcation level of proper hepatic artery and gastroduodenal artery, so it is not necessary to take hepatic arteries at a distal location for its maximal length as in LDLT.

After the left hepatic artery is identified, dissection is proceeded to the right side (of the hepatoduodenal ligament) to expose the left portal vein and a vessel loop is applied to it. The right side of the hepatoduodenal ligament is dissected to identify the right hepatic artery and a vessel loop is applied to it. Right and main portal veins located posterior to right hepatic artery are dissected and identified with vessel loops. Thereafter, the common hepatic duct is divided at its hilar end followed by meticulous hemostasis around the bile duct. As the common hepatic duct is divided, the right hepatic artery is identified on its course posteriorly. The right, left, and proper hepatic arteries are dissected proximally to the bifurcation level of the gastroduodenal artery from the common hepatic artery.

18.2 Installation of Veno-Venous Bypass

18.2.1 Installation Method

After mobilization of the liver and dissection around the hilum are completed and prepared for hepatectomy, the veno-venous bypass is set up for extracorporeal circulation during the anhepatic phase (from hepatectomy to implantation of graft liver). Initially, the pulse of the left femoral artery is identified on the left inguinal area and vertical skin incision around 3 cm is made medially to the left femoral artery and perpendicularly to the inguinal ligament (Fig. 18.1). The subcutaneous fatty layer (camper's fascia) is dissected to identify a great saphenous vein. The vessel loop is applied to the identified GSV (Fig. 18.2). There exist several small branches to GSV during dissection in the cranial direction, which should be all ligated and divided carefully. Meticulous ligation on lymphatics around the vessel is necessary during dissection to prevent complications including lymphocele. Further dissection in the cranial direction would reveal saphenofemoral junction encountering the femoral vein. Further dissection proximally to the saphenofemoral junction to expose the femoral vein is carried out, then vessel loop and vascular tourniquet are applied to the femoral vein after dissection from the surrounding connective tissues (Fig. 18.3). The femoral vein below and distal to the saphenofemoral junction is dissected and applied with a vessel loop. Meticulous care is required for the dissection of the posterior side of the femoral vein to not to injure small branches draining into the femoral vein on the posterior side because profuse bleeding and difficult hemostasis could occur. Distal femoral vein and GSV are fastened tightly with vessel loops to occlude blood flow. After all the vessels are dissected and separated, a vascular clamp is directly applied around the femoral vein distal to the saphenofemoral junction, and a fastened vessel loop is applied to GSV to occlude the entire inflow into the femoral vein (Fig. 18.4). The vertical incision on the femoral vein at 2 cm proximal to the saphenofemoral junction is made (Fig. 18.5), followed by the insertion of cannula sized around 24 Fr–28 Fr depending on the diameter of the femoral vein. At this moment, the opposite end of the inserted cannula is occluded with a tube clamp. Tip of the introduced cannula is placed around the left common iliac vein

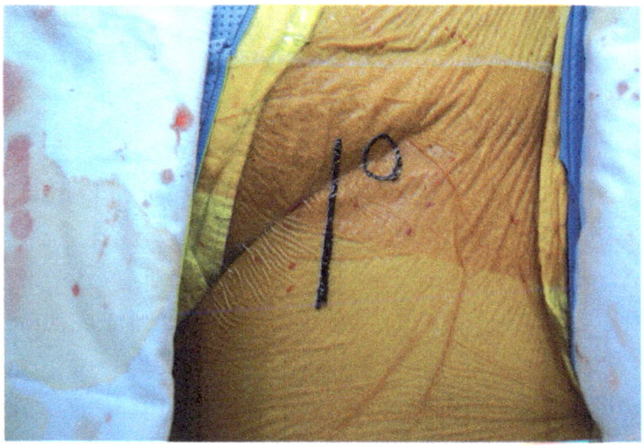

Fig. 18.1 Mark the imaginary route of femoral vein vertically around 3 cm medially to pulsating femoral artery

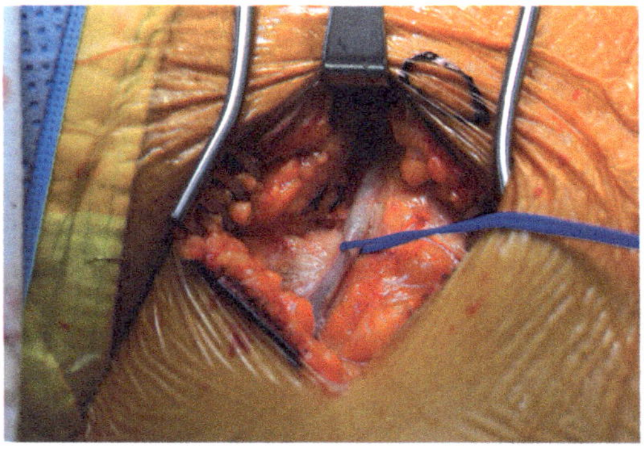

Fig. 18.2 Dissected GSV is positioned in the lateral traction with a vessel loop

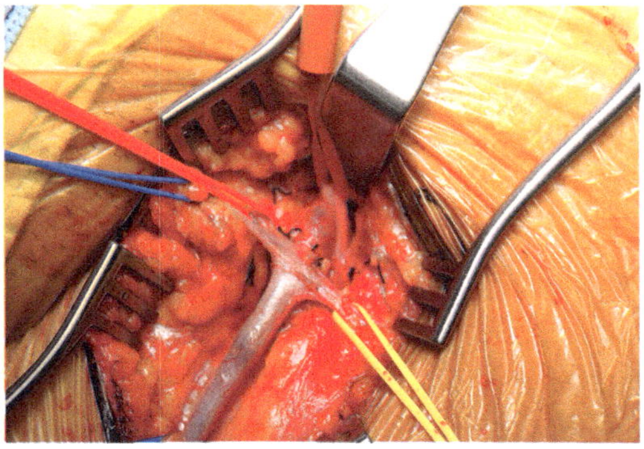

Fig. 18.3 Apply vascular tourniquet around the femoral vein proximal to the saphenofemoral junction

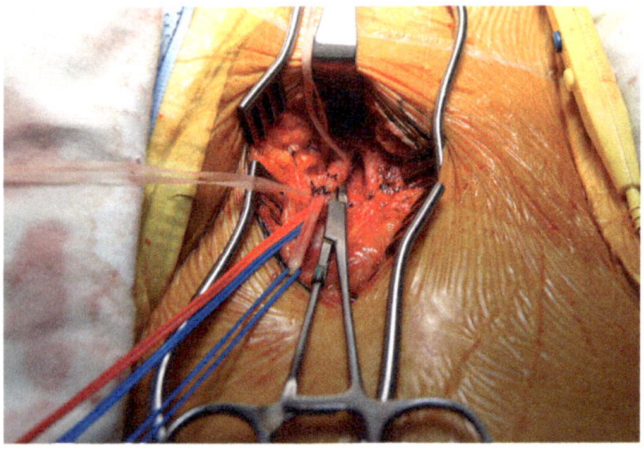

Fig. 18.4 GSV is vertically incised to make an entrance for a cannula into the femoral vein

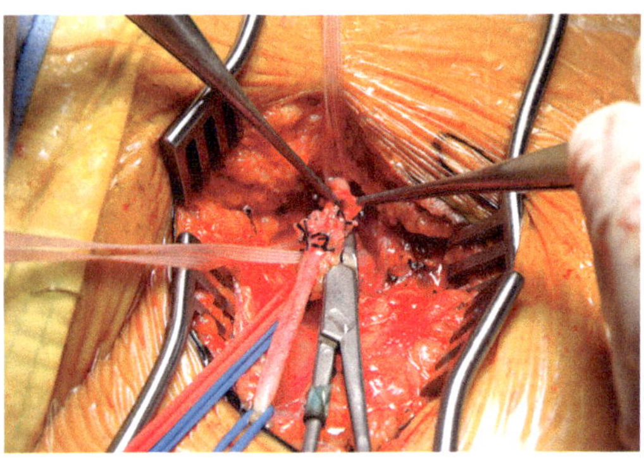

Fig. 18.5 Immediately before introducing the cannula into the femoral vein, blood flow from the distal part of the femoral vein is blocked using a vascular clamp

directly below the IVC and secured via the tightening of the vascular tourniquet applied [hung] beforehand. In adults, the proper length of the cannula inserted into the femoral vein is around 13–15 cm. The cannula is flushed with heparin to wash out remaining air bubbles inside and re-clamped with a tube clamp. The pump line is connected to the bypass machine and the return pump line is introduced to the catheter inserted into the internal jugular vein. Cannula inserted into the femoral vein is also connected to the pump line and veno-venous bypass is started after releasing the tube clamp (Fig. 18.6). The pump speed is maintained between 3000 and 3500 RPM (revolutions per minute) to keep blood flow from 0.8 to 1.0 L/min. For the bypass of portal flow, an RMI catheter is introduced into the main portal vein which is divided as high in the hilum as possible. In the case of well-developed portosystemic collateral, bypass from portal flow might not necessarily be needed.

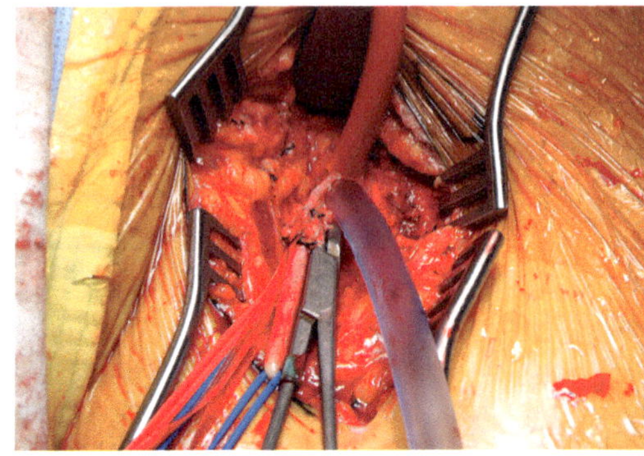

Fig. 18.6 The vascular tourniquet is applied at the appropriate location after the cannula [tube] is inserted into the femoral vein

18.2.2 Removal Method

After reperfusion of the transplanted liver, removal of the veno-venous bypass is carried out. At first, the pump line is disconnected by cutting the cannula between the two tube clamps applied to the distal end of the cannula, followed by turning off the pump machine. The pump line connected to the cannula inserted into the internal jugular vein is also disconnected. The cannula introduced into the femoral vein is removed after releasing the vascular tourniquet followed by tightening of the vascular tourniquet right after letting gush out of some blood from the femoral vein. Vascular clamp holding the distal femoral vein and vessel loops fastening GSV is released, followed by gushing out the stagnant blood and thrombus during clamping of the femoral vein, through compressing the thigh and leg distally. After removal of stagnant blood and thrombus, the incised part of the femoral vein is partially clamped with a vascular clamp and sutured.

18.2.3 Pros and Cons of Veno-Venous Bypass

18.2.3.1 Pros

During the anhepatic phase after total hepatectomy with resection of retrohepatic IVC after the suprahepatic IVC and the infrahepatic IVC are clamped, veno-venous bypass helps in maintaining hemodynamic stability and provides a longer anhepatic time for better surgical performance in implantation of the graft liver. Also, during the anhepatic phase, veno-venous bypass helps to reduce the incidence of post-transplant renal dysfunction by maintaining stable hemodynamic with sufficient blood flow to the kidney. The maintenance of mesenteric blood flow during the anhepatic phase can enable avoiding bowel congestion and edema.

18.2.3.2 Cons

Incidence of complications associated with veno-venous bypass has been reported around 10–30%, which includes unintended dislocation of the cannula, thrombosis in pump line with pulmonary embolism, air embolism, etc. Lymphocele, hematoma, infection, and nerve damage around the dissected GSV and femoral vein could also occur as complications. Additionally, total operation time might be prolonged due to the installation time for the veno-venous bypass.

18.3 Total Hepatectomy

After the installation of the veno-venous bypass is completed, total hepatectomy is done. At first, both the hepatic arteries are ligated and divided. The main portal vein is clamped and divided at the level of the right and left portal veins as high in the hilum as possible. Suprahepatic IVC and infrahepatic IVC are clamped and divided while taking care to retain as much as possible for sufficient length, and the diseased liver is removed (Fig. 18.7). The diameter of suprahepatic IVC is prepared and widened by opening the right, middle, and left hepatic veins into a common cloaca of the IVC (Fig. 18.8).

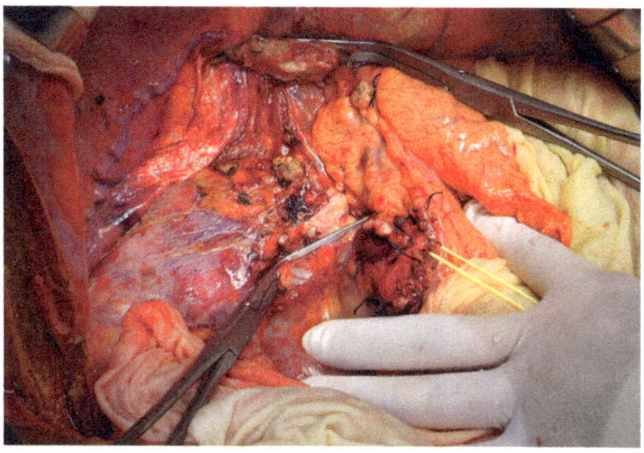

Fig. 18.7 Total hepatectomy is performed along with retrohepatic IVC

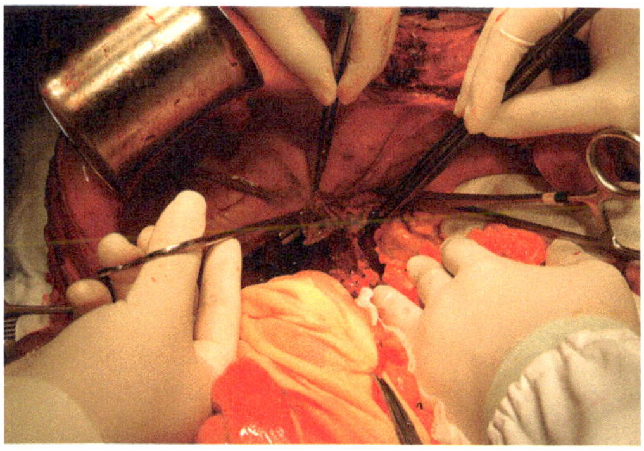

Fig. 18.8 Septa between the main hepatic veins entering suprahepatic IVC are cut and the diameter is widened

19 Implantation of the Deceased Donor Liver Graft

Young Kyoung You

Abstract

A longer ischemic time of more than 6 h has an obvious negative effect on the outcome of brain death liver transplantation. Liver graft procured at a geographically longer distance needs more time to recover graft function in general. Most centers prefer the piggyback technique for convenience. However, in some specific cases such as Budd-Chiari syndrome, extracorporeal circulation during the anhepatic phase has to be considered for the maintenance of hemodynamic stability.

Recipient hepatectomy followed by outflow (inferior vena cava) and portal vein reconstruction then reperfusion of the graft is performed under serious monitoring of an individual. Restoration of coagulation function of the liver varies according to the graft condition and arterial reconstruction of the graft required prior to control minor bleeders. Attempt to meticulous bleeding control before entire vascular reconstruction seems inefficient. Duct-to-duct anastomosis in biliary reconstruction is a general trend.

Y. K. You (✉)
Division of Hepatobiliary-Pancreas Surgery and Liver Transplantation, Department of Surgery, Seoul St. Mary's Hospital, College of Medicine, The Catholic University of Korea, Seoul, South Korea
e-mail: yky602@catholic.ac.kr

Keywords

Ischemic time · Brain death liver transplantation · Piggyback technique · Reperfusion Anhepatic · Coagulation · Duct-to-duct anastomosis

A longer ischemic time of more than 6 h has an obvious negative impact on the outcome of liver transplantation.

The Piggyback technique is the general trend.

19.1 Anastomosis of IVC (Inferior Vena Cava)

In the case of retrohepatic IVC removal, end-to-end reconstruction at both the parts of the IVC had to be made promptly to restore systemic circulation using 4-0 or 5-0 monofilament nylon. At this moment, veno-veno bypass procedure is unnecessary due to established porto-systemic collaterals in most of the end-stage liver diseases.

The anastomosis can be performed either end-to-side or side-to-side fashion. Occasionally end-to-side reconstruction has to be completed in the deep, narrow operation field. And recipient's suprahepatic IVC stump is prone to the withdrawal of the cross-clamp; therefore, side-to-side anastomosis techniques are rather preferred recently (Fig. 19.1). However, one might have difficulties in the operation field securement in the huge graft right liver.

H. C. Yu (ed.), *Hepato-Biliary-Pancreatic Surgery and Liver Transplantation*,
https://doi.org/10.1007/978-981-16-1996-0_19

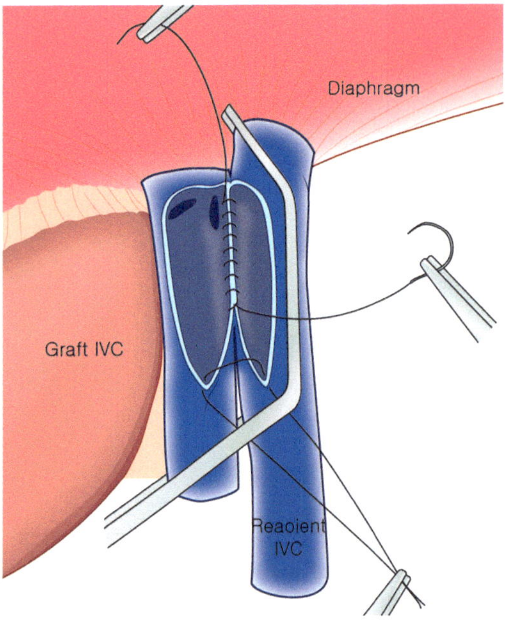

Fig. 19.1 Side-to-side anastomosis for graft and recipient inferior vena cava in liver transplantation

19.2 Anastomosis of the Portal Vein

Anastomosis under the accurate configuration of the portal axis is the key point of portal inflow securement. Another important issue is the avoidance of redundancy of both the parts of portal veins. Postoperative graft enlargement makes easy angulation of the anastomotic line, which might evoke the portal inflow disturbance.

Also, we need to make enough anastomotic growth factors to avoid mechanical stricture of the portal vein. Portal vein anastomosis is performed either with 6-0 or 5-0 monofilament nylon suture.

19.3 Reperfusion

Reperfusion is the highlight of liver transplantation. At this moment, aggressive monitoring and management by the anesthesiologists should be guaranteed. Not a few cases experience hemodynamic instability and cardiac dysrhythmia at this stage. Sometimes an episode of cardiac arrest could develop. Abrupt gushing materials such as cold preservation solution, various metabolites in the liver graft, and congested intestinal inflows to systemic circulation could evoke such kind of undesirable events.

If necessary, steroids and immunoglobulins are injected at this moment. Undetected hemostasis from the major vessels during the procurement and bench procedure should be identified immediately.

19.4 Anastomosis of the Hepatic Artery

Right after the control of bleeders from the vessels, management of minor bleeders and blood oozing focus should be postponed to the restoration of hepatic arterial supply. Perfect hemostasis could not be obtained despite all the efforts. After complete vascular reconstruction, all the efforts to attain hemostasis should be done. The arterial anastomosis can be performed at the junction of the gastroduodenal artery and common hepatic artery with minimal tissue dissection (Fig. 19.2). In case of insufficient arterial supply from the common hepatic artery or gastroduodenal artery because of various reasons such as severe atheromatic plaque, arterial denuding due to repeated previous arterial manipulation, etc., interposition graft from the infrarenal aorta could be the alternative method for reconstruction of the hepatic artery. Preventing kinking and excessive bending is an essential component of successful arterial

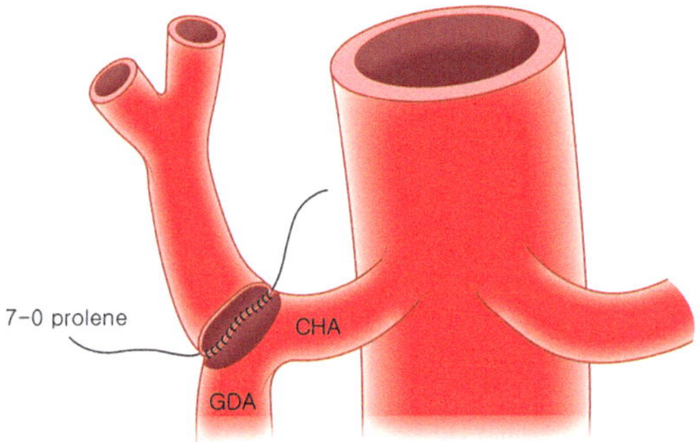

Fig. 19.2 The arterial anastomosis of graft liver at the junction of the gastroduodenal artery and common hepatic artery of the recipient in liver transplantation

reconstruction. Transmesocolic and retrogastric route is recommended for this purpose.

As the arterial interposition graft, the cadaveric iliac arterial graft of artificial graft such as PTFE or Dacron graft can be used.

19.5 Bile Duct Anastomosis

Duct-to-duct anastomosis has been widely accepted as a routine procedure in bile duct reconstruction during liver transplantation. In contrast to the bile duct to the enteric anastomosis, we expect fewer morbidities related to ascending cholangitis.

Furthermore, duct-to-duct reconstruction allows prompt endoscopic approach in postoperative complications. Monofilament continuous running suture materials are used in the anastomosis, and interrupted sutures can be selected in the anticipating stricture, but the outcomes of the bile duct stricture are reported similar to that of the continuous suture. T-tube is not recommended in general.

19.6 Addendum

The coagulation status of the recipient restores insidiously after successful implantation of the graft. Thorough hemostasis before abdominal wound closure has to be considered as an essential process in liver transplantation. Events of minor capsular injury during organ procurement procedure could progress to huge graft hepatic subcapsular hematoma or bleeding to free peritoneal space. Various hemostatic agents such as fibrin glue or gel, powder, and collagen patch coated with fibrinogen are effective in general. Transabdominal drainage tubes are placed in the dependent portion around the graft liver, subphrenic spaces, Morrison's pouch, and gastrohepatic junction. Drainage tubes are placed through the main wound rather than the stab wound to avoid bleeding at the stabbing area under improper hemostatic conditions of the recipient.

Meticulous layer by layer wound closure can make dead space free abdominal wound.

Part III

Living Donor Liver Transplantation

Donor Right or Extended Right Hemihepatectomy

20

Jae-Won Joh and Gyu-seong Choi

Abstract

Unlike conventional hepatic resection, donor surgery of living donor liver transplantation must preserve the flow of blood to the graft and the remaining liver. Resection should also maintain sufficient length to facilitate anastomosis during the recipient's surgery. Of course, the most important thing in surgery is the safety of the donor.

Keywords

Donor surgery · Right hepatectomy Extended right hepatectomy · Liver transplantation · Liver graft

20.1 Donor Selection

The donor must be medically healthy, including the psychiatric part, and must be willing to donate liver voluntarily. The donor must be of an age capable of making decisions, and the criteria for determining the age may vary from center to center. The degree of fatty liver should not be severe, and the donation would be considered inappropriate if the anatomical structure impairs the donor's safety. It is preferable to have no tumor or serious cardiovascular disease, the pure relationship between the donor and recipient should be proven, and the compatible ABO blood type should be appropriate. If the ABO blood type is incompatible, transplantation can be performed after pretreatment, but long-term results need to be considered.

20.2 Graft Selection

Although controversial, the minimum remaining liver volume to ensure the safety of the donor should be at least 30–35% of the total liver volume, and the remaining liver should not be associated with problems like congestion or ischemia. In order not to cause congestion in the remaining liver, the case of selecting an extended right hepatic resection in which the middle hepatic vein is excised together should be limited to the presence of another hepatic vein through which blood flow of segment 4 is drained. In a graft performed by conventional right hepatic resection, the venous blood flow to the anterior section may be blocked and the volume of the functioning parenchyma may be reduced depending on the anatomical structure. In this case, liver transplantation using a modified right liver graft in which

Supplementary Information The online version contains supplementary material available at https://doi.org/10.1007/978-981-16-1996-0_20.

J.-W. Joh (✉) · G.-s. Choi
Department of Surgery, Samsung Medical Center, Sungkyunkwan University School of Medicine, Seoul, South Korea

H. C. Yu (ed.), *Hepato-Biliary-Pancreatic Surgery and Liver Transplantation*,
https://doi.org/10.1007/978-981-16-1996-0_20

the branch of the middle hepatic vein is reconstructed using cryopreserved or artificial vessels can be selected.

20.3 Incision of Operation

As with conventional hepatectomy, the donor lies in the supine position, and one can fold both the arms or one arm toward the body as needed. Inverted T-shaped incision which is traditionally used in the right hepatic or enlarged right hepatic resection or midline extension from the bilateral subcostal incision, midline extension from the right subcostal incision, J-shaped incision, or inverted L-shaped incision is mainly used. Recently, there have been many young donors for living donor liver transplantation, and the incision tends to become smaller. So, there are cases where an upper midline incision or right subcostal incision is made. The selection of the incision may vary depending on the experience and preference of the operator, but the most important thing is the donor's safety and an appropriate surgical field of view that does not damage the graft. Also, the incision should be large enough to allow the graft to be taken out of the body. After securing the incision, an appropriate retractor is used to secure the field of view. The retractor can be selected differently depending on the operator's preference or the environment of the center. However, since the location of the liver is under the ribs, it is important to use a retractor that can secure the field of vision by sufficiently retracting the ribs toward the patient's head.

20.4 Liver Biopsy and Liver Mobilization

After laparotomy, the ligament of teres is excised followed by installing the retractor. The overall left and right ratio of the liver and the condition of the liver are visually checked, and liver biopsy for the frozen section is performed. Moving upward, separate the falciform ligament from the liver, checking the inferior vena cava (IVC) in the upper part of the liver, and dissect the groove between the right hepatic vein and the middle hepatic vein. The coronary and triangular ligaments between the right liver and the diaphragm are divided. From the top, the right hepatic vein is separated by ligating the IVC ligament starting under the origin of the right hepatic vein, and from the bottom, dissection is done to the groove between the caudate lobe and IVC. The donor's liver without a history of inflammation usually does not have adhesion with the surrounding organs, but if the right adrenal gland and hepatic parenchyma are adhered to each other, it is recommended to ligate the adrenal gland during separation from the liver to prevent bleeding. Although there is no particular problem in ligating and separating the small right inferior hepatic vein that meets while mobilizing the IVC and the right liver, ligation is recommended so that the right inferior hepatic vein of more than 5 mm should be delayed to the brink of liver extraction. This is because if these veins play an important role in the outflow of blood, it may be necessary to drain this flow by anastomosis with the recipient's IVC during transplantation. If these veins are ligated before parenchymal resection, congestion of the liver at the site can occur and damage the graft. The IVC ligament, which is located just below the right hepatic vein, surrounds the IVC, and careful dissection must be done because bleeding can occur if dissection goes the wrong way. If the length of the IVC ligament is long, suture ligation must be performed. When the right hepatic vein is exposed after full liver mobilization, a suspension umbilical tape is placed between the right hepatic vein and the middle hepatic vein (Fig. 20.1). This is for the hanging maneuver, which helps accurate parenchymal resection and reduces bleeding in the deep areas. If the frozen liver section examination reveals fatty liver, transplantation is decided based on the type of fatty liver (macrovesicular fatty liver), degree (more than 30%), size of the remaining liver, and the condition of the recipient.

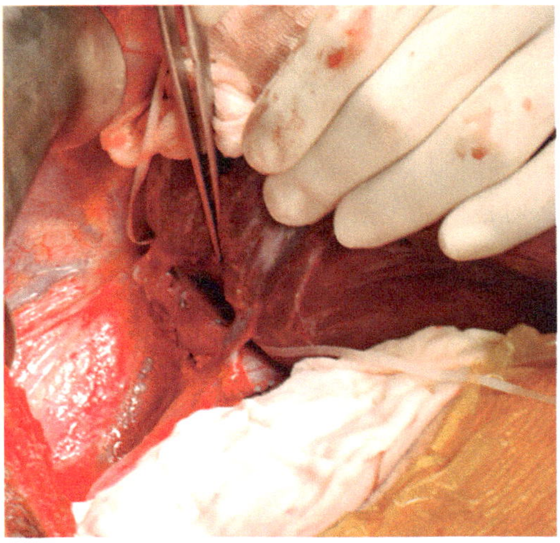

Fig. 20.1 The mobilization of the right liver with the preserved large right inferior hepatic vein. The suspension umbilical tape is placed

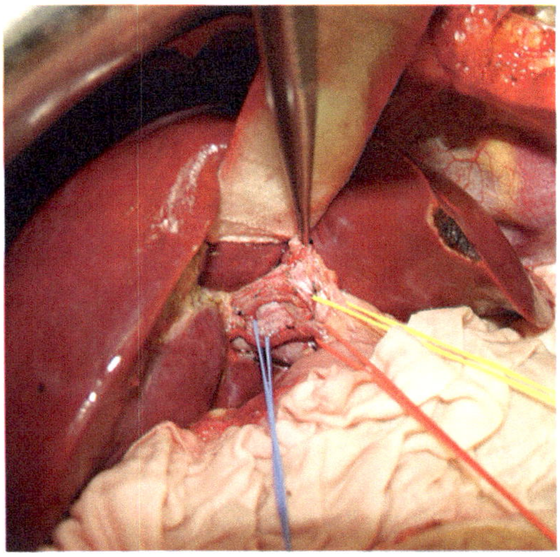

Fig. 20.2 After cholecystectomy, the right hepatic artery (red vessel loop), right portal vein (blue vessel loop), and common bile duct (yellow vessel loop) are exposed

20.5 Cholecystectomy and Dissection of the Hepatic Hilum

Cholecystectomy and dissection of the hepatic hilum should be performed while the anatomical structure is identified through preoperative examinations such as CT and MRCP. Because there may be cases with anatomical variations in the presence of the accessory duct running around the gallbladder, careful dissection of the gallbladder should be done. Intraoperative cholangiography may be performed to check the path of the bile duct and select the duct resection site. Careful dissection of the hepatic duct must be done along with checking the path of the common bile duct, common hepatic duct, and right hepatic duct. At this time, the tissue around the bile duct should be preserved to the maximum extent possible so that the blood flow in the bile duct is well maintained. The right hepatic artery must be dissected to a sufficient length until the middle or left hepatic artery appears and to the start of the intrahepatic level so that it is not damaged during the right bile duct resection. Depending on the anatomical variation, there may be a right hepatic artery on the right side of the common bile duct, or running in front of the common bile duct. Therefore, it is necessary to obtain sufficient information about this anatomy before surgery. The dissection and sufficient mobilization of the portal vein should be performed while the anatomical structure is identified by the preoperative examination. If necessary, the length of the portal vein can be sufficiently obtained by ligating a small branch running to the caudate lobe (Fig. 20.2).

20.6 Intraoperative Ultrasound

When the dissection of the hepatic hilum is complete, the border between the right and left lobe is checked while the blood flow in the right hepatic artery and the right portal vein is temporarily blocked using a vascular clamp (Fig. 20.3). After marking this boundary with an electric cautery device, the relationship between the middle hepatic vein and the parenchymal resection plane can be checked using ultrasound. The resection plane is located on the right side of the middle hepatic vein in case of performing a right hepatectomy, and the branch of the middle hepatic vein draining the anterior section can be confirmed by ultrasound (Fig. 20.3). The resection

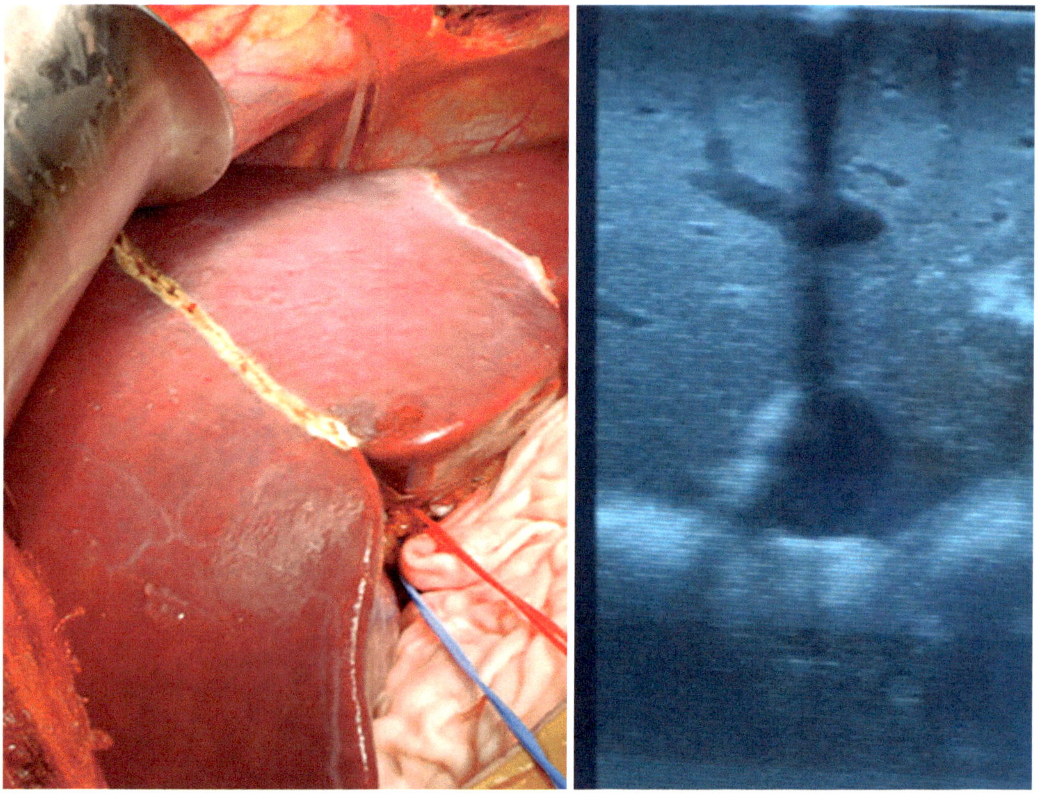

Fig. 20.3 After marking the boundary between the right and left lobes with vascular clamp and electric cauterization, the location of the resection surface and the middle hepatic vein branch is confirmed using ultrasound

surface should be on the left side of the middle hepatic vein in case of performing extended right hepatectomy, and it should be confirmed that another hepatic vein draining segment 4 exists. The resection line on the hilum side should be positioned slightly to the left than in conventional right hepatectomy to prevent the right hepatic duct from exfoliating too much.

20.7 Hepatic Parenchymal Resection

Before resecting the liver parenchyma, place the gauze behind the right liver so that the resection line is centered. When using a small incision especially, a midline incision, it is better to place the gauze and move the liver to the left rather than tilting the patient. Two or three pairs of towing threads are hung on both sides of the cutting line. If the liver is sufficiently lifted through this method, the resection is easy with the resection surface located higher than the heart which prevents the bleeding. Prepare to implement the Pringle's maneuver in case of unexpected bleeding, and start actual resection [1]. Parenchymal resection is performed using an ultrasonic dissector (Fig. 20.4). At this time, microbleeding can be prevented by using a bipolar coagulator for the resection surface and the surgical field of view can be better secured thereby making the operation more comfortable. In the case of right hepatectomy that does not include the middle hepatic vein, a branch of this vein measuring 5 mm or more that flows from the anterior section should be excised using a clip that can be removed and then restored on the bench procedure [2]. A beating middle hepatic vein can be identified at the graft side in case of extended right hepatic resection, or at the residual liver side in case of conventional right hepatic resection. This middle hepatic vein can guide the resection surface.

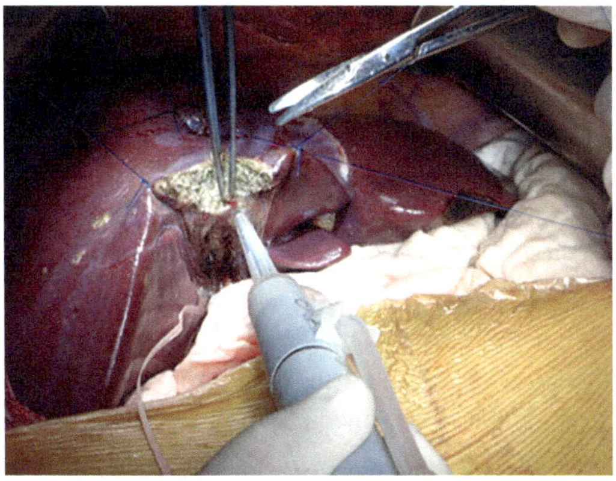

Fig. 20.4 Resect the parenchyma using an ultrasonic dissector (CUSA®) and cauterize the bleeding area on the resection surface using a bipolar coagulator

20.8 Resection of Hepatic Duct

When the hepatic parenchyma is sufficiently separated and the right hepatic duct is exposed, the duct is resected which may be assisted by intraoperative cholangiography (Fig. 20.5a). Before resection, the right hepatic artery and the right portal vein are pulled downwards using a vessel loop to prevent unexpected damage caused by sharp instruments used during resection (Fig. 20.5b). After setting the starting site of the right hepatic duct and a virtual resection line, the resection is started in a direction perpendicular to the right hepatic duct. Starting the resection on the right side of the right hepatic duct is unsuit-

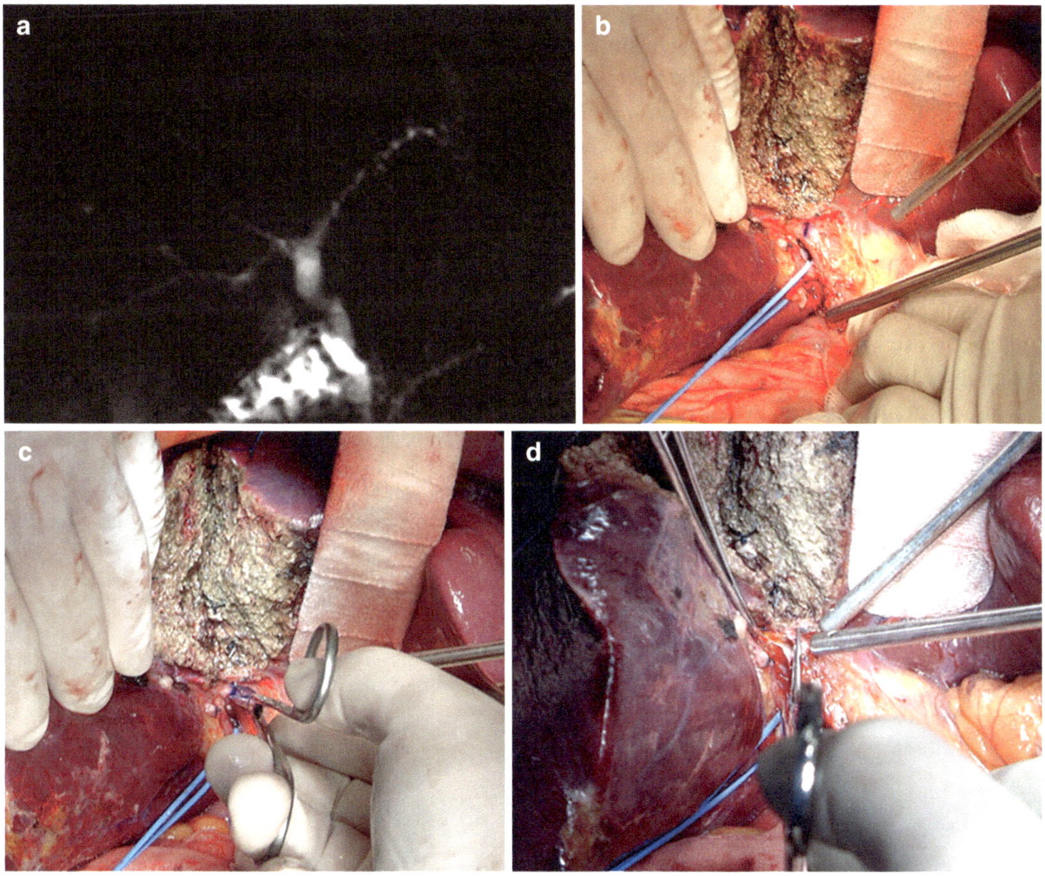

Fig. 20.5 (**a**) Bile duct variation (type C) confirmed by preoperative cholangiography. (**b**) Using a vessel loop, pull the right hepatic artery and right portal vein toward the leg. (**c**) The anterior direction of the hepatic duct (ventral direction of the donor) is excised perpendicularly. (**d**) Resection in the vertical direction of the running path of the right hepatic duct. (**e**) Closing the remaining bile duct with suture-ligation. The hepatic duct looks like a pig nose on the side of the graft

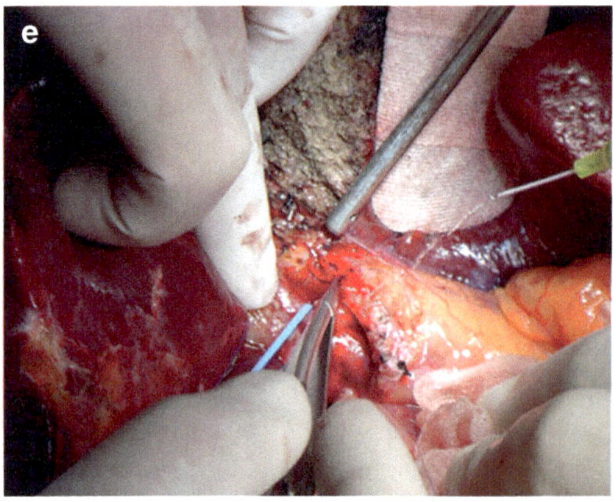

Fig. 20.5 (continued)

able because the early-branched anterior and posterior hepatic ducts can be resected separately. Start resection in the perpendicular direction, confirm the safety of the left hepatic duct and the direction of the anterior and posterior hepatic ducts, and then proceed with the total resection. The resection of the right hepatic duct is performed in a direction vertical to the driving direction of the duct in order to preserve blood flow around the duct to the maximum extent possible (Fig. 20.5c, d). It is better to use suture ligation rather than using electric cauterization for microbleeding which occurs at this time to preserve blood flow around the bile ducts (Fig. 20.5e).

20.9 Hanging Maneuver

After resection of the hepatic duct, the caudate lobe and the remaining deep hepatic parenchyma are resected after pulling out the suspension tape placed in advance above the right hepatic artery and portal vein. This not only reduces bleeding but also appreciably helps in accurate hepatic resection.

20.10 Extraction of the Graft

When the parenchymal resection is completed, the graft is extracted in a state ready for perfusion. Heparin is injected intravenously before vascular ligation. In some centers, heparin is injected during graft perfusion. If the preserved right inferior hepatic vein exists, it is resected first. At this time, bite the IVC sufficiently with a vascular clamp to obtain a vein of sufficient length. The vessels are ligated or clamped and then resected in the order of the right hepatic artery, the right portal vein, and the right hepatic vein. After the graft is handed over to the perfusion team, the blood vessels bitten by the vascular clamp are suture-ligated.

References

1. Park JB, Joh JW, Kim SJ, et al. Effect of intermittent hepatic inflow occlusion with the Pringle maneuver during donor hepatectomy in adult living donor liver transplantation with right hemiliver grafts: a prospective, randomized controlled study. Liver Transpl. 2012;18:129–37.
2. Akamatsu N, Sugawara Y, Kaneko J, et al. Effects of middle hepatic vein reconstruction on right liver graft reconstruction. Transplantation. 2003;76:832–7.

21 Donor Left Hemihepatectomy

Kyung-Suk Suh and Suk Kyun Hong

Abstract

During donor hepatectomy in living donor liver transplantation, donor's safety and graft quality preservation must be ensured at the same time. There are several tips and pitfalls to consider in donor left hepatectomy. Recently, minimally invasive techniques including pure laparoscopic technique have increasingly been adopted for major donor hepatectomy.

Keywords

Donor hepatectomy · Living donor liver transplantation · Left hepatectomy Laparoscopy · Minimally invasive

21.1 Incision and Exposure

For left hepatectomy, the Mercedes-Benz incision was preferred traditionally. However, an inverted L incision has now come to be used more frequently. Further, the functional and cosmetic needs of donors have recently led to increased use of the minimally invasive donor hepatectomy.

21.2 Liver Mobilization

The falciform ligament is dissected from the liver and up toward the inferior vena cava in order to expose the middle and left hepatic veins. Next, the space between the right and middle hepatic veins is dissected to expose the inferior vena cava. The left liver is then dissected from the diaphragm while dissecting the coronary ligament using electrocautery. The left triangular ligament at the end of the left liver is dissected from the diaphragm.

The left lateral section of the liver is moved to the right using a malleable retractor. The lesser sac is exposed while applying traction on the stomach in the direction of 5 o'clock. If the left hepatic artery branches off the left gastric artery, caution must be taken not to damage the vessel. The left lateral section is flipped right, while the hepatogastric ligament is dissected to expose the ligamentum venosum located between the caudate lobe and the left lateral section. The ligamentum venosum is then ligated and divided near the left hepatic vein. The tissues surrounding the left hepatic vein are dissected cleanly to prepare for the hanging tape to pass between the middle and left hepatic vein trunk and the inferior vena cava.

Supplementary Information The online version contains supplementary material available at https://doi.org/10.1007/978-981-16-1996-0_21.

K.-S. Suh (✉) · S. K. Hong
Department of Surgery, Seoul National University College of Medicine, Seoul, South Korea
e-mail: kssuh@snu.ac.kr

H. C. Yu (ed.), *Hepato-Biliary-Pancreatic Surgery and Liver Transplantation*,
https://doi.org/10.1007/978-981-16-1996-0_21

Tip: Before mobilizing the left liver, place gauze under the left liver toward the diaphragm to reduce the risk of damaging the intestines or the spleen with electrocautery and to facilitate the dissection of the liver from the diaphragm. The first assistant can also press on the patient's intestines backward and to the left with a malleable retractor in order to facilitate visualization during ligation of the left triangular ligament.

21.3 Placement of the Hanging Tape

The right-angle clamp is placed between the right and middle hepatic veins. The end of the clamp is inserted into the space between the left hepatic vein and the inferior vena cava to create a tunnel for the hanging tape (Fig. 21.1a). If enough space has not been created in one direction, insert the right-angle clamp toward the opposite direction to secure enough space. Once the tunnel has been created, hold the tape sling at the end of the right-angle clamp and pass it between the right hepatic vein and the middle hepatic vein as well as under the middle and left hepatic veins (Fig. 21.1b); the hanging tape should pass above the inferior vena cava. As there is risk of massive bleeding from inferior vena cava damage, the right-angle clamp should be manipulated carefully and slowly.

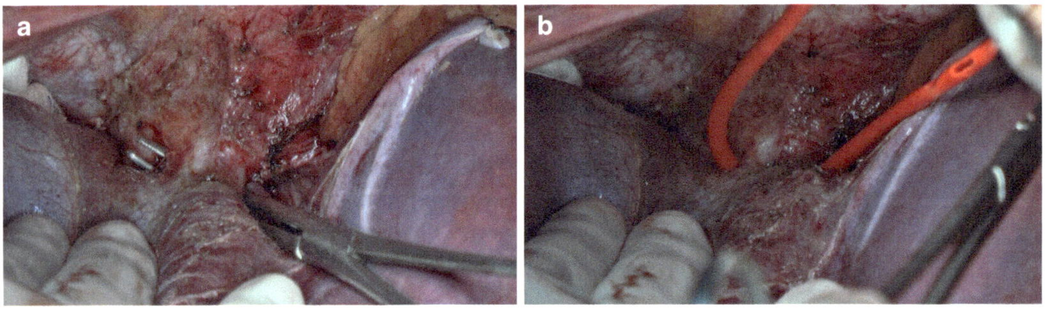

Fig. 21.1 Preparing for the hanging maneuver. (**a**) A clamp between the left hepatic vein and the inferior vena cava. (**b**) A nelaton tube between the right hepatic vein and the middle hepatic vein as well as under the middle and left hepatic veins

21.4 Cholecystectomy

This is not much different from regular cholecystectomy. Ensure that the remaining cystic duct has sufficient length so that the course of the biliary duct can be confirmed using a probe or so that a contrast agent can be injected into the biliary duct for intraoperative cholangiogram.

21.5 Hilar Dissection and Demarcation for Transection

Confirm any changes in the hepatic artery, portal vein, or bile duct in preoperative computed tomography (CT) and magnetic resonance imaging (MRI) before proceeding with surgery. To begin, dissect away the tissues surrounding the left hepatic artery to confirm where the left hepatic artery bifurcates off the common hepatic artery. Carefully dissect the tissues to avoid damage to the hepatic artery. In addition, be careful to prevent heat damage to the artery from excessive use of electrocautery. Dissect the surrounding tissues around the middle hepatic artery to expose it. Divide the lesser sac and expose the caudate lobe, then ligate the exposed branches of the portal vein that enter the caudate lobe. Once the tissues are surrounding the left hepatic artery and the posterior aspect of the middle hepatic artery, the left portal vein is easily exposed.

Unlike the crimson color of the surface of the right liver, the left liver can change to a dark red color with the temporary blockage of inbound blood flow. This turns into a border between the left and right liver. Mark this border on the surface of the liver using electrocautery and use it as a reference line for the resection of the left liver. This border will enter between the right and left hepatobiliary ducts. Subsequently, release the vessel loop or vascular clamp to maintain perfusion into the liver during liver resection.

Tip 1: Palpate intraoperatively to obtain a general overview of the course of the right, left, and middle hepatic arteries.

Tip 2: Temporarily ligate the left and middle hepatic arteries and left portal vein using vessel loops or vascular clamps to observe the change in color of the left liver.

21.6 Resection of the Liver Parenchyma

Use CUSA® (Cavitron Ultrasonic Surgical Aspirator) to dissect the liver parenchyma along the border between the left and right sides of the liver. Follow the midplane of the liver carefully while avoiding Gleason branches to easily dissect the parenchyma. Ligate any middle hepatic vein branches draining the right liver along the resection plane. Dissect the parenchyma around the hilum to expose the hilar plate.

Tip: Use ultrasound to periodically confirm the position of the middle vein and ensure that the resection plane is not skewed toward the right of the middle vein.

21.7 Resection of the Left Bile Duct

Pass the probe into the long tail of the remnant cystic duct from cholecystectomy to locate the border between the right and left bile ducts (Fig. 21.2). After applying a tagging suture, make a small incision to the distal left bile duct. Re-confirm the location of the branches of the left and right bile ducts before proceeding with complete division of the left bile duct. Use continuous

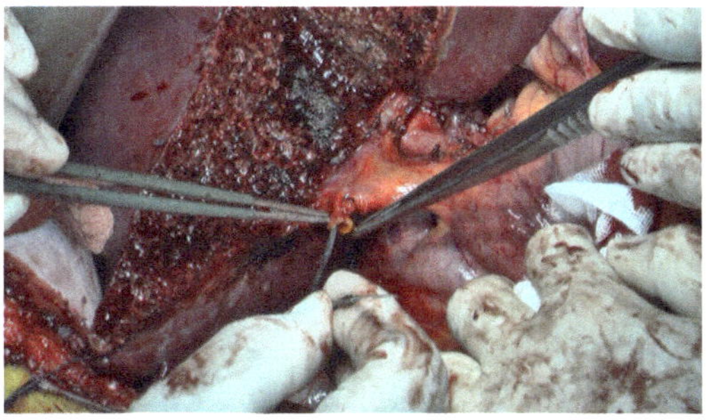

Fig. 21.2 Bile duct probing

suturing with nonabsorbable sutures to close the stump of the bile duct to prevent distortion of the bile duct and leakage of bile fluids. Finally, separate and ligate the branches of the portal vein and dissect and ligate the hilum gradually.

Tip 1: Apply superior-inferior traction on the suture site of the bile duct during suturing to prevent distortion of the bile duct.

21.8 Resection of the Remaining Liver Parenchyma

Bring the lower end of the hanging tape out superior to the left hepatic artery and portal vein and use the hanging maneuver to dissect the liver parenchyma (Fig. 21.3). As there are multiple Gleason branches that cross the resection plane of the caudate lobe, make sure to ligate them carefully. Visualize the vessel structures by adequately dissecting the tissues surrounding the inferior vena cava, the middle hepatic vein, and the origin of the left hepatic vein.

Tip: As the remaining liver parenchyma is located deep within the abdominal cavity, using the hanging maneuver can reduce bleeding and keep the resection plane of the liver parenchyma straight.

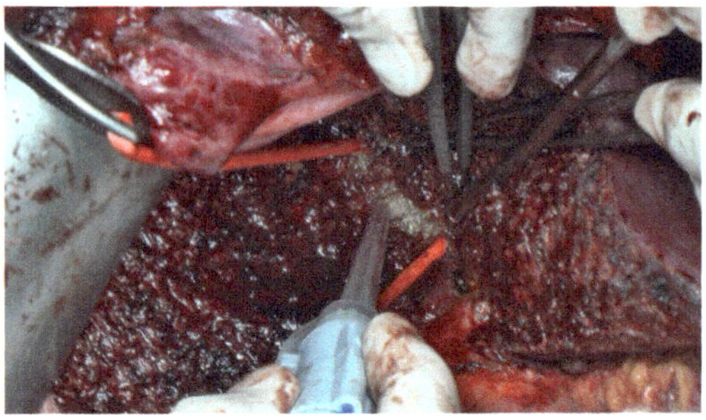

Fig. 21.3 Transecting liver parenchyma in the deep portion

21.9 Vessel Dissection and Liver Retrieval

Ligate the left hepatic artery at the point where the left hepatic artery diverges from the proper hepatic artery. Divide the left hepatic artery and confirm regurgitant flow. If the middle hepatic artery originates from the right hepatic artery, dissect the middle hepatic artery near its origin and divide it. Use a vascular stapler or a vascular clamp to divide the left hepatic vein as closely as possible to the inferior vena cava. Leave the hepatic artery, portal vein, and hepatic vein on the graft side as long as possible without damaging the vascular structure of the donor.

Tip 1: When dividing the portal vein, apply a vascular clamp vertically to avoid narrowing of the left portal vein.

Tip 2: Hold the surface of the liver with gauze to avoid damage or slipping when removing the graft from the abdominal cavity of the donor.

21.10 Bench Operation

The left liver graft should be perfused using organ preservation fluid that has been chilled to approximately 4 °C through the portal vein. A syringe filled with this preservation fluid can be used to irrigate the left hepatic artery and the left bile duct. The structures of the blood vessel and biliary duct can be confirmed in this way, and the graft can be trimmed to optimize anastomosis.

21.11 Pure Laparoscopic Donor Hepatectomy

Until very recently, living donor hepatectomy has been performed under conventional laparotomies. Compared to conventional laparotomies, laparoscopic surgery leads to better cosmetic outcomes, shorter hospital stays, and less pain. Further, various studies have shown that postoperative complication rates are reduced in laparoscopic surgery. Along with these benefits, due to the increased experience and knowledge in laparoscopic surgery in the era of striving toward minimally invasive surgery, pure laparoscopic donor hepatectomy is also being performed at some centers.

Laparoscopic surgery differs from traditional surgery in that the position of the trocar is fixed, and the operator visualizes the field from the patient's lower limb area (caudal view). Manipulating the scope to obtain views from various angles is particularly important in laparoscopic hepatectomy because of the relatively small space available for instrument manipulation. To maximize the visualization and depth of perception, a 3D flexible laparoscopy is preferred. To make the border between the right and the left liver more prominent and find a safe area for resection through real-time confirmation of the location of the bile duct, indocyanine green near-infrared fluorescence can be used (Fig. 21.4). Following the resection, the graft can be removed using an incision made horizontally above the pubic symphysis, which can be covered by underwear and is therefore esthetically preferable.

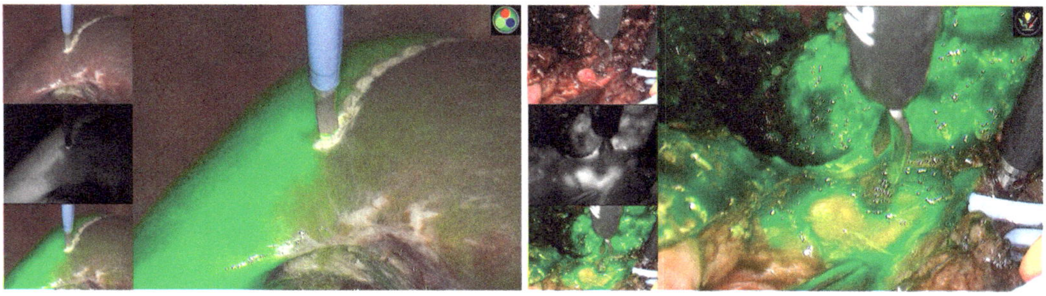

Fig. 21.4 Usage of indocyanine green near-infrared fluorescence

Living Donor Liver Graft Back-Table Procedure

22

Choon Hyuck David Kwon and Gyu-seong Choi

Abstract

Trimming is performed with a focus on the reconstruction of blood flow. If two or more portal veins or bile ducts are present due to anatomical variations, venoplasty or ductoplasty can be performed at the back-table to combine them. In this chapter, we will introduce a method of reconstructing the blood flow of the graft and explain the reconstruction of the portal vein and bile duct with anatomical variations. The reconstruction method may differ depending on the preferences of the surgeon and the transplantation institute.

Keywords

Living donor liver graft · Back-table procedure · Hepatic vein reconstruction · Portal vein reconstruction · Biliary reconstruction Venoplasty · Ductoplasty

22.1 Hepatic Vein Reconstruction

The goal of hepatic vein reconstruction is to prevent congestion of the graft by preventing obstruction of the venous outflow.

22.1.1 Securing Blood Flow in the Anterior Section of the Modified Right Liver Graft

The outflow of the anterior section of the liver that drains into the middle hepatic vein is reconstructed in the modified right liver graft. The method of reconstruction differs depending on the kind of vascular graft used (Fig. 22.1). When using a cryopreserved vein, the direction of the vein should be checked before anastomosis to ensure that the valve does not interfere with blood flow. As in veno-venous anastomosis, the anastomosis should be prevented from narrowing the outflow by providing appropriate growth factor (Fig. 22.2).

Supplementary Information The online version contains supplementary material available at https://doi.org/10.1007/978-981-16-1996-0_22.

C. H. D. Kwon (✉) · G.-s. Choi
Department of General Surgery, Digestive Disease & Surgery Institute, Cleveland Clinic, Cleveland, OH, USA

H. C. Yu (ed.), *Hepato-Biliary-Pancreatic Surgery and Liver Transplantation*,
https://doi.org/10.1007/978-981-16-1996-0_22

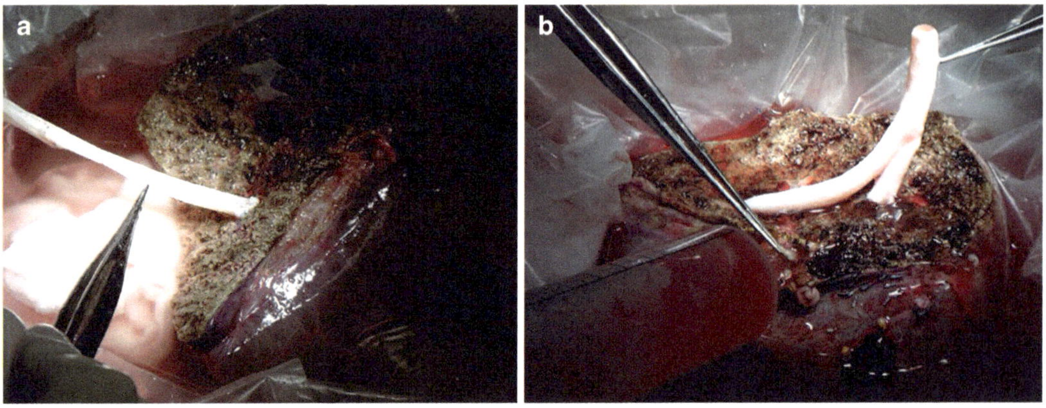

Fig. 22.1 (**a**) Reconstruction of the middle hepatic vein using cryopreserved vein. (**b**) Reconstruction of the middle hepatic vein using cryopreserved artery

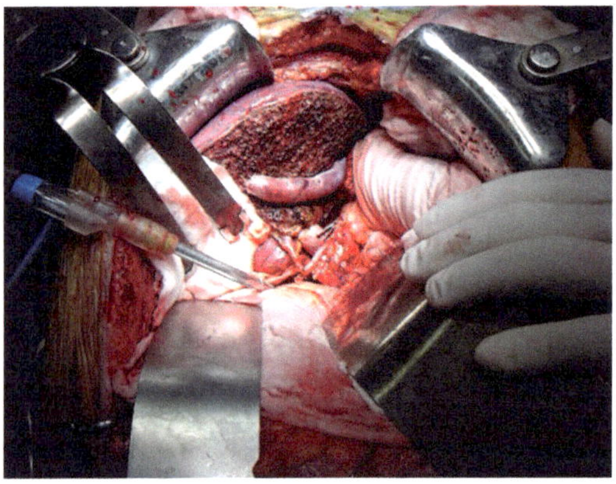

Fig. 22.2 Reconstructed vascular graft connected to recipient

22.1.2 Middle Hepatic Vein Reconstruction of Extended Right Liver Graft

There is a method of reconstructing the middle hepatic vein that involves increasing the length using a vascular graft similar to a modified right liver graft, while another method involves reconstructing the middle and right hepatic veins into one. In this case, it is recommended to use a vein graft to place a bridge connecting the middle and right hepatic veins. Vein grafts can also be used to make an enclosed fence to perform anastomosis around the blood vessels. The commen trunk of the right hepatic vein and reconstructed mddile hepatic vein are, then, anastomosed to the inferior vena cava of the recipient (Fig. 22.2).

22.1.3 Reconstruction of Blood Flow in Left Liver Graft

The middle and left hepatic veins may appear respectively depending on the anatomical variation in an extended left liver graft. In addition, a conventional left liver graft may have more than one vein. In this case, since the distance between the middle and left hepatic veins is small, the two veins are connected by angioplasty which directly anastomoses the adjacent walls of the two veins.

22.1.4 Reconstruction of the Large Right Inferior Hepatic Vein

In the case of right inferior hepatic venous resection involving a portion of the vena cava in donor surgery, an anastomosis can be performed directly on the vena cava of the recipient. However, if the right inferior hepatic vein is short, it should be reconstructed using a vein graft or another vascular graft. If the distance from the right hepatic vein of the recipient to the right inferior hepatic vein of the graft is not large, then the two veins can be reconstructed using a bridge or fence vein graft.

22.2 Portal Vein Reconstruction

Portal vein reconstruction is not common in partial liver transplantation. In the case of type II, wherein the portal vein is triangulated, or type III, wherein the posterior portal vein branches earlier, two portal veins appear if the right liver is used.

22.2.1 Reconstruction Using the Recipient's Portal Vein

If the distance between the two portal veins is far, the recipient's portal vein can be obtained in a Y-shape and used for reconstruction. In this case, the anastomosis should be performed by calculating the direction of the blood flow to the two portal veins. If one portal vein is bent or narrowed, more blood can flow to the other portal vein, which can in turn prevent blood from flowing into the narrowed portal vein. Shortening the inside of both the portal veins and slightly lengthening the outside is a way to prevent the direction of blood flow from being distorted.

22.2.2 Reconstruction Using Vein Graft Due to Short or Variation in the Recipient's Portal Vein

When using a Y-shaped graft, if the recipient's portal vein is short due to thrombus or has variations, or if there is a large size discrepancy between the two portal veins, blood may only flow to one side. There is a way to connect a sufficiently large vein graft that serves as a bridge between the two portal veins to form them into one, then connect it to the portal vein (Fig. 22.3).

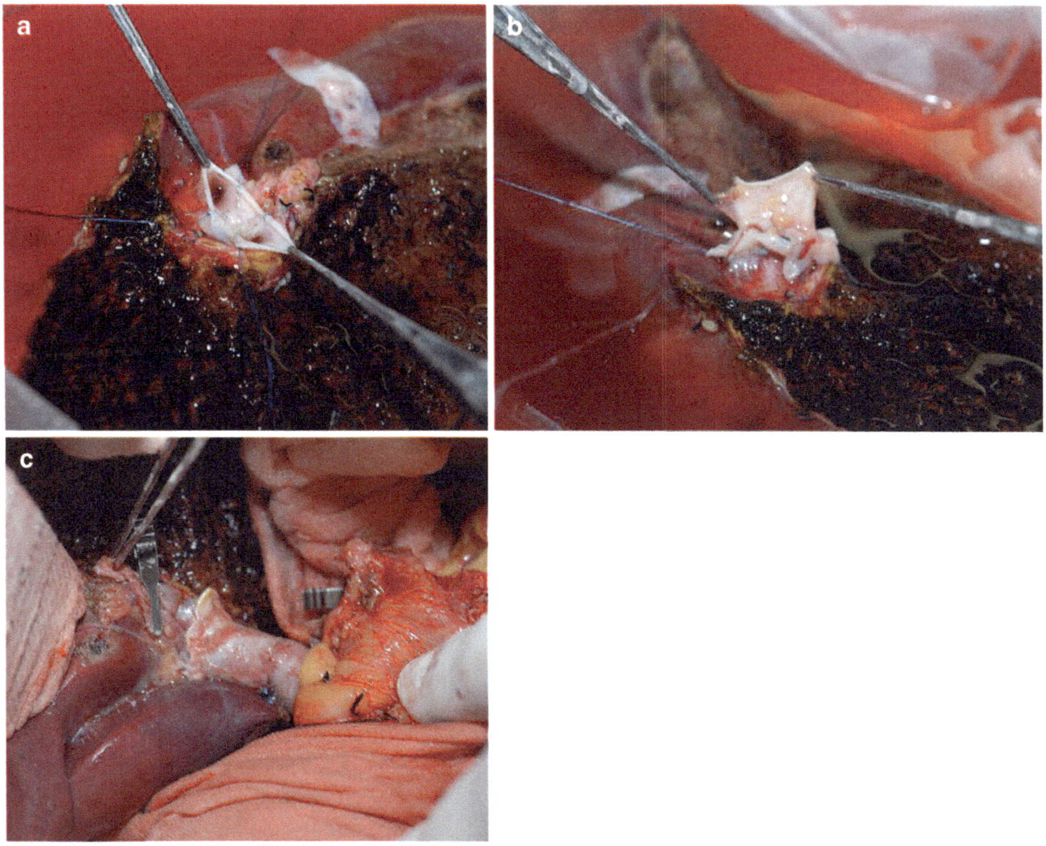

Fig. 22.3 (**a**) Process of connecting two portal veins into one using a vein graft. (**b**) Process of reconstructing the portal vein using the recipient's portal vein. (**c**) Reconstructed portal vein after reperfusion

22.3 Biliary Reconstruction

If more than one bile duct of the graft appears, it can either be anastomosed individually or made into one. The size of the two bile ducts should not be significantly different, and they should be at a distance that can be pulled to an appropriate value. When two bile ducts of similar size are made into one, connecting the 12 o'clock point and 6 o'clock point of the bile duct narrows the bile duct, which may interfere with the bile duct anastomosis. Instead, it is better to anastomose the 2 o'clock with 10 o'clock points and the 4 o'clock with 8 o'clock points.

Middle Hepatic Vein Reconstruction of Right Liver Graft

23

Dong-Sik Kim

Abstract

Reconstruction of the middle hepatic vein is an important part of the procedure using a modified right lobe graft. Various modifications are available depending on the specific situation of the graft and the availability of vascular grafts. It is generally recommended that tributaries larger than 5 mm in diameter be reconstructed. In this chapter, basic concepts and technical tips are discussed and an example is provided in the form of a video clip.

Keywords

Vascular graft · Patency · Cryopreserved iliac vein · Cryopreserved iliac artery · PTFE

Supplementary Information The online version contains supplementary material available at https://doi.org/10.1007/978-981-16-1996-0_23.

D.-S. Kim (✉)
Division of HBP Surgery and Liver Transplantation, Department of Surgery, Korea University College of Medicine, Seoul, South Korea
e-mail: kimds1@korea.ac.kr

23.1 Overview

The most commonly used type of graft in living donor liver transplantation (LDLT) using the right lobe is the modified right lobe graft. In consideration of donor safety, the middle hepatic vein is allowed to remain on the donor side to prevent congestion in the remnant left lobe. The middle hepatic vein for the graft is reconstructed on the back-table to prevent congestion in the anterior section. Through this reconstruction of the middle hepatic vein, the outcomes of LDLT using the right lobe could be significantly improved [1].

Venous congestion in the right anterior section has been shown to have an important effect on the regeneration of the graft [2]. Therefore, the reconstructed vein must remain functional during the initial two-week period after surgery while the regeneration of the graft occurs rapidly. Stenosis or obstruction of the middle hepatic vein graft accompanied by an increase in transaminase is recommended to be managed through an interventional procedure.

23.2 Judgment on the Necessity of Reconstructing the Middle Hepatic Vein

The reconstruction of the middle hepatic vein depends on the extent to which the venous blood from the right anterior section is drained into it.

H. C. Yu (ed.), *Hepato-Biliary-Pancreatic Surgery and Liver Transplantation*,
https://doi.org/10.1007/978-981-16-1996-0_23

Therefore, the preoperative computed tomography of the donor should be closely reviewed to obtain the sizes and locations of the tributaries, particularly V5 and V8, that drain into the middle hepatic vein. During donor surgery, if the right hepatic artery is blocked with a bulldog clamp after the parenchyma and tributaries of the middle hepatic vein have been cut, the degree of congestion in the right anterior section can be directly checked [3]. The graft to recipient weight ratio (GRWR) of the graft or the degree of steatosis may also be considered. In general, reconstruction is recommended when the diameter of the tributary entering the middle hepatic vein is 5 mm or more.

23.3 Blood Vessels Used for Reconstruction

Various blood vessels have been used to reconstruct the middle hepatic vein. Because the process involves reconstructing the venous system with low blood pressure, vascular grafts that can reflect the original characteristics of the middle hepatic vein that deliver the lower pressure state of the right atrium and the central vein more than the durability of the blood vessel are preferred, such as cryopreserved iliac vein. However, its supply is limited. Good results have been reported using alternatives such as cryopreserved iliac arteries, a greater saphenous vein from the recipient, a left portal vein taken from the removed recipient's liver, or an artificial vein such as polytetrafluoroethylene (PTFE) [4–6].

23.4 Technical Considerations for Reconstruction

The goal of reconstruction is to maintain the blood flow naturally, but each liver graft has different locations of the openings of the tributaries of the middle hepatic vein exposed on the cut surface, and they may also have different numbers. Further, the positional correlation with the right hepatic vein, the existence of the right inferior hepatic vein, the type of blood vessel graft to be used for reconstruction and the physical properties thereof, and the location of the branch already existing in the blood vessel graft should all be considered together. In addition, there is a difference in the reconstruction method depending on whether the right hepatic vein and the middle hepatic vein are anastomosed separately or as a single one at the time of anastomosis, thus necessitating close communication between team members.

The anastomosis should be initiated after considering the overall design in front of the liver graft and the vessel graft to be used for reconstruction such that a natural angle can be formed in order to avoid twisting or folding of the vessel graft.

23.5 Anastomosis Tips (See Video 23.1)

1. The blood vessels are arranged according to the design previously thought of. It does not matter if the blood vessel to be used is a type that maintains the lumen itself, such as an artery or PTFE, but if the material is large and cannot maintain its lumen by itself, such as an iliac vein, distortion of the vessel graft that occurs while placing and determining the anastomosis position can be minimized by filling the lumen with heparinized saline.
2. If a vein is used as a vessel graft for reconstruction, check if there are any valves inside, and remove any found.
3. The order of the tributaries to be anastomosed to the vessel graft needs to be determined in consideration of the location and direction of the recipient's middle hepatic vein stump. The order needs to be determined to avoid any suffering in anastomosis from the previously made anastomosis. If the tributaries are not lined up straight, it is convenient to start the anastomosis from the one located in the middle.
4. Hang the 6-0 prolene double-arm suture at both ends of the opening of the tributary to be anastomosed following the direction of the blood vessel to be reconstructed.

5. Make a hole in the wall of the vessel graft with a diameter equal to or slightly larger than the inner diameter of the tributary. At this time, if using artery or PTFE, do not make a simple incision, but cut it out in a circle.
6. Using the inner thread of a 6-0 prolene double-arm suture that has been previously hung, pass the needle from the inside to the outside of the vessel graft and tie it.
7. Using the thread on the far side from the operator, suture in an over-and-over manner while moving toward the operator. During this process, be careful not to tear the blood vessel or narrow the lumen by pulling the thread too hard.
8. When approaching the other end, the last stitch needs to be placed very close to the originally hung thread, and then a knot must be made outside the lumen.
9. Turning over the vessel graft in the opposite direction, the anastomosis line on the opposite side should be placed in front.
10. Check the anastomosis you just made from the inside.
11. After repeating the process in (6–8), cut the thread. Be careful not to accidentally include the other side in this process. If there is any difficulty stemming from the narrow lumen, placing a dilator in the vessel graft helps prevent mistakes.
12. Repeat steps (4) to (11) while matching the direction and distance to the next tributary to be anastomosed.

23.6 In the Case of Anastomosis of Right Hepatic Vein and Reconstructed Middle Hepatic Vein as a Single Orifice

If the right hepatic vein and the reconstructed middle hepatic vein are made into one opening, the bench surgery time is longer, but all the veins can be anastomosed at once, thereby avoiding congestion in the right anterior section from immediately after reperfusion to until the end of the reconstruction of the middle hepatic vein; sometimes, this allows unnecessary bleeding from the cut surface or venous reconstruction site to be avoided. Further, by artificially making the anterior side of the middle hepatic vein bulge, the outflow of the right hepatic vein becomes enlarged, thus reducing the risk of outflow obstruction that can occur as the liver regenerates and rotates [7].

At this time, the anterior side of the right hepatic vein and the posterior side of the reconstructed middle vein are sutured very close to each other to prevent loosening, while the anterior side of the reconstructed middle hepatic vein is 1.5–2 times wider than the back, making it swell naturally due to the pressure of the vena cava after reperfusion. This can have the effect of widening the lumen of the entire anastomosis (see Video 23.1).

23.7 Reconstructed Middle Hepatic Vein after Reperfusion

1. After the reconstruction of the middle hepatic vein using a cryopreserved iliac vein, the vascular graft was anastomosed to the confluence of the middle and left hepatic vein (Fig. 23.1).

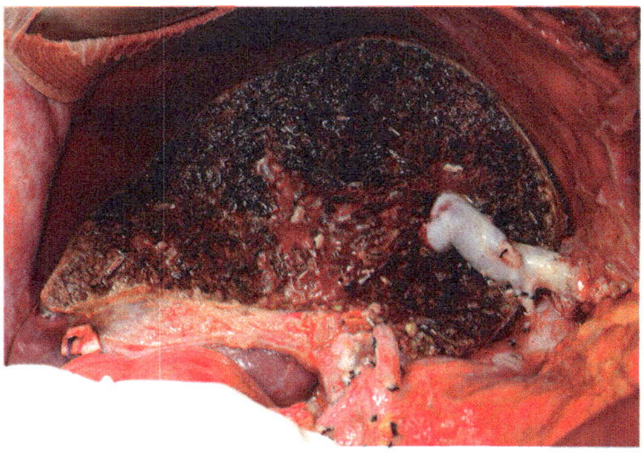

Fig. 23.1 Reconstruction of the middle hepatic vein and anastomosis to the recipient's middle-left hepatic vein confluence using a cryopreserved iliac vein. Care should be taken during anastomosis to ensure that the reconstructed middle hepatic vein is not distorted when blood flow is resumed

2. Outcome after anastomosis of the middle and right hepatic vein of the graft as a single orifice using the cryopreserved iliac vein (Fig. 23.2).
3. Anastomosis after reconstruction of the middle hepatic vein using PTFE (Fig. 23.3).

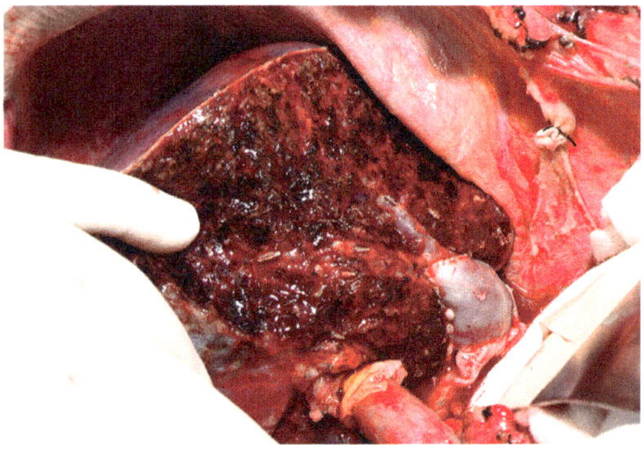

Fig. 23.2 Using a cryopreserved iliac vein, the opening of the middle and right hepatic veins is made into a single orifice, while the anterior wall is designed to be large and connected to the vena cava (see Video 23.1)

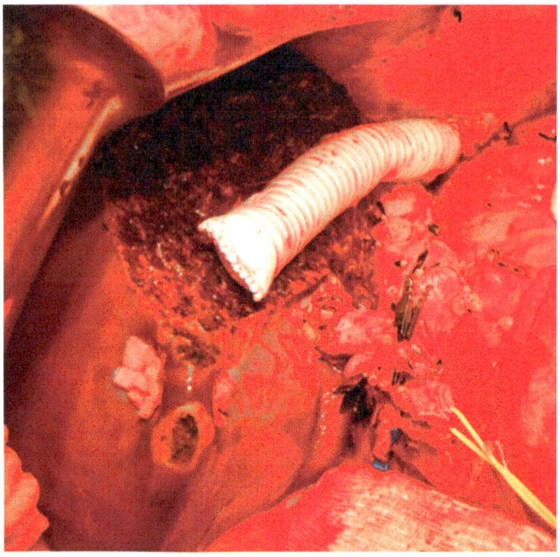

Fig. 23.3 Reconstruction of the middle hepatic vein using an artificial graft

References

1. Lee S, Park K, Hwang S, Lee Y, Choi D, Kim K, et al. Congestion of right liver graft in living donor liver transplantation. Transplantation. 2001;71(6):812–4.
2. Chen HL, Tsang LL, Concejero AM, Huang TL, Chen TY, Ou HY, et al. Segmental regeneration in right-lobe liver grafts in adult living donor liver transplant. Clin Transpl. 2012;26(5):694–8.
3. Hwang S, Lee SG, Park KM, Kim KH, Ahn CS, Lee YJ, et al. Hepatic venous congestion in living donor liver transplantation: preoperative quantitative prediction and follow-up using computed tomography. Liver Transpl. 2004;10(6):763–70.
4. Hwang S, Lee SG, Ahn CS, Park KM, Kim KH, Moon DB, et al. Cryopreserved iliac artery is indispensable interposition graft material for middle hepatic vein reconstruction of right liver grafts. Liver Transpl. 2005;11(6):644–9.
5. Hwang S, Jung DH, Ha TY, Ahn CS, Moon DB, Kim KH, et al. Usability of ringed polytetrafluoroethylene grafts for middle hepatic vein reconstruction during living donor liver transplantation. Liver Transpl. 2012;18(8):955–65.
6. Cattral MS, Greig PD, Muradali D, Grant D. Reconstruction of middle hepatic vein of a living-donor right lobe liver graft with recipient left portal vein. Transplantation. 2001;71(12):1864–6.
7. Sugawara Y, Makuuchi M, Akamatsu N, Kishi Y, Niiya T, Kaneko J, et al. Refinement of venous reconstruction using cryopreserved veins in right liver grafts. Liver Transpl. 2004;10(4):541–7.

Recipient Total Hepatectomy

24

Kwang-Woong Lee and Jaehong Jeong

Abstract

Recipient total hepatectomy is an important step for a successful liver transplantation. Specifically, in order to reduce biliary complications, precise anatomical knowledge and delicate surgical skills are required when handling the hepatic hilum. Further, in living donor liver transplantation, various approaches are required depending on the situation of the donor surgery and the quality of the graft. Therefore, various techniques should be applied depending on the specific situation of the donor and the recipient

Keywords

Liver transplantation · Recipient hepatectomy Benign biliary stricture · High hilar dissection Portal vein thrombosis

Supplementary Information The online version contains supplementary material available at https://doi.org/10.1007/978-981-16-1996-0_24.

K.-W. Lee (✉)
Department of Surgery, College of Medicine, Seoul National University, Seoul, South Korea

J. Jeong
Soon Chun Hyang University Hospital, Bucheon, South Korea

24.1 Introduction

Recipient total hepatectomy is the process of removing the existing diseased liver for liver transplantation (LT), and it requires rapid and accurate surgery, as there are many collateral vessels and a major bleeding tendency due to cirrhosis, along with sufficient anatomical knowledge for successful vascular and biliary reconstruction of the graft. In the case of living donor LT in particular, when the hilar structures are dissected, they should be peeled to as long a length as possible to obtain a bile duct, a hepatic artery, and a portal vein of sufficient lengths. It is also very important to avoid injury to the vessels supplied to the biliary tract during biliary dissection. The incidence of biliary complications after living donor LT has been reported to range from 8.4% to as much as 35.8% [1]. In an effort to narrow this wide range, a “High Hilar Dissection (HHD)” was introduced in which, rather than dissecting the structures of the hepatic hilum separately to supply sufficient blood flow to the bile duct, the hepatic hilum was cut all at once at the intrahepatic level [2]. In this chapter, we will introduce some techniques while ultimately focusing on the process of dissecting hepatic hilum.

H. C. Yu (ed.), *Hepato-Biliary-Pancreatic Surgery and Liver Transplantation*,
https://doi.org/10.1007/978-981-16-1996-0_24

24.2 Surgical Method

24.2.1 Incision

In general, the combination of a sub-costal incision with a central upper incision is widely used to secure the field of view, and even an inverted L-shaped incision may ensure a sufficient field of view. Severe cirrhosis may occasionally cause severe bleeding during the skin incision due to the development of collateral vessels, and caution is required during this incision. If the ligament teres is reopened, the portal pressure will increase when it is ligated during the incision, so care should be taken to avoid injuring it.

24.2.2 Mobilization of the Liver

After the three hepatic vein inlets are sufficiently dissected, mobilization of the left liver is performed first. The left coronary and triangular ligament are cut while pulling down the left liver. At this time, the left triangular ligament should be ligated. Next, the lesser omentum is incised and the left liver is fully mobilized. Then, the right coronary and triangular ligament are cut while pulling down the right liver, and the hepatorenal ligament is cut afterward. At this point, the bare area is dissected to expose the right side of the inferior vena cava. The short hepatic vein between the inferior vena cava and the liver is sequentially ligated and cut from caudal to cranial, and from right to left. In this process, it is not necessary to forcibly treat the short hepatic veins located on the left side of the inferior vena cava, and it is safe to treat them after cutting the right hepatic vein, which provides sufficient vision. Finally, when the middle and left hepatic veins are cut after the liver is completely separated from the inferior vena cava, the recipient total hepatectomy is considered to be complete.

24.3 Handling of the Hepatic Hilum

24.3.1 Classical Hilar Dissection Technique

Since vessels and bile duct of sufficient length are required for successful anastomosis of the graft, it is important to dissect each structure as long as possible. In particular, during biliary dissection, it is very important to prevent damage to the blood vessels supplied to the bile duct to reduce the biliary complications, and it is also important to secure a sufficient length to avoid tension during biliary anastomosis. First, the hepatoduodenal ligament is palpated to check the location of the hepatic artery, after which the left side of the hepatoduodenal ligament is dissected to expose the proper and left hepatic arteries. The proper hepatic artery is completely peeled off, then encircled with a vessel loop. Next, the origin of the right hepatic artery is identified, the right hepatic artery is encircled with a vessel loop, and then the left and right hepatic arteries are dissected to a sufficient length. During this process, excessive pulling of the arteries should be avoided as it may increase the risk of arterial thrombosis due to intimal injury. As the right hepatic artery is dissected, the portal vein is exposed. Next, the portal vein is carefully dissected along the portal wall and encircled with a vessel loop. The bile duct is also sufficiently dissected and encircled with a vessel loop. Then, each structure is dissected to the liver as much as possible to facilitate anastomosis (Fig. 24.1).

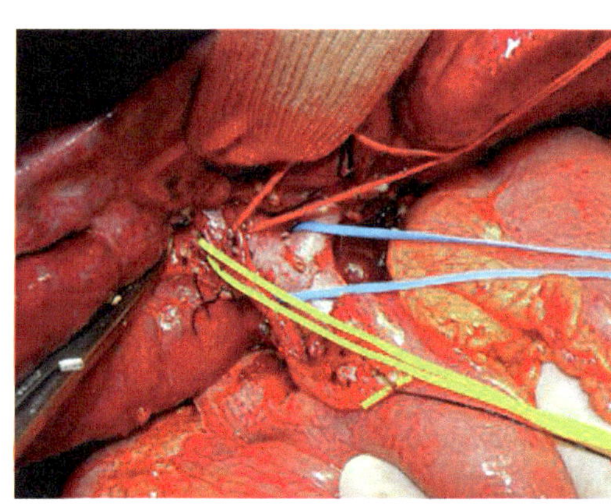

Fig. 24.1 Classical hilar dissection

24.3.2 High Hilar Dissection Technique (HHD)

Without individually dissecting the hepatic hilum, the entire hepatoduodenal ligament is blocked with a sufficiently large vascular clamp, then the hilar plate is dissected to cut both glissonean pedicles over the second-order level. When clamping the entire hepatoduodenal ligament, care should be taken to avoid damage to the hepatic artery, and it should be clamped cephalad as much as possible. The greatest advantage of HHD is that it can secure a healthy bile duct in which blood vessels are not damaged with sufficient length, which is beneficial during bile duct anastomosis (Fig. 24.2). In addition, since the portal vein can be obtained at the level of the second branch, when the donor's portal vein has two separate openings in the living donor LT, the recipient's portal vein can be used as a Y-graft. This makes it possible to overcome the twisting phenomenon in portal vein anastomosis.

24.3.3 Modified High Hilar Dissection Technique

24.3.3.1 Whole Flow Preserving HHD

Depending on the circumstances, donor surgery may be delayed. In this case, the application of HHD is limited. The biggest drawback of HHD is that it can cause severe portal hypertension, which blocks the whole portal flow, in turn leading to intestinal congestion, metabolic derangement, or bleeding. In particular, in the case of poorly developed collateral vessels, the degree of portal hypertension is more severe, and it may be impossible to close the abdomen. To overcome these shortcomings, a method of performing HHD while maintaining portal flow was introduced by Soejima et al. [3]. This is a method of sufficiently dissecting only the portal vein while leaving the bile duct and hepatic artery intact in the handling of hepatic hilum, and it is important to dissect along the portal vein wall. If both portal veins are sufficiently detached from the surrounding tissues, the bile duct and hepatic artery can be cut at the highest possible level. Since blood flow through both portal veins is wholly preserved, it is possible to flexibly respond to various situations that can arise during the donor surgery.

24.3.3.2 Left Flow Preserving HHD

Left flow preserving HHD is a procedure that only takes advantage of the above-described HHD and whole flow HHD techniques [4]. First, only the right glissonean pedicle is clamped, then cut over the second-order level (Fig. 24.3). The main advantage of this technique is that it can secure a healthy biliary tract of a similar enough length to that of HHD, with another advantage

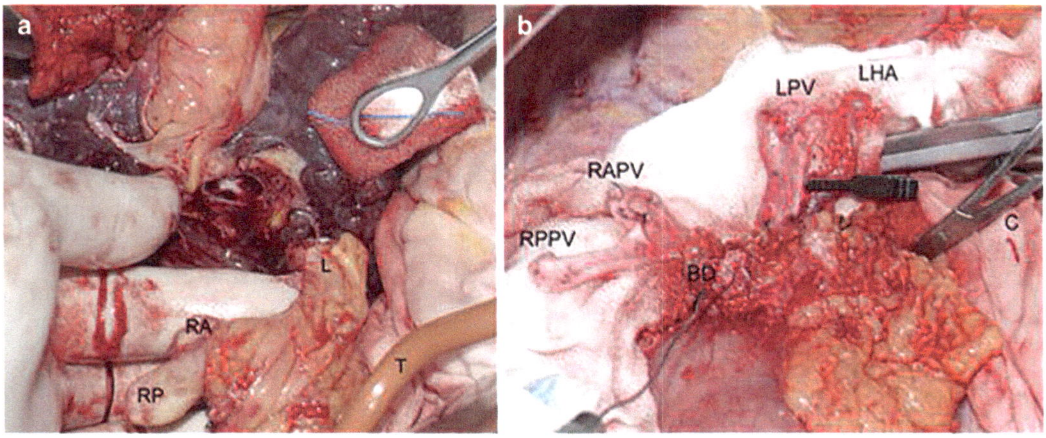

Fig. 24.2 High hilar dissection. (**a**) Glissonean pedicles at the second order. (**b**) Complete dissection of each structure after HHD

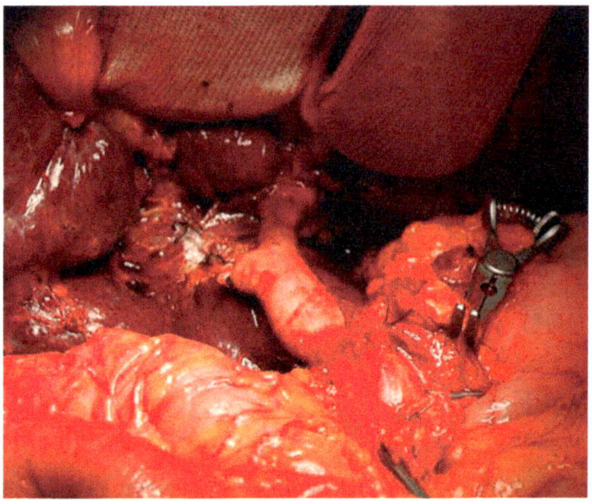

Fig. 24.3 Left flow preserving HHD

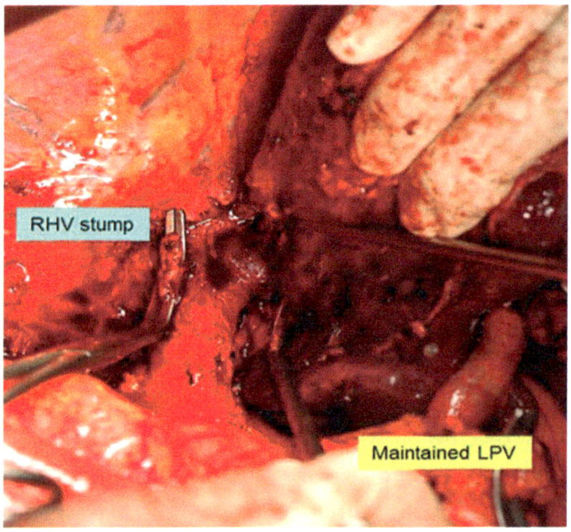

Fig. 24.4 Complete separation from inferior vena cava with left flow preserving HHD

being that it can cut the right hepatic vein, so it can safely handle the short hepatic vein located on the left side of the inferior vena cava with excellent visibility (Fig. 24.4). In addition, since the blood flow to the liver is maintained through the left portal vein, the middle and left hepatic veins, it can flexibly cope with situations that may arise during the donor surgery.

24.4 Portal Vein Thrombectomy

Portal vein thrombus is often found in patients with advanced liver cirrhosis, and short segmental thrombus can be easily removed through the careful eversion of the portal vein. It is not necessary to completely remove the thrombus, and careful manipulation is required as the weakened portal vein wall may tear. Occasionally, portal vein thrombosis may develop to the superior mesenteric vein, in which case, after opening the lesser sac by incising the greater omentum, dissecting between the lower border of the pancreas and the mesentery of transverse colon can lead to exposure of the superior mesenteric vein. If the dissecting of the superior mesenteric vein is sufficient, the superior mesenteric vein is then encircled with a vessel loop. Finally, venotomy is performed to carefully remove the thrombus.

24.5 Coping with and Prevention of Bleeding during Surgery

As mentioned above, since most cases are accompanied by cirrhosis, there is a tendency for the recipients to bleed easily due to the development of collateral vessels and coagulopathy. In some cases, the inferior phrenic artery is exposed in the right bare area. If hemostasis is performed with an electric cauterizer in response to bleeding here, delayed bleeding may occur, so it is safe to suture ligation with 4-0 prolene. Massive bleeding may occur during the cutting of the short hepatic vein, in which case, compulsorily attempting ligation without sufficient visibility can cause more severe bleeding. Therefore, the safe approach is to first press the bleeding site with a finger and block the blood flow to the liver, then dissect the surrounding area to secure space, and finally suture the bleeding site from the inferior vena cava.

24.6 Conclusion

Recipient total hepatectomy is not simply a procedure for removing diseased liver, but it is a preliminary step toward transplanting a new liver, so it must be flexibly performed according to the specific situations of the donor and the recipient. The acceptable anhepatic time varies depending on the degree of development of collateral vessels and the delay in donor surgery, and the technique used to dissect the hepatic hilum may vary depending on the condition of the bile duct and vessels of the donor, or its location if there is liver cancer. Therefore, various techniques of the procedure should be applied depending on the situation, and proper communication with the donor operator is essential.

References

1. Chok KS, Lo CM. Systematic review and meta-analysis of studies of biliary reconstruction in adult living donor liver transplantation. ANZ J Surg. 2017;87(3):121–5.
2. Lee KW, Joh JW, Kim SJ, Choi SH, Heo JS, Lee HH, et al. High hilar dissection: new technique to reduce biliary complication in living donor liver transplantation. Liver Transpl. 2004;10(9):1158–62.
3. Soejima Y, Fukuhara T, Morita K, Yoshizumi T, Ikegami T, Yamashita Y, et al. A simple hilar dissection technique preserving maximum blood supply to the bile duct in living donor liver transplantation. Transplantation. 2008;86(10):1468–9.
4. Shehta A, Jeong J, Lee KW, Lee JM, Hong SK, Cho JH, et al. A tailored strategy for recipient hepatectomy: left portal flow preserving high hilar dissection. J Gastrointest Surg. 2019;23(12):2466.

Reconstruction of Hepatic Vein and Portal Vein

25

Deok-Bog Moon and Sung-Gyu Lee

Abstract

To ensure a successful liver transplantation (LT), one must secure adequate hepatic arterial and portal inflow, as well as good outflow through the hepatic veins (HVs).

Wide HV outflow can be achieved through pertinent HV venoplasty of the liver graft at the back-table and of the recipient in vivo. These procedures not only allow for a wide anastomotic opening of the HV to be made, but they also enable easy and safe HV anastomosis, even under a bad operative visual field. As a result, the technical complications of hepatic venous outflow can be minimized.

In the case of single graft LDLT, the recipient's right or left portal vein (PV) is not typically used for PV reconstruction; instead, bifurcation of the main PV is preferred to avoid redundancy and stenosis. In the case of dual graft LDLT, the long-length recipient's right and left PV should be kept intact during hilar dissection, so they can be used for PV reconstruction of both grafts. At this time, we should try to further reduce the risk of PV twisting by maintaining good alignment during anastomosis.

D.-B. Moon · S.-G. Lee (✉)
Division of Hepatobiliary Surgery and Liver Transplantation, Department of Surgery, Asan Medical Center, University of Ulsan College of Medicine, Seoul, South Korea
e-mail: mdb1@amc.seoul.kr; sglee2@amc.seoul.kr

Keywords

Hepatic vein · Venoplasty · Portal vein Anastomosis · Back-table operation · LDLT

25.1 Reconstruction of Hepatic Vein

To ensure a successful liver transplantation (LT), one must secure adequate hepatic arterial and portal inflow, as well as good outflow through the hepatic veins (HVs). Wide HV outflow can be achieved by pertinent HV venoplasty of the liver graft at the back-table and of the recipient in vivo, then the congestion-induced dysfunction of the implanted liver graft can be minimized [1].

25.1.1 Back-Table Procedures

25.1.1.1 Modified Right Lobe Graft

Augmentation HV venoplasty should be performed when the right hepatic vein (RHV) is not large enough for a diameter exceeding 3–4 cm. While there are several types of RHV venoplasty, the most common type involves a longitudinal incision of the inferior corner of RHV including hepatic parenchyma, followed by augmentation patch venoplasty using the recipient's bisected great saphenous vein (GSV) after dilatation with hydrostatic pressure; this is also the most reliable method when no homologous vas-

H. C. Yu (ed.), *Hepato-Biliary-Pancreatic Surgery and Liver Transplantation*,
https://doi.org/10.1007/978-981-16-1996-0_25

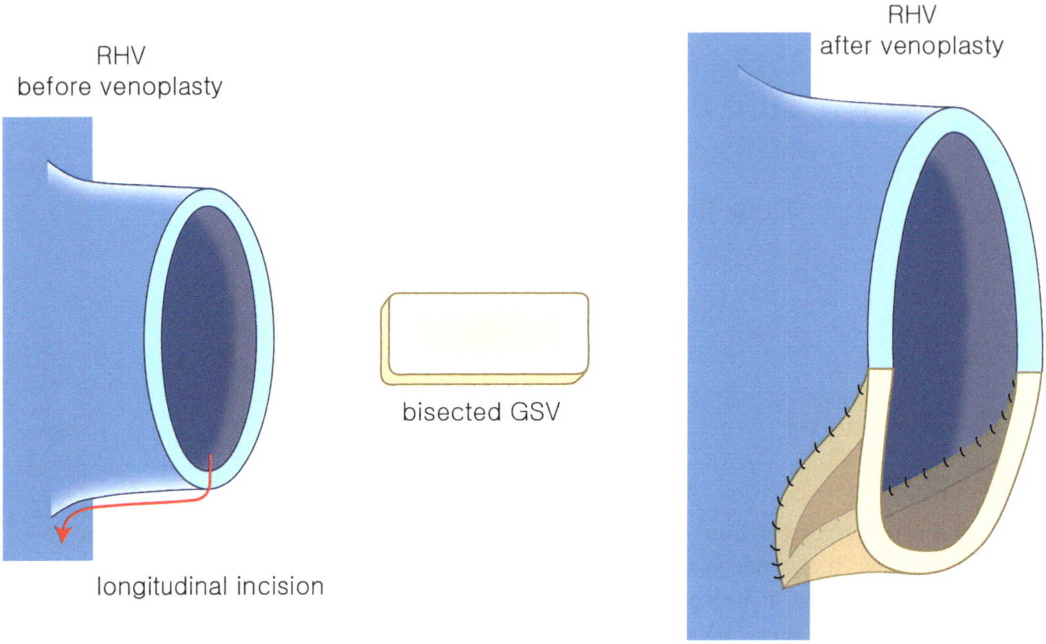

Fig. 25.1 Venoplasty of right hepatic vein (RHV) at the back-table. First, a longitudinal incision was made into the parenchyma at the inferior corner, then augmentation venoplasty was performed using a bisected great saphenous vein (GSV) patch. *RHV* right hepatic vein, *GSV* great saphenous vein

cular graft can be obtained from the deceased organ donor [2, 3]. Hence, we can make a more than 4 cm-sized large RHV at the back-table and minimize the risk of HV stenosis or kinking, which can occur as a result of the post-transplant-enlarged liver graft related mostly to regeneration or, less commonly, acute rejection (Fig. 25.1). The recipient's re-canalized paraumbilical vein and cadaveric iliac vein can be used as alternative vascular patches for HV venoplasty, and cadaveric arteries or PTFE artificial vascular grafts are used in rare situations as well. The operative techniques do not differ much among the various types of vascular patches, and in this study, we primarily describe the method of venoplasty using bisected GSV.

When procuring the liver graft laparoscopically, we often encounter a liver graft with too short of an HV stump from the parenchymal surface, and its anastomosis cannot be performed safely without venoplasty at the back-table. In this inconvenient situation, using a combination of previously described augmentation venoplasty and the additional neo-vascular stump formation of RHV using a vascular-patch fence can help us perform wide and easy RHV anastomosis (Fig. 25.2).

When the modified right lobe graft has two or more short HVs that are larger than 5 mm in diameter, we should reconstruct them in the same way as the sizable middle HV branches [4, 5]. In the case of a single short HV, the previously described augmentation patch venoplasty is required to avoid venous outflow disturbance. Compared to the right HV, we need to be more cautious about the condition of the vascular wall in regard to whether or not it has a weak portion and too short of a stump length; when it does have both of these characteristics, an incision including the hepatic parenchyma should be made along the weak portion, and patch venoplasty or vascular fence should be performed to make a short HV with a wide opening and adequate stump length.

In the case of two or more short HVs, separate anastomosis is sometimes performed when two short HVs are wide apart and have sufficiently large diameters. However, technical errors may arise when there is a space discrepancy between

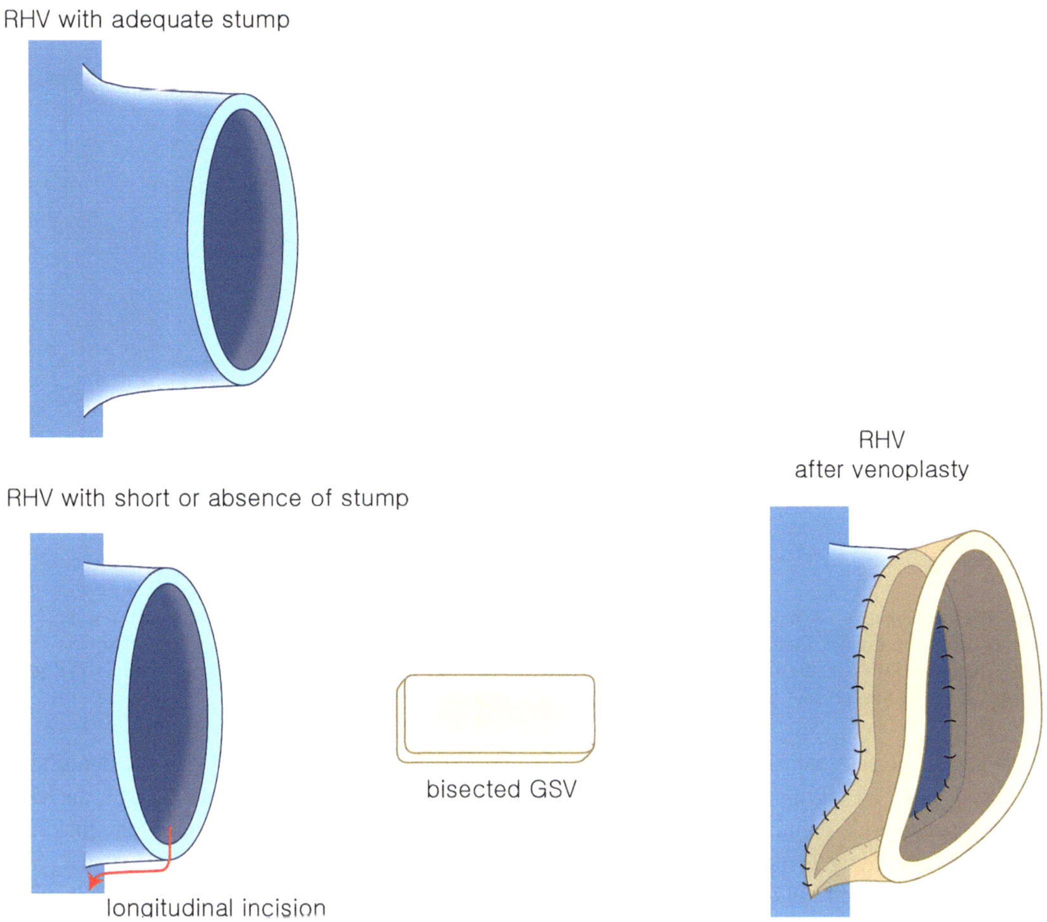

Fig. 25.2 Venoplasty of RHV with a short stump or even no stump at the back-table. First, a longitudinal incision was made into the parenchyma at the inferior corner, then a neo-vascular stump was made with fencing of bisected GSV. Hence, the newly formed RHV has a wide diameter and sufficient stump length. *RHV* right hepatic vein, *GSV* great saphenous vein

the recipient's right upper quadrant after total hepatectomy and the donor's liver graft, and subsequent outflow disturbances occur more frequently when the regeneration of the liver graft displaces the inferior vena cava and aggravates kinking of the short HVs. To avoid those problems, one solution is to make a wide common HV opening from the multiple short HVs at the back-table through the combination of augmentation patch venoplasty and vascular fencing [6]. This procedure can help us perform easy and simple anastomosis in the recipient while reducing the risk of venous outflow disturbance (Fig. 25.3).

25.1.1.2 Extended Right Lobe Graft

Back-table procedures for both right and middle HVs are necessary to secure good venous outflows. When separate anastomosis of RHV and MHV is prepared, the procedures are almost the same for the modified right lobe graft, and they refer to a previous description [4]. The only precaution that must be taken is to ensure that the MHV stump has an adequate length, which can be accomplished using an interposition vascular graft for tension-free and easy anastomosis with the recipient's common trunk of middle and left HV.

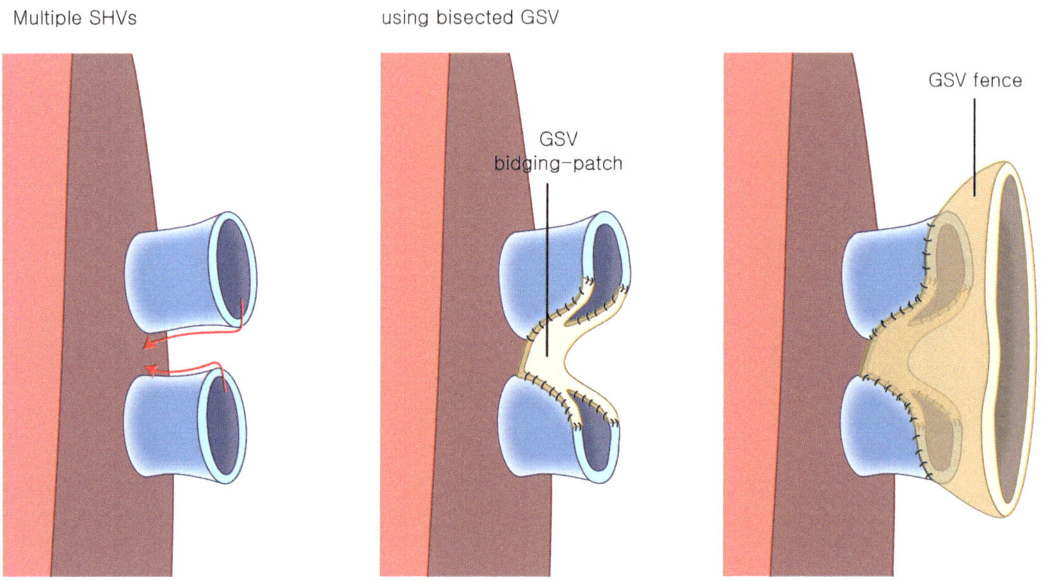

Fig. 25.3 Venoplasty of multiple short hepatic veins (SHVs) at the back-table. First, longitudinal incisions are made between SHVs in the same manner as the venoplasty of RHV. Second, the SHVs are connected by a bridging patch of bisected GSV, and finally, a wide single SHV opening is made by fencing of bisected GSV. *SHV* short hepatic vein, *RHV* right hepatic vein, *GSV* great saphenous vein

When single anastomosis of RHV and MHV is prepared using an all-in-one method, we should make a single wide common HV opening at the back-table according to the following steps [7]: First, bridging patch venoplasty should be performed between RHV and MHV, after which a vascular fence using bisected GSV or other vascular patch should be attached to the common opening, except for the posterior wall of RHV, to lengthen the anterior wall of the opening. This not only allows us to perform easy and safe anastomosis by decreasing the tension of anastomosis, but also reduces the risk of outflow obstruction by forming a big pouch toward the superior, inferior, and anterior sides of anastomosis (Fig. 25.4). The Hong Kong group does not perform bridging venoplasty and vascular fencing of the anterior wall, but only makes a triangular-shaped common opening between RHV and MHV with approximation corner sutures at the superior and inferior sides along with an additional transverse incision including the hepatic parenchyma followed by continuous approximation sutures [8]. At a basic level, we share the creation of a single common opening between RHV and MHV with that method. However, when we procure the extended RL graft and leave a big segment 4 HV in the donor side, which drains into the MHV trunk nearby, the RHV and MHV are a wide distance apart, and making a common opening without a bridging vascular patch is difficult and can lead to a disastrous situation, such as tearing of the vascular wall and prevention of anastomosis related to the excessive tension during implantation (Fig. 25.5).

25.1.1.3 Left Lobe Graft

A left lobe graft may have a higher chance of venous outflow disturbance when used for a single or dual graft living donor liver transplantation (LDLT), because such situations offer an inadequate atmosphere to stably support the liver graft. Hence, HV augmentation venoplasty at the back-table is essential to reduce the complication of venous outflow.

In cases of pediatric LDLT, HV of the left lobe graft from an adult living donor is typically large enough for the recipient's HV, and augmentation venoplasty at the back-table is not usually required. However, a single large common HV opening should be made by dividing the vascular septum between RHV, MHV, and left hepatic vein (LHV) in the pediatric recipient.

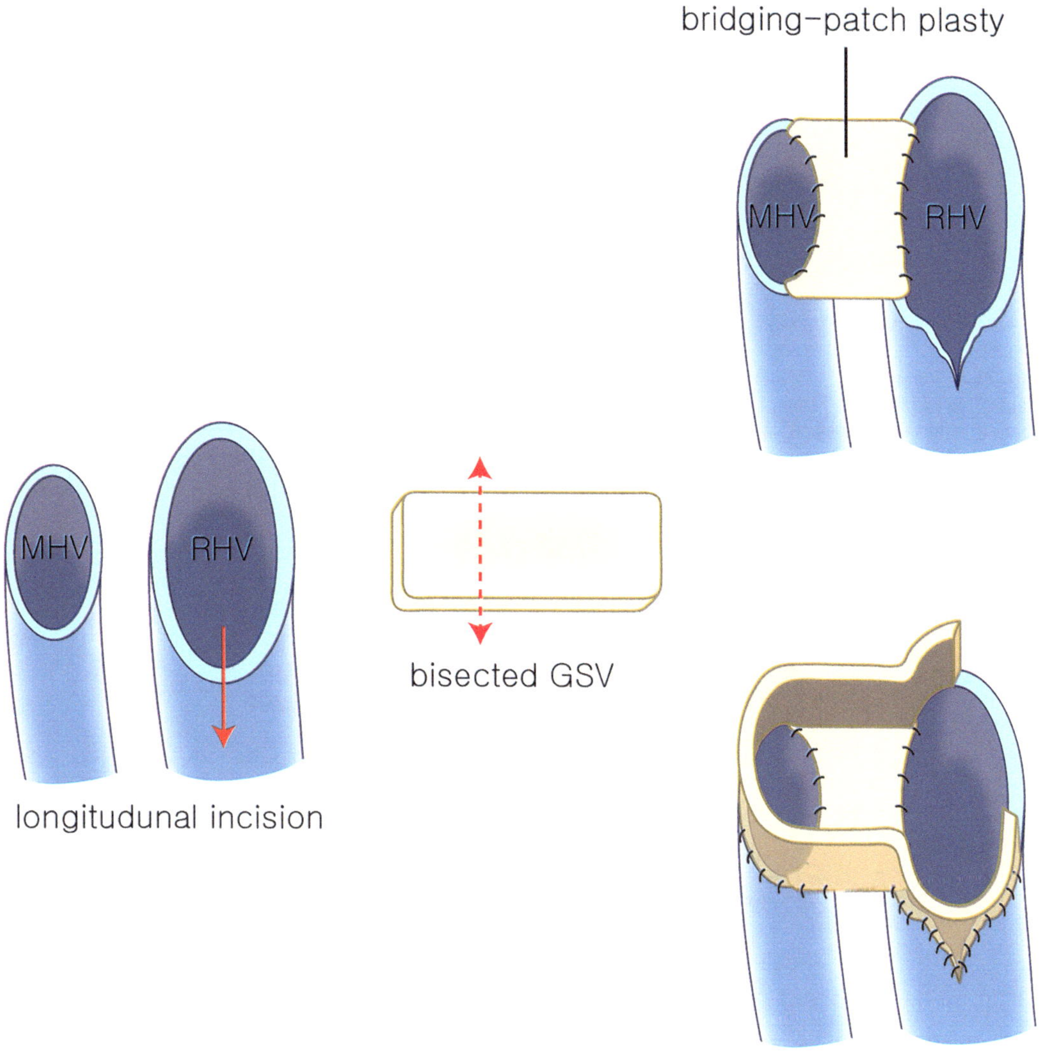

Fig. 25.4 Venoplasty between RHV and middle hepatic vein (MHV) of extended right lobe graft at the back-table. First, a bridging patch with bisected GSV is placed between RHV and MHV, and a longitudinal incision of the inferior corner of the RHV is made. Second, a single wide common opening of RHV and MHV is made by fencing of bisected GSV. *RHV* right hepatic vein, *MHV* middle hepatic vein, *GSV* great saphenous vein

In the case of an adult single left lobe graft LDLT, it is very important to perform wide HV anastomosis to decrease the post-transplant hepatic venous outflow disturbances. In the recipient's side, we should use the common HV opening after dividing the septum between RHV, MHV, and LHV. Correspondingly, the HV of the left lobe graft should be enlarged to match the recipient's large common HV opening through HV augmentation venoplasty at the back-table using bisected GSV or other vascular patches [1]. We may incise the corner of the MHV side or both the MHV and LHV sides, then perform augmentation venoplasty. When the recipient's common HV opening is too large compared to the HV of the left lobe graft, or when the HV stump of the left lobe graft is too short for comfortable anastomosis, we prefer to additionally perform combined fencing to the HV of the left lobe graft, and a large HV opening with an HV stump of a sufficient length can be made for wide and easy anastomosis (Fig. 25.6).

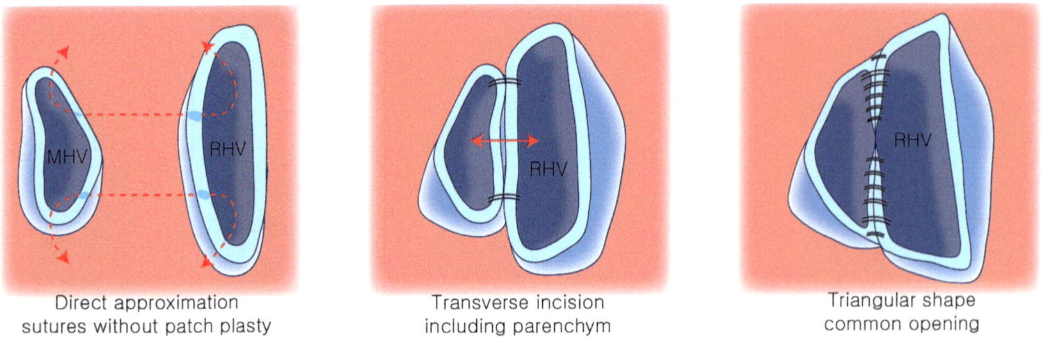

Fig. 25.5 Venoplasty of extended right lobe graft at the back-table by the Hong Kong group. First, direct approximation sutures are placed without a vascular patch between RHV and MHV, then a transverse incision including hepatic parenchyma is performed at the midpoint of the approximation line. Finally, a triangular-shaped common opening is made using continuous sutures of the approximation line, but it lacks an adequate stump length for a common hepatic vein opening, except for the posterior wall of RHV. *RHV* right hepatic vein, *MHV* middle hepatic vein

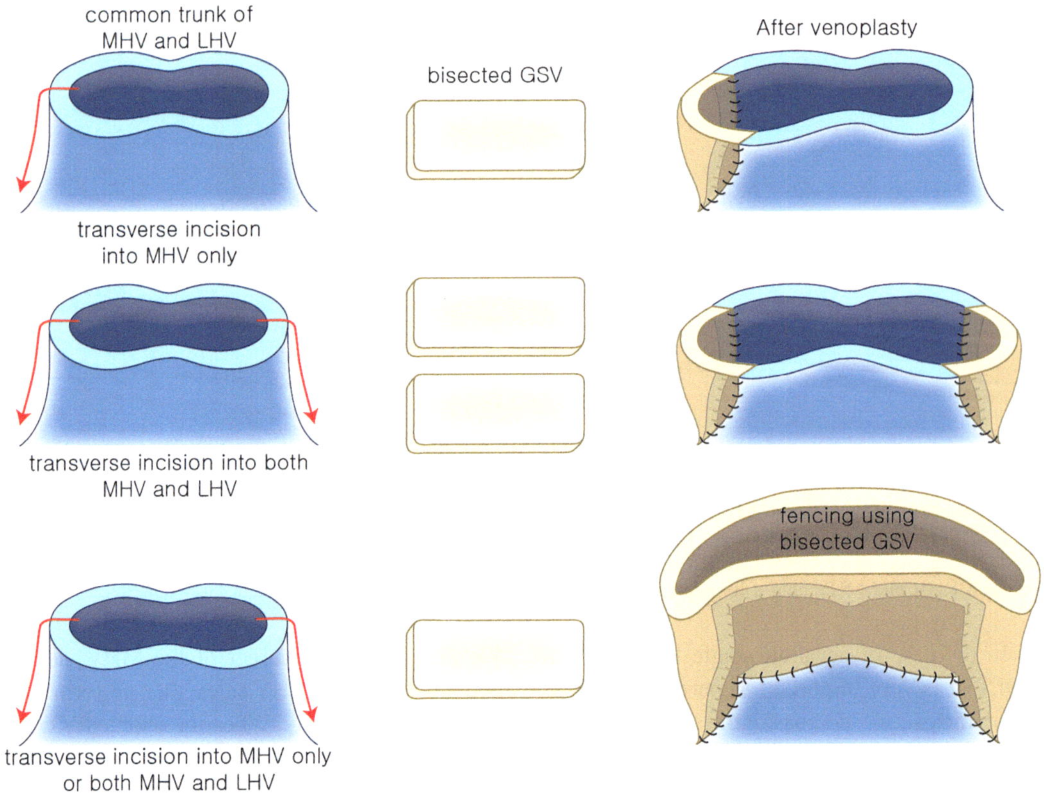

Fig. 25.6 Venoplasty of middle and left hepatic veins (LHV) common opening of left lobe graft at the back-table. Augmentation venoplasty can either be conducted only at the MHV side or at both the MHV and LHV sides. Additional fence to the hepatic vein (HV) using bisected GSV is useful for making a wide common HV opening with an adequate stump length when the stumps of HV are too short and/or multiple HV openings come out. *MHV* middle hepatic vein, *LHV* left hepatic vein, *HV* hepatic vein, *GSV* great saphenous vein

In the case of dual graft LDLT using two left lobes [9, 10], we perform augmentation HV venoplasty to both left lobe grafts, and the transverse diameter of the middle and left HV common opening should be made to have a length exceeding 3 cm by using a vascular patch or fencing [1].

25.1.2 Recipient Operation

To achieve good hepatic venous outflow, we need to perform pertinent venoplasty to each of the recipient's RHV, middle and left HV common opening, and inferior vena cava (IVC), in the same way as the back-table operation of the donor liver graft. These procedures make it possible to not only make a wide anastomotic opening of the HV, but also perform easy and safe HV anastomosis, even under a bad operative visual field. As a result, we can minimize the technical complications of hepatic venous outflow [1].

25.1.2.1 Modified Right Lobe Graft

Upon completion of the back-table operation, the HVs of the modified right lobe graft including RHV, more than 5 mm-sized short HVs, and interposing vascular grafts of more than 5 mm-sized MHV branches should all be reconstructed in the recipient. Basically, we should make the HV openings in the recipient wider than those of the donor's liver graft. In the case of RHV, a longitudinal incision is commonly made in the inferior corner RHV including the IVC wall to adjust the size of the donor's RHV [2] (Fig. 25.7). When the right lobe graft is larger than the recipient's right upper quadrant space after total hepatectomy, or when the locations of HV inflow between RHV of the liver graft and the recipient's RHV are different than the cross-section line of the recipient's IVC, a longitudinal incision of the inferior corner of the recipient's RHV is often not enough by itself to secure good RHV outflow. As an alternative measure, the combination of a transverse incision of the anterior wall of RHV and a longitudinal incision of the inferior corner of RHV including the IVC wall allows us to convert the elliptical RHV opening to an oval shape, and subsequently reduce the risk of outflow disturbance of RHV. However, this method is not safe, because there is a risk of a disastrous event related to the excessive tension during RHV anastomosis as well as the tearing of its vascular wall. Patch venoplasty including vascular fence

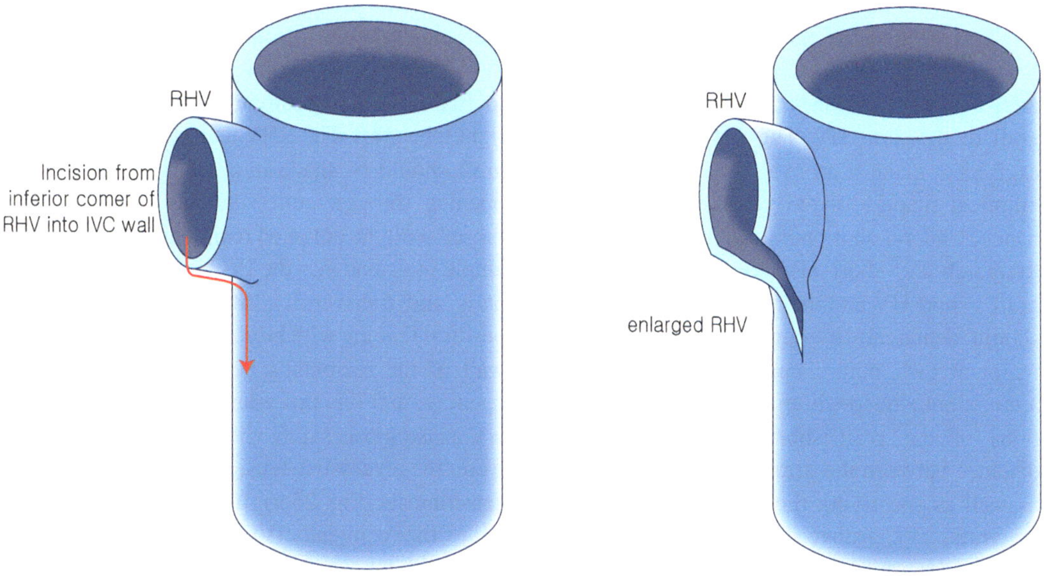

Fig. 25.7 Venoplasty of recipient's RHV before engraftment. Longitudinal incision only including the inferior vena cava (IVC) wall is performed at the inferior corner of RHV. *RHV* right hepatic vein, *IVC* inferior vena cava

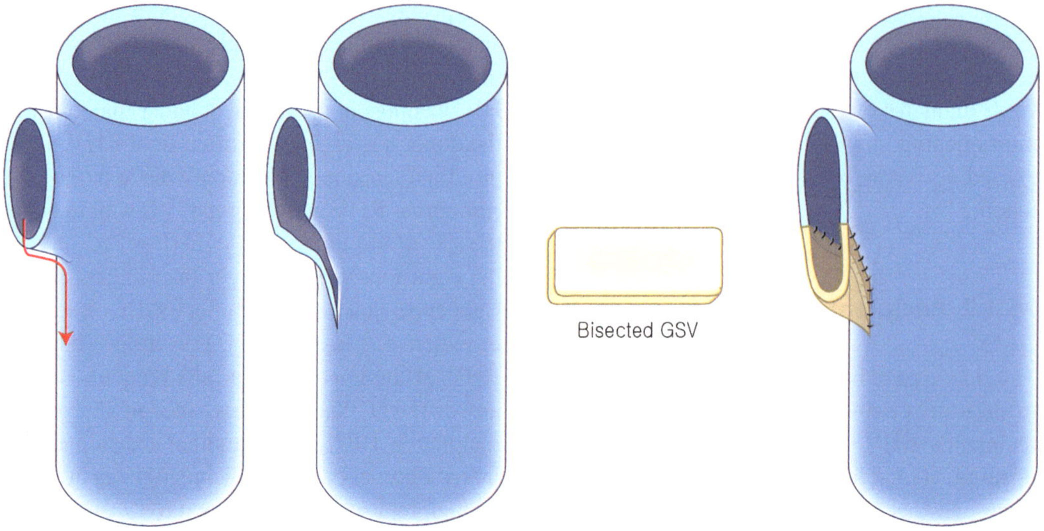

Fig. 25.8 Venoplasty of recipient's RHV using bisected GSV-patch before engraftment. First, we make a large HV opening with a longitudinal incision including the IVC wall at the inferior corner of RHV, and then we make a new RHV opening with an adequate stump length using bisected GSV-patch venoplasty to the inferior corner of the incised RHV. *RHV* right hepatic vein, *GSV* great saphenous vein, *HV* hepatic vein, *IVC* inferior vena cava

with bisected GSV or other vascular materials might help substantially mitigate those risks. As a result, the newly made large recipient's RHV opening has an adequate stump length with a healthy vascular wall at the lower half of the anterior wall and the lower 1/2 or 1/3 of the posterior wall, and we can therefore easily and safely perform wide RHV anastomosis (Fig. 25.8).

Short HV anastomosis should be performed at the corresponding location of the recipient's IVC after a larger incision in the IVC wall than the graft of the short HV. The IVC wall should be excised to make it an oval shape rather than an elliptical shape to avoid venous outflow disturbance. Under a poor operation field, it is difficult to match the short HV location between the graft's short HV and the recipient's IVC, and we should demarcate its corresponding site at the recipient IVC before engraftment in consideration of both the longitudinal and transverse locations of the graft short HV. Measuring the distance between the graft's RHV and short HV as well as specifying the transverse location of the graft's IVC groove might help the anastomosis at the appropriate site.

The MHV interposition graft draining segment 5 and 8 hepatic veins are typically anastomosed to the recipient's middle and left HV common opening [4]. For a recipient who has previously had hepatocellular carcinoma, intrahepatic duct stones, or other related conditions, left-sided hepatectomy is often impracticable, because LHV is absent and because MHV can frequently not be accurately obtained. Under those conditions, the MHV interposition graft can be anastomosed with the anterolateral wall of the recipient's IVC. However, we prefer single HV anastomosis to two separate anastomoses such as extended right lobe graft. The RHV and MHV interposition graft should be made into a large common HV opening through quilt venoplasty, then anastomosed with the enlarged recipient's RHV through ample incisions into the IVC wall both longitudinally and transversely. At this time, we should perform fencing with bisected GSV to the anterior wall of the recipient's newly made wide RHV opening, and this procedure can help us perform HV anastomosis safely without the risk of tearing from the excessive tension that occurs during anastomosis (Fig. 25.9). In addition, total clamping of the recipient's IVC, including RHV longitudinally or transversely, along with the application of veno-venous bypass, can often be beneficial for the operative procedure.

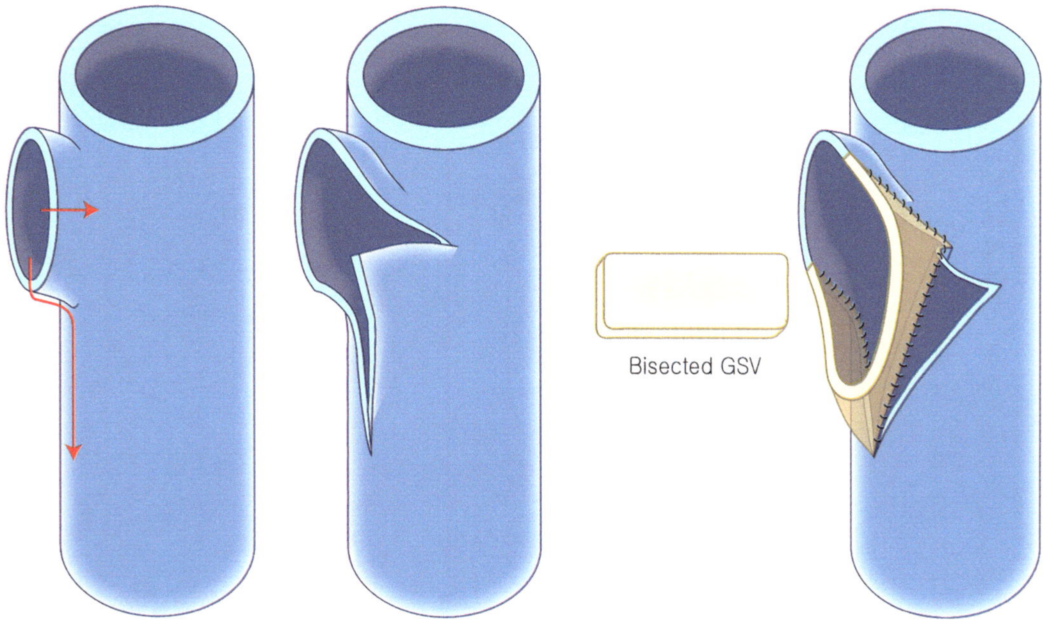

Fig. 25.9 Venoplasty of recipient's RHV using bisected GSV-patch after additional transverse incision. First, we perform both longitudinal and transverse incisions including the IVC wall at the inferior corner and the mid-portion of the anterior wall of RHV, respectively, to make an oval-shaped wide HV opening. Then, additional bisected GSV-patch venoplasty can give the new large RHV an adequate stump length. *RHV* right hepatic vein, *GSV* great saphenous vein, *IVC* inferior vena cava, *HV* hepatic vein

25.1.2.2 Extended Right Lobe Graft

In the case of separate anastomoses of RHV and MHV, the method of HV anastomosis is the same as that for the modified right lobe graft [3].

In the case of single anastomosis, after making a common HV opening between RHV and MHV of the liver graft at the back-table, we should clamp the recipient's IVC longitudinally, including RHV and MHV, or clamp the recipient's both supra- and infrahepatic IVC, including all three HVs under veno-venous bypass. In consideration of the longitudinal and transverse diameters of the graft's common HV opening, we can incise the recipient's RHV into the IVC wall longitudinally and transversely, and the Hong Kong group routinely makes a triangular-shaped HV opening without patch plasty after excision of the IVC wall [8]. To make an anastomosis while maintaining the natural course of the graft's MHV, a transverse incision of the recipient's RHV anterior wall should be made into MHV. When the liver graft is too big for the recipient's right upper quadrant space after total hepatectomy, the transverse incision should be extended into the recipient's LHV for the graft's MHV to maintain its course more naturally. Bisected GSV fencing to the newly made large HV opening in the recipient can avoid disastrous events resulting from the tearing of its anastomosis related to the undue tension during anastomosis, and the dome-shape contour of HV anastomosis after perfusion can secure good HV outflow regardless of any post-transplant morphologic changes related to regeneration of the liver graft or its swelling due to acute rejection (Fig. 25.10).

25.1.2.3 Left Lobe Graft

Similar to the right lobe graft positioning at the right upper quadrant space orthotopically, we implant the left lobe graft orthotopically, but it is typically leaning toward the right upper quadrant

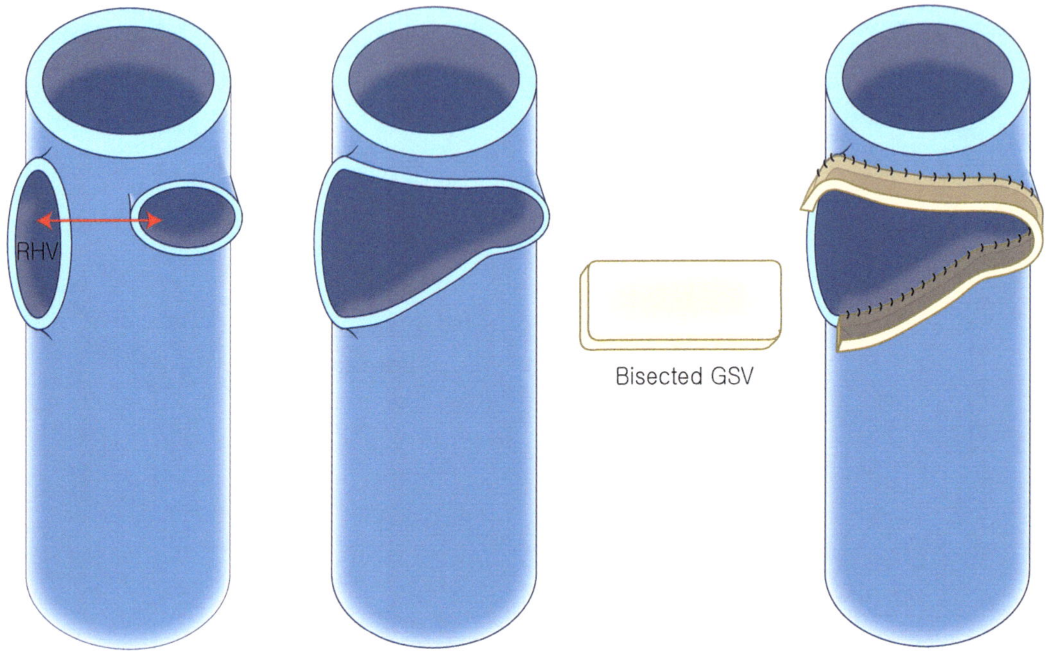

Fig. 25.10 Venoplasty of recipient's HVs before engraftment of extended right lobe graft. First, a new large common hepatic opening is made by a transverse incision from the recipient's RHV to the middle and left HV common trunk. Then, vascular fence using bisected GSV except for the posterior wall of RHV is made to avoid excessive tension during anastomosis and to create a dome-shape wide HV outflow. *HV* hepatic vein, *RHV* right hepatic vein, *GSV* great saphenous vein

space due to its empty space. This may result in twisting of HV anastomosis, and severe outflow disturbance can occur.

As a countermeasure, we should make a large common HV opening including all three major HVs of the recipient by dividing the septum between RHV, MHV, and LHV under supra- and infrahepatic IVC clamping with veno-venous bypass, then performing anastomosis with the enlarged common HV opening of the left lobe graft with bisected GSV patch venoplasty or fencing at the back-table. This kind of maximally enlarged HV anastomosis can minimize the twisting effect depending on the position change of the left lobe graft. The transverse diameter of the recipient's RHV-MHV-LHV common opening is large, at around 4–5 cm in length, but the transverse diameter of the graft's MHV-LHV common opening after patch venoplasty alone is often not sufficiently large to anastomose with the recipient's RHV-MHV-LHV common opening, and it might be necessary to perform a size reduction venoplasty of the recipient's RHV-MHV-LHV common opening to ensure size matching and safe anastomosis; this can be accomplished by suturing the divided septal wall between RHV and MHV in both the anterior and posterior sides, which can also form an HV stump with an adequate length.

When we performed an augmentation HV venoplasty using both a vascular patch and fencing in the left lobe graft at the back-table, its transverse diameter was already sufficiently enlarged for direct anastomosis with the recipient's RHV-MHV-LHV common opening, and there was no need to perform an additional procedure on the recipient side.

As an additional measure to reduce HV outflow disturbance, we placed a tissue-expander in the right upper quadrant space to support the left lobe graft. This was intended to prevent excessive tilting of the left lobe graft toward the right side.

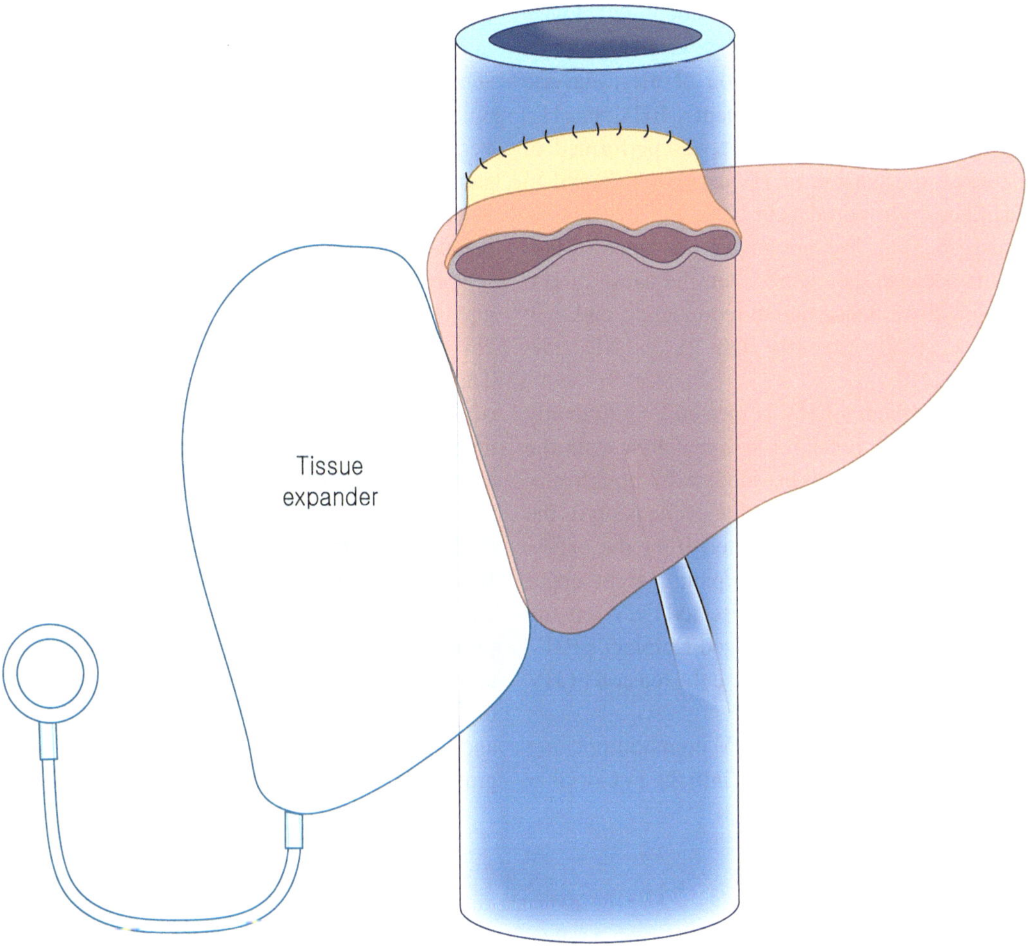

Fig. 25.11 Tissue-expander into the right upper quadrant space to support the left lobe, which prevents excessive tilting of the left lobe graft toward the right side and helps maintain good HV outflow

In addition, to maintain good HV outflow, we began to deflate the tissue-expander step-by-step after 1 week, but retained it for 2–3 weeks until HV anastomosis could not be deformed any further with the aid of graft regeneration and the formation of perihepatic adhesion (Fig. 25.11).

25.1.2.4 Dual Liver Graft

Compared to single graft LDLT, dual graft LDLT requires a longer operation time, particularly in anhepatic phase. Under supra- and infrahepatic clamping, we should perform augmentation venoplasty at both RHV and MHV-LHV of the recipient after transverse and/or longitudinal incision toward the IVC wall to accommodate the already enlarged HV openings of the grafts through augmentation venoplasty at the back-table [10]. During long anhepatic phase, which completely blocks the portal and systemic venous return, veno-venous bypass is necessary to maintain stable vital signs and to prevent mesenteric congestion. The absence of veno-venous bypass can infrequently result in postoperative severe or even necrotizing pancreatitis related to mesenteric congestion; in which case one should not hesitate to apply veno-venous bypass when there is complete blockage of portosystemic venous return.

Two Left-Sided Liver Grafts

In consideration of a good operation field, we should start HV anastomosis from the right-sided graft positioning in a 180° counterclockwise rotation, then apply a 90°clockwise rotation. In the early period, interposition of the cadaveric iliac vein between the recipient's RHV and HV of the right-sided liver graft was performed to decrease the tension of HV anastomosis and to facilitate right portal vein (PV) and BD anastomosis [9, 11]. We no longer use interposition grafts because they were often the cause of HV outflow disturbance due to redundancy, and they did not actually affect the right PV and BD anastomosis [10].

The recipient's RHV is incised longitudinally at the inferior corner for size-matching with the enlarged HV of the right-sided graft through augmentation venoplasty. If extensive tension of the HV reconstruction is expected from the excessively large size of the recipient's right upper quadrant space, additional bisected GSV fencing to the lower half of the enlarged recipient's RHV might be beneficial to decrease the tension of HV anastomosis.

The recipient's MHV-LHV common opening typically needs to be incised into the IVC wall at the corner of the MHV side, after which augmentation venoplasty using bisected GSV patch should be performed for size-matching with the enlarged HV of the left-sided graft with a transverse diameter of more than 3 cm. When the stump length of the MHV-LHV common opening is too short and the HV anastomosis is anticipated to be difficult, we should perform vascular fencing including patch venoplasty to the recipient's enlarged MHV-LHV opening to make the HV stump have an adequate length (Fig. 25.12). This procedure guarantees that the anastomosis of HV will proceed safely without tearing under a poor operation field and even in the presence of extreme tension during anastomosis.

Right- and Left-Sided Liver Grafts

Both liver grafts are orthotopically positioned, and the same reconstruction methods described previously are respectively used for the right- and left-sided liver grafts. We begin by performing reconstruction of HVs including RHV, SHV, and MHV interposition grafts of the right-sided graft, then proceed with anastomosis HV of the

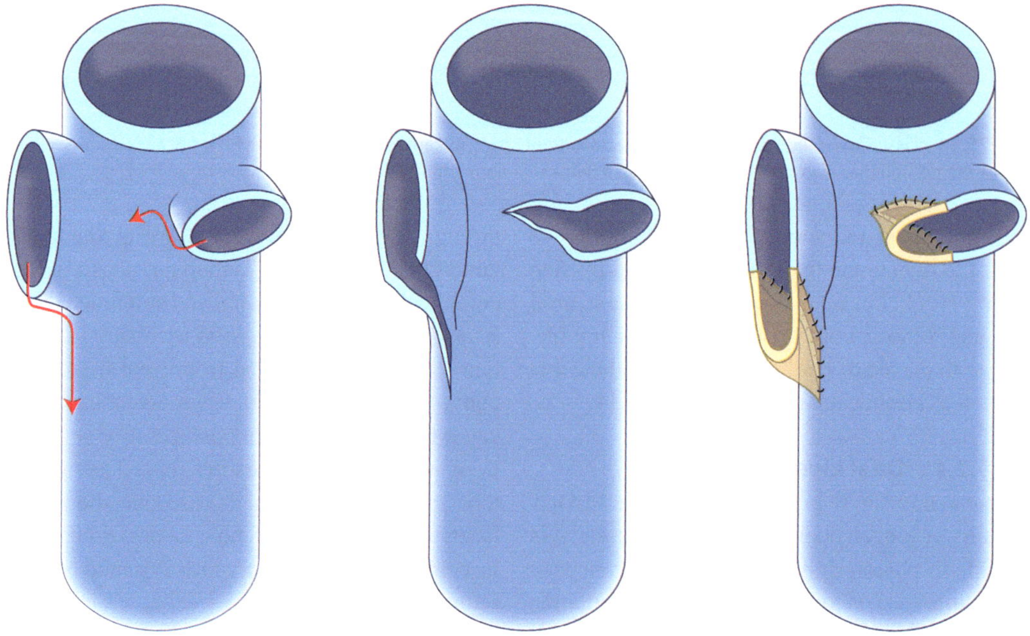

Fig. 25.12 Venoplasty of recipient's HVs before implantation of dual-graft using two left-sided grafts. Incisions are made at the inferior corner of RHV and the right corner of the middle and left HV common trunk. Then, vascular patch venoplasty and/or fencing are performed at both HVs using bisected GSV. *HV* hepatic vein, *RHV* right hepatic vein, *GSV* great saphenous vein

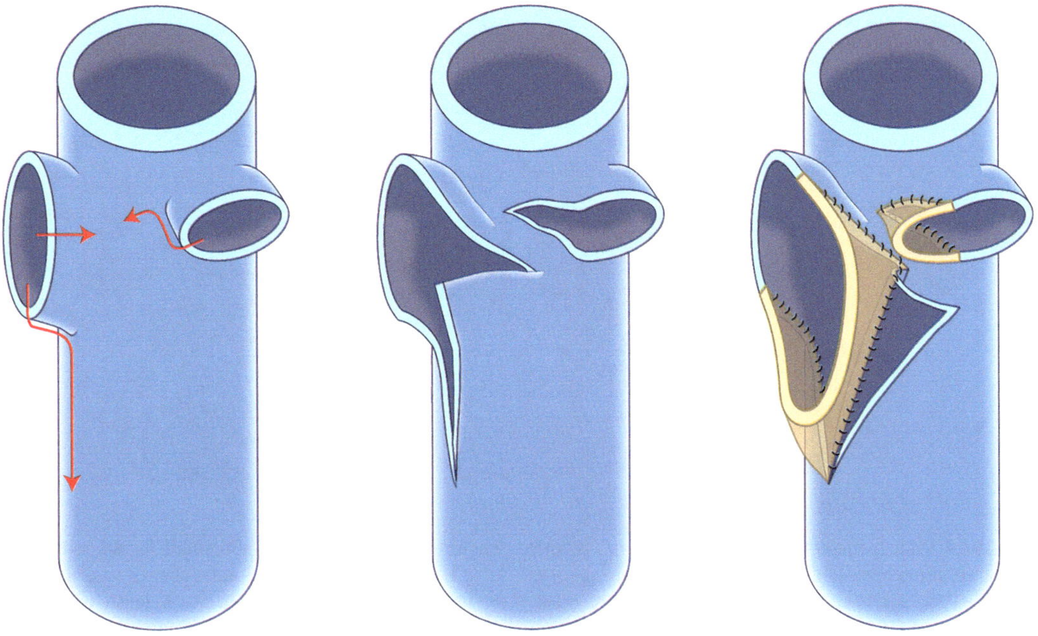

Fig. 25.13 Venoplasty of recipient's HVs before implantation of dual-graft using right- and left-sided grafts. In RHV, we make longitudinal and transverse incisions at the inferior corner and the mid-point of anterior wall, respectively. In the middle and left HV common trunk, we also make a transverse incision at the right-side corner to make wide HV openings. Then, vascular patch venoplasty and/or fencing are performed at both HVs using bisected GSV. *HV* hepatic vein, *RHV* right hepatic vein, *GSV* great saphenous vein

left-sided graft to the recipient's MHV-LHV common trunk. The important difference in reconstruction compared to the two left-sided liver grafts lies in how the MHV interposition graft is reconstructed, because the MHV interposition graft cannot be anastomosed to the recipient's MHV-LHV common trunk. It can be reconstructed to the anterior wall of the IVC after a longitudinal incision or excision, but we currently prefer to perform single anastomosis between the large common HV opening of the right-side graft through quilt venoplasty at the back-table and by enlarging the recipient's RHV through ample incision into the IVC wall longitudinally and transversely (Fig. 25.13).

25.2 Reconstruction of Portal Vein

In the case of single graft LDLT, the recipient's right or left PV is not usually used for PV reconstruction, as main PV is preferred, to avoid redundancy and stenosis. In the case of dual graft LDLT, we should keep the recipient's right and left PV intact during hilar dissection and use them for the PV reconstruction of both grafts. To reduce the risk of PV twisting, we perform anastomosis of each of the medial and lateral corners of the recipient's right and left PVs with the medial and left corners of each of the PVs of both grafts when based on the recipient's coronal plane.

PV of the procured partial liver graft often comes out with a paper-thin wall and/or too short of a stump, and the recipient's PV is often excessively enlarged and thick-walled under longstanding portal hypertension. The severe discrepancy between the graft's and recipient's PV during anastomosis may cause embarrassing events such as tearing or technical difficulties. For safe and easy PV anastomosis in those situations, we should perform PV re-enforcement by placing bisected GSV over the weakened PV wall of the graft and/or making a funnel-shaped

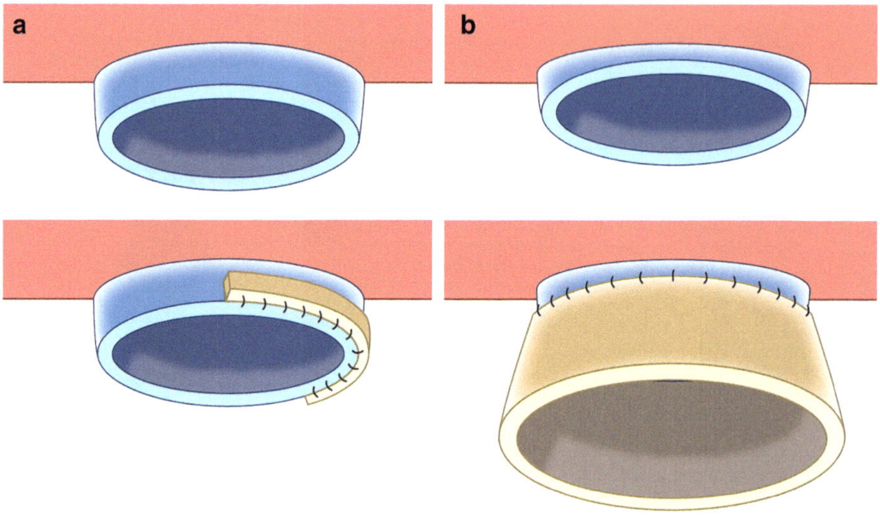

Fig. 25.14 Management of the portal vein (PV) of the liver graft at the back-table. (**a**) When the wall of the PV is paper-thin, we need to perform PV re-enforcement using bisected GSV to avoid tearing of the wall during anastomosis. (**b**) When the stump of PV is too short, or when the diameter of PV is too small for the recipient's large PV, we need to make a funnel-shaped vascular fencing using bisected GSV to obtain a sufficiently wide opening that is thick-walled and that has an adequate stump length. *PV* portal vein, *GSV* great saphenous vein

vascular fencing of the graft PV to have a wide opening that is thick-walled and that has an adequate stump length at the back-table (Fig. 25.14).

When PV thrombosis and/or stenosis are present in the recipient, we should first try to perform thrombectomy while taking extreme caution to keep the PV wall intact. However, when thrombectomy is not feasible for keeping the PV wall intact, we prefer to leave it alone, then measure the intraluminal diameter at the expected anastomotic site of the recipient's PV. If the diameter is small, with a size of less than 1 cm, PV plasty should be performed using bisected GSV or other vascular patches to enlarge the recipient's PV diameter to avoid anastomotic stenosis [12] (Fig. 25.15).

In contrast to pediatric LDLT, effective thrombectomy or plasty through the whole length of PV in adult LDLT is often not possible, particularly for intrapancreatic PV, due to periportal inflammatory changes that occur under severe portal hypertensive state. Hence, we should perform intraoperative cine-portogram (IOP) after engraftment to identify the residual PV thrombosis and/or stenosis, along with co-existing sizable portosystemic collaterals, which can be possible routes for lethal post-transplant portal flow steal [12, 13]. By using IOP, we can perform not only ballooning or stent placement to the residual PV thrombosis and/or stenosis, but also surgical interruption or embolization of the sizable portosystemic collaterals.

25.2.1 Right Lobe Graft

The donor's first-order PV branches including right and left PV typically ramify from main PV, but the second-order PV branches in the right lobe graft, including right anterior and posterior PV, often ramify directly from main PV without common trunk of right PV, such as type 2 or 3 PV variations. In the case of the procurement of a right lobe graft in a donor with type 2 or 3 PV variations, nostril-shaped or two separate PV openings entering into each of the right anterior and posterior sectors come out. At the back-table, we can make a single PV opening by using the recipient's PV Y-graft, and safe and easy PV anastomosis is possible during implantation [14]. However, when we cannot obtain a healthy recipient's PV Y-graft to pre-existing PV steno-

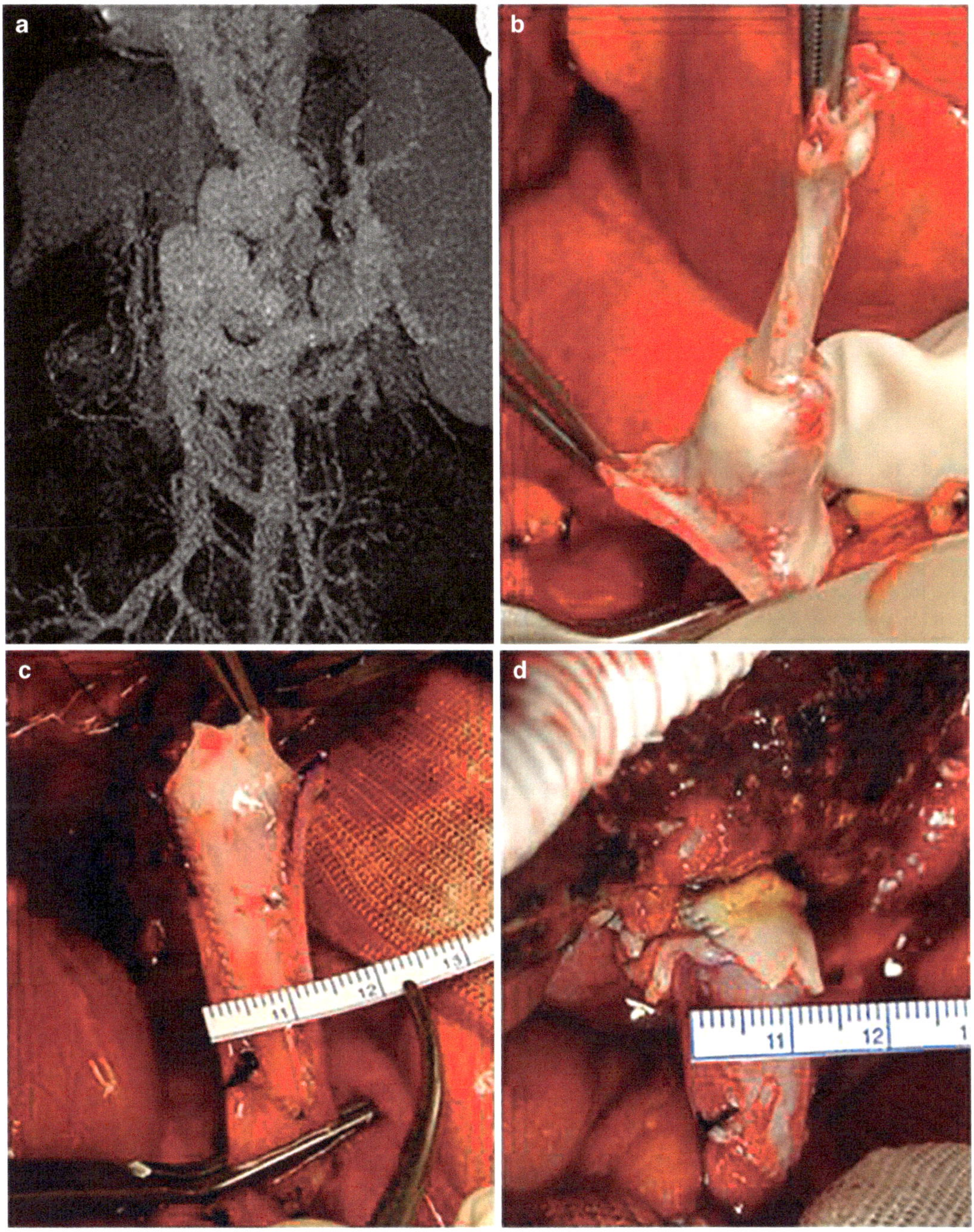

Fig. 25.15 Management of PV obstruction or stenosis. (**a**) The recipient had severe PV stenosis and a large coronary vein as portosystemic collaterals. (**b**) Organized PV thrombus was removed by eversion thrombectomy. (**c**) We performed PV plasty using bisected GSV because PV was still stenotic even after thrombectomy, but intrapancreatic PV was not amenable to PV plasty due to periportal inflammatory changes occurring under severe portal hypertensive state. (**d**) PV anastomosis was performed without stenosis at the anastomosis, but the residual stenosis of intrapancreatic PV was relieved by intraoperative PV stenting and interruption of coronary vein under the guidance of intraoperative cine-portogram (IOP). *PV* portal vein, *GSV* great saphenous vein, *IOP* intraoperative cine-portogram

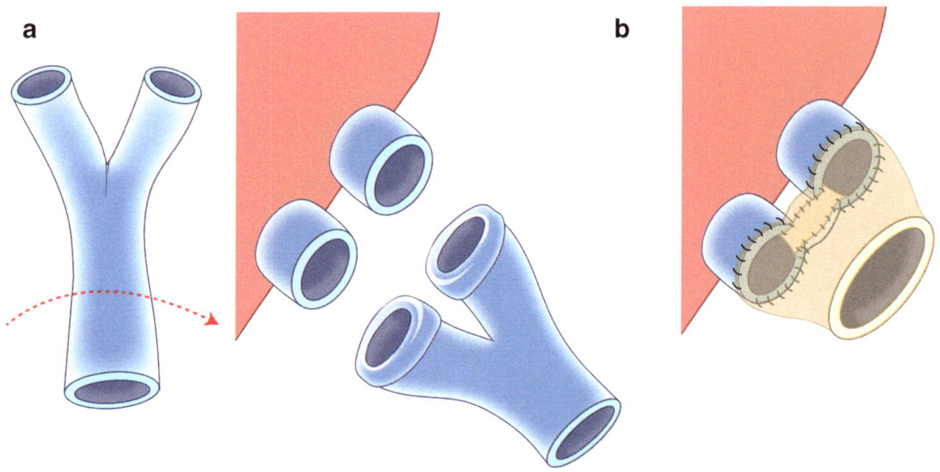

Fig. 25.16 Management of multiple PV openings of the right lobe graft, such as type 2 or 3 PV, at the back-table. (**a**) When nostril-shaped or two separate PV openings come out, a PV single opening is made using the recipient's PV Y-graft. At the time of Y-graft anastomosis to the graft PVs, both medial sides should be everted as much as possible, while both lateral sides should not be everted as much. Hence, the anastomotic openings are enlarged while the distance between PV bifurcation is minimized, and we can thereby avoid kinking of the reconstructed PV Y-graft. (**b**) When a healthy recipient's PV Y-graft is not available due to pre-existing PV stenosis or thrombosis, a single PV opening with an adequate stump can be made by bridging between the two PV openings of the liver graft and then additional fencing using the recipient's bisected GSV patch or a fresh cadaveric iliac vein Y-graft. *PV* portal vein, *GSV* great saphenous vein

sis or thrombosis, we should make a single PV opening with the recipient's bisected GSV bridge and fence, or a fresh cadaveric iliac vein Y-graft [15] (Fig. 25.16).

25.2.2 Left Lobe Graft

The left PV of the graft is relatively small compared to the right PV, and the chance of anastomotic stenosis of the PV is also high. Hence, performing PV anastomosis with closer sewing and while providing growth factor at the time of completion is helpful for reducing the risk of anastomotic stenosis. The right and left corners of the PV stump of the graft can be decided by the transverse direction to the umbilical portion of the left PV, and we can easily access them by opening the tips of the Mixter clamp after having inserted it into the umbilical portion of the left PV.

In the recipient, the right and left corners of the main PV should be decided by the recipient's coronal plane. After the right and left corner sutures are placed between the LPV of the graft and the recipient's MPV, we can perform PV anastomosis without the risk of twisting of PV anastomosis. When the recipient has a small anterior-to-posterior depth between the abdominal wall and the spine, the reconstructed PV of the left lobe graft might be compressed and become stenotic in an orthotopic position. In that situation, we should place the left lobe graft in the right-side tilting position toward the spacious right upper quadrant space to avoid PV compression. However, we should also insert a tissue-expander into the right upper quadrant space to support the left lobe graft and to avoid twisting of the vascular structures including HV and PV, which might be related to excessive right-side tilting of the left lobe graft.

25.2.3 Dual Lobe Grafts

In the case of dual graft LDLT using both right and left lobe grafts, the methods of PV anastomosis are basically the same as those used in the PV reconstructions of the right and left lobe grafts, respectively. In the recipient, each of the right and left corners of the right and left PVs can be determined by the recipient's coronal plane, similar to the single LDLT. Marking with a sterilized pen might be helpful to ensure that anastomosis is performed correctly without twisting. In addition, the length of each of the recipient's right and left PV to the anastomotic sites of each PV of the liver graft should be short to avoid the presence of excessive tension during PV anastomosis. In the graft side, each of the right and left corners of the right and left PV can be demarcated using the same method used in each single graft LDLT.

In the case of dual graft LDLT using two left lobe grafts, we should be particularly careful when performing right PV anastomosis to the right-sided graft, because the right-sided graft is positioned based on a 180° counterclockwise rotation followed by a 90° clockwise rotation status. However, the determinations of the right and left corners of the PV stump of the right-sided graft (inverted left lobe graft) can be made using the same method used for single left lobe graft LDLT. Both corners of the PV stump of the inverted left lobe graft can be determined by the transverse direction to the umbilical portion of the left PV, and we can perform right PV anastomosis with minimal risk of PV twisting.

References

1. Lee SG. A complete treatment of adult living donor liver transplantation: a review of surgical technique and current challenges to expand indication of patients. Am J Transpl. 2015;15(1):17–38.
2. Hwang S, Lee SG, Ahn CS, Moon DB, Kim KH, Sung KB, et al. Morphometric and simulation analyses of right hepatic vein reconstruction in adult living donor liver transplantation using right lobe grafts. Liver Transpl. 2010;16(5):639–48.
3. Gyu Lee S, Min Park K, Hwang S, Hun Kim K, Nak Choi D, Hyung Joo S, et al. Modified right liver graft from a living donor to prevent congestion. Transplantation. 2002;74(1):54–9.
4. Lee SG. Techniques of reconstruction of hepatic veins in living-donor liver transplantation, especially for right hepatic vein and major short hepatic veins of right-lobe graft. J Hepato-Biliary-Pancreat Surg. 2006;13(2):131–8.
5. Lee S, Park K, Hwang S, Lee Y, Choi D, Kim K, et al. Congestion of right liver graft in living donor liver transplantation. Transplantation. 2001;71(6):812–4.
6. Hwang S, Lee SG, Park KM, Kim KH, Ahn CS, Moon DB, et al. Quilt venoplasty using recipient saphenous vein graft for reconstruction of multiple short hepatic veins in right liver grafts. Liver Transpl. 2005;11(1):104–7.
7. Hwang S, Lee SG, Ahn CS, Moon DB, Kim KH, Ha TY, et al. Outflow vein reconstruction of extended right lobe graft using quilt venoplasty technique. Liver Transpl. 2006;12(1):156–8.
8. Lo CM, Fan ST, Liu CL, Wong J. Hepatic venoplasty in living-donor liver transplantation using right lobe graft with middle hepatic vein. Transplantation. 2003;75(3):358–60.
9. Lee S, Hwang S, Park K, Lee Y, Choi D, Ahn C, et al. An adult-to-adult living donor liver transplant using dual left lobe grafts. Surgery. 2001;129(5):647–50.
10. Song GW, Lee SG, Moon DB, Ahn CS, Hwang S, Kim KH, et al. Dual-graft adult living donor liver transplantation: an innovative surgical procedure for live liver donor Pool expansion. Ann Surg. 2017;266(1):10–8.
11. Lee SG, Hwang S, Park KM, Kim KH, Ahn CS, Lee YJ, et al. Seventeen adult-to-adult living donor liver transplantations using dual grafts. Transplant Proc. 2001;33(7–8):3461–3.
12. Moon DB, Lee SG, Ahn CS, Hwang S, Kim KH, Ha TY, et al. Section 6. Management of extensive nontumorous portal vein thrombosis in adult living donor liver transplantation. Transplantation. 2014;97(Suppl 8):S23–30.
13. Moon DB, Lee SG, Ahn C, Hwang S, Kim KH, Ha T, et al. Application of intraoperative cine-portogram to detect spontaneous portosystemic collaterals missed by intraoperative doppler exam in adult living donor liver transplantation. Liver Transpl. 2007;13(9):1279–84.
14. Hwang S, Lee SG, Ahn CS, Kim KH, Moon DB, Ha TY, et al. Technique and outcome of autologous portal Y-graft interposition for anomalous right portal veins in living donor liver transplantation. Liver Transpl. 2009;15(4):427–34.
15. Hwang S, Ha TY, Song GW, Jung DH, Moon DB, Ahn CS, et al. Conjoined unification Venoplasty for double portal vein branches of right liver graft: 1-year experience at a high-volume living donor liver transplantation center. J Gastrointest Surg. 2016;20(1):199–205.

26 Hepatic Artery Anastomosis

Chul-Soo Ahn

Abstract

Hepatic Arterial Anastomosis is the most important procedure in living donor liver transplantation. For optimal stump function, it is critical to ensure meticulous and atraumatic dissection of hepatic hilum in both the donor and recipient operations. A partial graft artery is small and thin, especially with multiple arteries. Therefore, a precise anastomotic technique is required for safe anastomosis with a surgical microscope or loupes. In the recipient hilar dissection, each of the arterial stumps is identified up to at least the second branches for size matching with the donor arterial stumps. Interrupted or continuous anastomotic techniques are commonly used with several modifications. For stumps that are too short, the backwall first technique is useful, and this was done here without stump rotation. It is preferable to subject all graft arterial stumps to anastomosis if possible. Following anastomosis, doppler ultrasonography is performed to evaluate the patency. In the case of arterial thrombosis, early re-anastomosis with different health inflow is essential for graft saving.

C.-S. Ahn (✉)
Division of Hepatobiliary Surgery and Liver Transplantation, Department of Surgery, Asan Medical Center, University of Ulsan College of Medicine, Seoul, South Korea
e-mail: ahncs@amc.seoul.kr

Keywords

Living donor liver transplantation · Hepatic artery · Anastomosis · Right gastroepiploic artery

26.1 Introduction

Hepatic Arterial Anastomosis (HAA), known as the most important procedure in living donor liver transplantation, is closely and directly related to the perioperative or postoperative results after transplantation. In living donor liver transplantation, persistent portal high pressure may occur as a result of the small graft size precluding arterial blood flow, which may in turn increase arterial complications. It is necessary to use anastomotic techniques to achieve optimal results. After applying a surgical microscope in hepatic artery anastomosis, the arterial complications rates are significantly decreased [1]. The microscope provides precise and meticulous anastomosis with its sufficient magnification, but a long training period is required for a surgeon to become familiar with this technique. Recently, high magnification loupes have begun replacing surgical microscopes in certain cases with comparable results. In addition, their indications are increasing as their experiences are increasing [2].

H. C. Yu (ed.), *Hepato-Biliary-Pancreatic Surgery and Liver Transplantation*,
https://doi.org/10.1007/978-981-16-1996-0_26

26.2 Graft Artery

The size of a graft arterial stump is smaller than those of whole liver grafts, and its mean diameter is less than 3 cm (1–4 cm) [3]. More than 40% of the left lobe grafts and 5% of the right lobe grafts had multiple hepatic arteries [4, 5]. Although graft hepatic artery stumps from a healthy donor represent the highest tissue quality, they have thin and weak arterial walls and make anastomosis difficult. During a graft harvest, the arterial stump should be cut without tension to safely preserve the arterial intima of both sides [3]. In the case of multiple arteries, the nondominant stump should be cut first to evaluate the backflow from its stump with the intact dominant artery. In general, the recessive arterial stump is reconstructed or ligated according to its back-bleeding quality after dominant stump reconstruction. However, reconstructions of all feasible arterial stumps are preferable for several reasons. For one, they restore the original anatomic blood supply. As each stump of a multiple artery graft is smaller and has a higher risk of complication, multiple anastomosis may save the graft if one artery is thrombosed. It can sometimes be difficult to identify the dominant stump, and the nondominant stump may be located deeper, making its reconstruction difficult or impossible if the dominant one has been reconstructed.

26.3 Recipient Artery

Minimizing arterial injury is the most important consideration during recipient hilar dissection. Severe fibrosis and collateral vessels developed from cirrhosis make the dissection of hilar structure difficult. By hyperdynamic circulation, particularly with portal hypertension, the hepatic artery becomes stiffer with intimal hypertrophy or edema despite an increase in the diameter [6]. This pathologic condition makes the arterial wall fragile and vulnerable to injury during hilar dissection. Preoperative arterial intimal injury by TACE and radiation are risk factors for arterial thrombosis or stricture.

During dissection, extensive traction of the vessel should be avoided to prevent intimal injury. It is important to identify all hepatic arteries (left, middle, and right HA) up to their second branches for size matching with the donor arterial stump [7]. After removing the recipient liver, a vascular clamp should be placed at the proximal portion of the recipient arterial stump. If the clamp is applied at the distal portion, the tiny intimal tear during hilar dissection would worsen with forceful and pulsatile blood flow, which would result in transmural thrombosis in the stump. When all recipient arterial stumps are injured, several arteries are used alternatively; the right gastroepiploic artery is the most commonly used because it is easy to mobilize with sufficient length and it can supply sufficient blood flow.

26.4 Anastomosis Techniques

There are several important factors for the selection of the inflow stump in the recipient, including sufficient and pulsatile blood flow from the stump, intimal tearing or thrombus or mural calcification by inspection, and size-matching between two stumps. Less than a twofold size discrepancy is considered safe for direct anastomosis. All connective tissues outside of adventitia, which is potent thrombogenic material, should be trimmed to make the anastomotic site round and smooth before suturing. The anastomotic site in the recipient is located deep inside and moves up and down with heartbeats and respiration. An approximator clamp, an atraumatic double-armed clamp moving on a side bar, is an essential instrument for HAA, as it substantially facilitates the procedure by providing orientation and tension-free anastomosis (Fig. 26.1). Nylon, which is stronger than prolene, is a preferable suture material with an arterial diameter from 7.0 to 10.0. During anastomosis, the needle should go through the whole thickness of the arterial wall with the right angle. Partial, not including intima, or oblique suture may result in transmural hematoma or intimal folding, which may in turn result in inner wall narrowing. When the intima is thickened or divided from adventitia, an upward forceps can be used to lift up the whole arterial wall (Fig. 26.2).

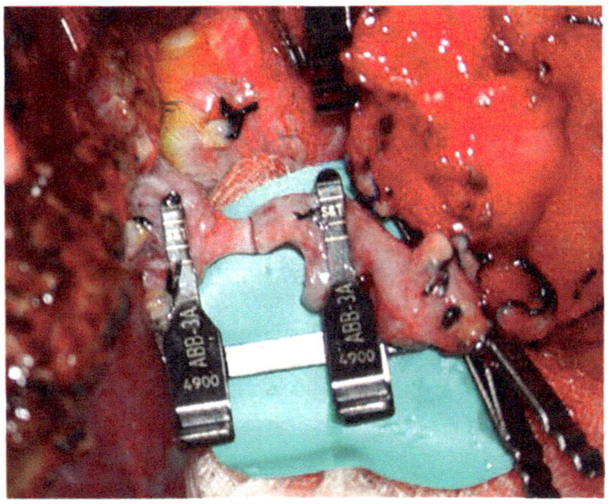

Fig. 26.1 After complete removal of periadventitial tissue, all arterial stumps were approximated for tension-free anastomosis using a double-armed clamp

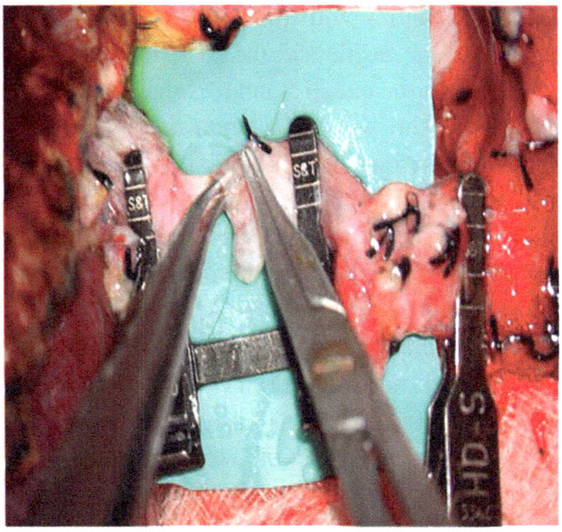

Fig. 26.2 The upward forceps were inserted into the vascular lumen and used to lift up its wall to facilitate full-thickness suturing. This technique is very useful when there is a thickened arterial wall with hypertrophy or intimal edema and when the intimal layer is separated from the adventitial layer

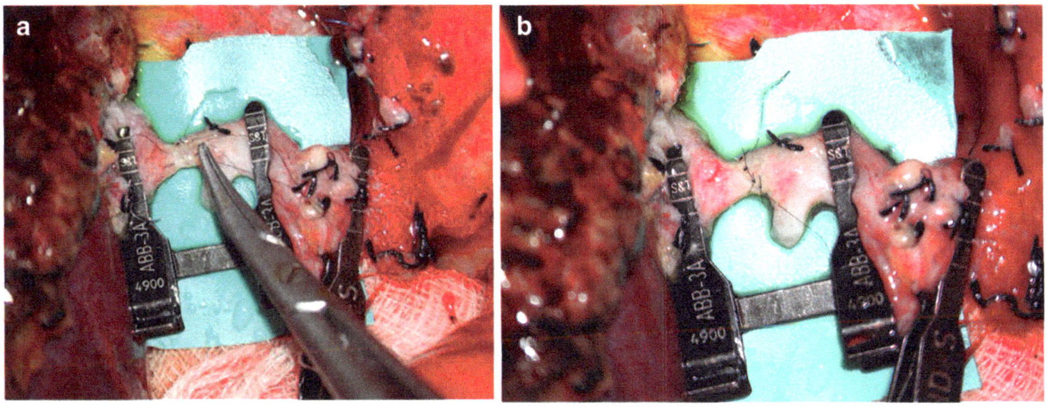

Fig. 26.3 Sutures were placed in the middle of each of the stitches untied (**a**), and after evaluating the full thickness and free backwall and confirming correct suture placement, all remnant sutures were tied (**b**)

Two types of anastomotic techniques are commonly used: interrupted or continuous. Various combined procedures of these are applicable in certain conditions. The interrupted suture technique starts with two stay sutures at the two lateral edges of the vessels. Following sutures are placed in the middle of each of the stitches untied to allow easy inspection of the posterior wall. After evaluating the full thickness suture and free backwall and confirming correct suture placement, all remnant sutures are tied at least three times (Fig. 26.3). Then, the approximator is rotated and the same sutures are repeated on the posterior wall, which is now the anterior position after the rotation. The continuous suture technique is easier and faster than the interrupted suture technique, but it has limitations such as a small artery or suboptimal arterial stump, intimal edema, or detachment. The backwall first technique is used when the donor hepatic arterial stump is too short for rotation and when the recipient arterial stump is fragile or diseased such that the rotation might result in further damage [8]. After the first stay suture, the interrupted technique begins with the donor side from the outside to the inside and the recipient side from the inside to the outside, and it is tied with a knot outside of the wall. The anterior wall is performed in the routine fashion described above.

Recently, cases of arterial reconstruction using surgical loupes rather than microscopic equipment are increasing due to their convenience with comparable results [2, 9]. However, to date, they have been applied in selective cases with sufficient size and healthy arterial stumps. The method using surgical loupes has attracted criticism for the resulting biliary complication and anastomotic stricture [10].

After anastomosis, doppler ultrasonography is performed immediately to demonstrate the patency of anastomosis. In the case of acute arterial thrombosis, though it is rare, early re-anastomosis with different healthy inflow is essential for graft saving.

In conclusion, atraumatic hilar dissection in both the donor and recipient operations ensures that all of the stumps are healthy. The use of precise and meticulous anastomotic techniques with suitable modification under sufficient magnification is essential for arterial anastomosis. Further, for the survival of the graft or the patient, early detection and early re-anastomosis are needed in acute arterial thrombosis.

References

1. Mori K, Nagata I, Yamagata S, et al. The introduction of microsurgery to hepatic artery reconstruction in living-donor liver transplantation—its surgical advantages compared with conventional procedures. Transplantation. 1992;54:263–8.
2. Li PC, Thorat A, Leng LB, Yang HR, et al. Hepatic artery reconstruction in living donor liver transplantation using surgical loupes: achieving low rate of hepatic arterial thrombosis in 741 consecutive recipients-tips and tricks to overcome the poor hepatic arterial flow. Liver Transplant. 2017;23:887–98.
3. Ahn CS, Lee SG, Hwang S, et al. Anatomic variation of the right hepatic artery and its reconstruction for living donor liver transplantation using right lobe graft. Transplant Proc. 2005;37:1067–9.
4. Ahn CS, Hwang S, Moon DB, et al. Right gastroepiploic artery is the first alternative inflow source for hepatic arterial reconstruction in living donor liver transplantation. Transplant Proc. 2012;44:451–3.
5. Uchiyama H, Harada N. Dual hepatic artery reconstruction in living donor liver transplantation using a left graft with 2 hepatic arterial stumps. Surgery. 2010;147:878–86.
6. Balci D, Ahn CS. Hepatic artery reconstruction in living donor liver transplantation. Curr Opin Organ Transplant. 2019;24:631–6.
7. Harada N, Yoshizumi T, Uchiyama H, et al. Impact of hepatic artery size mismatch between donor and recipient on outcomes after living-donor liver transplantation using right lobe. Clin Transpl. 2019;33:e13444.
8. Lee CF, Lu JC, Zidan A, et al. Microscope-assisted hepatic artery reconstruction in adult living donor liver transplantation—a review of 325 consecutive cases in single center. Clin Transpl. 2017;31:e12879.
9. Yagi T, Shinoura S, Umeda Y, et al. Surgical rationalization living donor liver transplantation by abolition of hepatic artery reconstruction under a fixed microscope. Clin Transpl. 2012;26:877–83.
10. Ikegami T, Yoshizumi T, Uchiyama H, et al. Hepatic artery reconstruction in living donor liver transplantation using surgical loupes: achieving low rate of hepatic arterial thrombosis in 741 consecutive recipients-tips and tricks to overcome the poor hepatic arterial flow. Liver Transplant. 2017;23:1081–2.

27 Biliary Reconstruction

Bong-Wan Kim

Abstract

The duct-to-duct anastomosis is now the standard procedure for biliary reconstruction and has better outcomes than the hepaticojejunostomy reconstruction in living donor liver transplantation (LDLT). There are some technical principles that help to minimize biliary complications after duct-to-duct anastomosis such as intraoperative cholangiography, tension-free and fine anastomosis, avoiding electrocautery on duct openings, and duct-to-mucosa anastomosis. External biliary stenting using small catheter might help to reduce bile leakage and ductoplasty for multiple graft ducts could facilitate duct-to-duct anastomosis.

Keywords

Living donor liver transplantation · Duct-to-duct anastomosis · Biliary complication

Supplementary Information The online version contains supplementary material available at https://doi.org/10.1007/978-981-16-1996-0_27.

B.-W. Kim (✉)
Division of Hepatobiliary Surgery and Liver Transplantation, Department of Surgery, Ajou University School of Medicine, Suwon, South Korea
e-mail: drbwkim@ajou.ac.kr

27.1 Chapter Outline

The usefulness of duct-to-duct biliary reconstruction in living donor liver transplantation was first reported by Azoulay et al. in 2001 [1]. Since then, it has been widely used as a standard biliary procedure in almost all transplantation centers [2]. However, when the recipient's biliary tract cannot be spared, or when the condition of the bile duct is not histologically suitable for anastomosis, Roux-en-Y hepaticojejunostomy must be performed. The essential techniques for a successful duct-to-duct biliary reconstruction while minimizing postoperative complications are summarized below.

27.2 Method

1. Cholangiography should be performed during donor hepatectomy

   In some hospitals, the structure of the biliary tract of the graft liver is analyzed using preoperative MR cholangiography. However, the use of intraoperative cholangiography can generally provide more accurate information on the intrahepatic biliary tract structure than MR cholangiography. By performing this procedure, it is possible to grasp the exact cutting position of the biliary tract of the graft liver while avoiding damage to the biliary tract of the graft liver, and therefore preventing the

H. C. Yu (ed.), *Hepato-Biliary-Pancreatic Surgery and Liver Transplantation*,
https://doi.org/10.1007/978-981-16-1996-0_27

occurrence of biliary complications after donor hepatectomy.

2. Ischemic damage to the graft's and recipient's biliary tracts must be avoided

   To avoid ischemic damage to the graft liver and to the biliary tract, hemostasis should be performed around the bile duct through suture ligation using small sutures of at least 6–0, rather than electrocautery. When cutting the biliary tract, it is also contraindicated to use electric cauterization, and sharp Metzenbaum scissors must be used for cutting. Due to the cauterization, the subserosal capillaries should not be grossly present. In addition, bleeding of the small arterioles should be observed on the cutting surface of the graft's and recipient's bile ducts. If ischemic damage of the recipient's biliary tract is suspected, or if bleeding is not observed on the cut surface due to poor bile duct condition, Roux-en-Y hepaticojejunostomy should be promptly performed instead of reconstruction.
3. When there are multiple bile duct openings on the cut edge with small distances between them, ductoplasty can be performed to combine them into a single orifice during the back-table procedure. However, the bile ducts must be separately anastomosed to the recipient's bile duct when undue tension is expected due to a large distance between them. Generally, ductoplasty is considered safe if the distance between the two bile ducts is less than 7 mm.
4. In a duct-to-duct biliary reconstruction, tension should be avoided at the anastomosis of bile ducts. Excessive tension on the anastomosis typically occurs as a result of the short preparation of the recipient's biliary. By contrast, the recipient's biliary tract should not be left too long, since it may bend after anastomosis. The biliary tract of the recipient should be cut with a Metzenbaum scissor to an optimal length.
5. The duct-to-duct biliary reconstruction may be performed by an end-to-end anastomosis for a single bile duct. If two anastomoses are required, the end-to-end anastomoses can be performed separately to the recipient's right and left hepatic ducts. Alternatively, an end-to-end anastomosis and an end-to-side anastomosis may be implemented to the recipient's common bile duct, or a second anastomosis may be performed at the recipient's cystic duct. Biliary anastomosis between the bile duct(s) of the graft liver and the recipient's biliary tract should be performed with sutures of 6–0 or finer. The bile duct suture can be performed by either continuous or interrupted suture manner or by a continuous suture on the posterior wall and interrupted sutures on the anterior wall. The selection of the anastomotic procedure depends on the preference and proficiency of the transplantation center, and there are no known differences in the postoperative outcomes of the different anastomotic procedures. However, the principle of the suture manner is to not leave a thread knot in the biliary tract and to ensure that the suture interval is tight and delicate, not exceeding 1 mm. In terms of suture material selection, prolene is regarded to be better than a PDS due to the reduced inflammation it causes, and the use of a fine suture technique with a 7-0 or 8-0 suture was reported to minimize biliary stricture [3].
6. In living donor liver transplantation, the size of the bile duct of the graft liver is relatively small, measuring approximately 5 mm in diameter, and there is a considerable disparity with the size of the recipient's bile duct opening, which is approximately 10 mm in diameter. This discrepancy can typically be overcome by duct-to-mucosa anastomosis, through which the graft bile duct is sewn to the mucosal layer of the recipient's bile duct [4, 5]. This is not only useful for overcoming the size discrepancy between the graft and recipient bile ducts, but it can also enable expansion growth of the graft's bile duct.
7. Each transplantation center has its own preference of inserting an external catheter with a size between 3- and 4-Fr into the biliary tract, also known as "external biliary stenting". External biliary stenting can decompress the intraluminal pressure of the biliary tract after LT, which can prevent post-transplant bile

leakage, and which allows for postoperative cholangiography to be easily performed if necessary [6]. In the case of a living donor liver transplantation using thc right lobe graft, it is desirable that the biliary catheter be inserted into the graft's posterior duct after passing through the anastomosis site from a common bile duct, because the right posterior duct is more angulated in anatomical position. The insertion of an internal biliary catheter without the role of decompression is not recommended because the stent can be easily dislodged and translocate to an unwarranted site in the biliary tract.

27.3 Conclusion

In living donor liver transplantation, biliary complications can be minimized by abiding the principles described above, and by using delicate and proficient techniques for biliary reconstruction. In addition, the biliary reconstruction technique can be differentially modified and developed for logical and rational reasons for each transplantation center or surgeon, which is thought to further reduce the occurrence of postoperative biliary complications.

References

1. Azoulay D, Marin-Hargreaves G, Castaing D, ReneAdam BH. Duct-to-duct biliary anastomosis in living related liver transplantation: the Paul Brousse technique. Arch Surg. 2001;136(10):1197–200. https://doi.org/10.1001/archsurg.136.10.1197.
2. Ishiko T, Egawa H, Kasahara M, Nakamura T, Oike F, Kaihara S, et al. Duct-to-duct biliary reconstruction in living donor liver transplantation utilizing right lobe graft. Ann Surg. 2002;236(2):235–40. https://doi.org/10.1097/00000658-200208000-00012.
3. Lin TS, Concejero AM, Chen CL, Chiang YC, Wang CC, Wang SH, et al. Routine microsurgical biliary reconstruction decreases early anastomotic complications in living donor liver transplantation. Liver Transpl. 2009;15(12):1766–75. https://doi.org/10.1002/lt.21947.
4. Kim BW, Bae BK, Lee JM, Won JH, Park YK, Xu WG, et al. Duct-to-duct biliary reconstructions and complications in 100 living donor liver transplantations. Transplant Proc. 2009;41(5):1749–55. https://doi.org/10.1016/j.transproceed.2009.02.097.
5. Kim SH, Lee KW, Kim YK, Cho SY, Han SS, Park SJ. Tailored telescopic reconstruction of the bile duct in living donor liver transplantation. Liver Transpl. 2010;16(9):1069–74. https://doi.org/10.1002/lt.22116.
6. Hong SY, Hu XG, Lee HY, Won JH, Kim JW, Shen XY, et al. Long-term analysis of biliary complications after duct-to-duct biliary reconstruction in living donor liver transplantations. Liver Transpl. 2018;24(8):1050–61. https://doi.org/10.1002/lt.25074.

Part IV

Cholecystectomy

Laparoscopic Cholecystectomy (3–4 Ports Method)

28

Sang Mok Lee

Abstract

Laparoscopic cholecystectomy (LC) is a surgical method that is considered the gold standard for the treatment of symptomatic GB stones, and it is recognized as an alternative to open cholecystectomy (OC). Although LC is a very safe operation, one must be familiar with all the different instruments used in a LC, and one should be able to perform an OC on top of acquiring the basic techniques needed for laparoscopic surgery (LS). The most serious complication of LS is bile duct injury. To minimize the risk of bile duct injury, widening Calot's triangle and taking a critical view of safety are the most important steps, along with avoiding thermal injury.

A variety of technical variations for LC have recently been introduced to minimize the invasiveness while reducing the size and number of ports to improve the cosmetic and postoperative outcomes.

Supplementary Information The online version contains supplementary material available at https://doi.org/10.1007/978-981-16-1996-0_28.

S. M. Lee (✉)
Department of Surgery, Kyung Hee University College of Medicine, Seoul, South Korea
e-mail: hbplapa@khu.ac.kr

Keywords

Laparoscopic cholecystectomy · Laparoscopic surgery · Critical view of safety · Bile duct injury · Technical variations

28.1 Introduction

Because of the advantages of laparoscopic surgery (LS), laparoscopic cholecystectomy (LC) is a surgical method that is considered the gold standard for the treatment of symptomatic GB stones, and it is recognized as an alternative to open cholecystectomy (OC) according to the surgeon's experience and skills with various instruments. Although LC is a very safe operation, it is performed using instruments that are restricted in use and make it so that the surgeon cannot feel by touch, and it therefore requires experience and has limitations in indications. This means that surgeons have to choose between OC or LC to map out a strategy before surgery. Since LC is an operation that uses many kinds of instruments, one must be familiar with all the instruments, and they should also be able to do simple first aid in the event of instrumental problems.

H. C. Yu (ed.), *Hepato-Biliary-Pancreatic Surgery and Liver Transplantation*,
https://doi.org/10.1007/978-981-16-1996-0_28

Recently, a variety of technical variations for LC have been introduced to minimize the invasiveness while reducing the size and number of ports to improve cosmetic and postoperative outcomes. Here, I would like to explain the surgical method of LC with three or four ports in terms of the technical aspects involved.

28.2 Preoperative Preparation

You should have a good understanding of the anatomical structure of the hepatobiliary system, you should be able to perform an OC, and you must have fully acquired the basic techniques of LS [1].

1. Make sure the preoperative diagnosis is correct.
2. Prior to surgery, identify past medical history and clinical patterns, then conduct various examinations and confirm inflammation, fibrosis, and anatomical variation around the gallbladder via imaging.
3. Check the combined diseases and the medicine currently being taken, and ensure that the patient is able to undergo general anesthesia. It is particularly important to confirm the use of anticoagulants.
4. Insert the Foley catheter only if the operation is expected to be prolonged. It is recommended to selectively insert the nasogastric tube only if the stomach or duodenum is highly dilated after forming pneumoperitoneum to the point of potentially interfering with the surgery.
5. The operating table should be remotely adjustable and suitable for performing intraoperative cholangiography during LC.

28.3 Anesthesia

General anesthesia and endotracheal intubation are recommended.

28.4 Patient's Posture and Arrangement of Equipment and Personnel

1. Patient's posture—the left arm is lowered to the torso and the right arm is extended to 90° for easy installation and management of the IV and A line.
2. Place a monitor on each side of the patient. The monitor located on the right side of the patient is attached with a CO_2 insufflator and optic equipment for both the operator and the camera assistant.
3. Both the operator and the camera assistant should be on the left side of the patient, while the first assistant should be on the right side of the patient.

28.5 Surgical Techniques

1. Creation of CO_2 Pneumoperitoneum

   The patient is placed in a mild Trendelenburg position. A small periumbilical incision is made according to the patient's status and the surgeon's preference as well as cosmetic considerations following one of two techniques: a closed technique or an open technique. I prefer the closed technique using a Veress needle.

   (1) Closed Technique Using a Veress Needle

      (a) Skin incision: A 1 cm skin incision is made vertically along the crease inside the navel or horizontally along the crease outside of the navel. The vertical incision is easier but has a larger cosmetic effect.

      (b) Insertion of the Veress needle: After skin incision, bluntly dissect the subcutaneous fat with scissors or clamps to expose the fascia and grasp the abdominal wall on either side of the umbilicus; both the skin and the fascia should be penetrated by breast clamps or towel clips to lift the abdominal wall. After lifting the abdominal wall, the Veress needle, held gently as if one were throwing a dart, is inserted into the abdominal cavity through the fascia and the peritoneum, where a characteristic popping sensation can be felt.

(c) Verification of location and patency of the Veress needle: These are respectively verified by repeated irrigation of clear normal saline in and out of the peritoneal cavity (syringe test), and by the dropped normal saline in the translucent herb of the Veress needle being drawn into the peritoneal cavity when the abdominal wall is lifted (drop test).

(d) Creation of pneumoperitoneum: After insertion of the Veress needle, CO_2 gas insufflation begins at a low flow rate (1–3 L/min) while watching the intra-abdominal pressure and insufflating flow rate. Once the abdomen has expanded to a certain extent, you should hear a tympanic sound when percussing the abdomen. The flow rate and the intra-abdominal pressure may increase without necessarily indicating a problem. However, if there is a sudden intra-abdominal pressure rise or asymmetric abdominal expansion, the gas insufflation should be stopped and the cause should be investigated. When the intra-abdominal pressure reaches the preset limitation (12–15 cm H_2O), the Veress needle should be removed.

(2) Closed Technique

Skin incision and exposure of the fascia are the same as in the closed technique. When the fascia is exposed, hold either side of the fascia with Kelly clamps and open the fascia while checking the preperitoneal fat or the peritoneum. Then, with the peritoneum elevated, cautiously open it with a finger or a scalpel and perform a pair of lateral stay sutures including the peritoneum and the fascia.

To verify a safe opening into the peritoneal space, insert the fifth finger and palpate the region around the opening.

2. Insertion of Trocars

After removing the Veress needle, insert a 10 mm disposal trocar into the peritoneal cavity while lifting the abdominal wall. While holding the end of the trocar deep in the palm of the hand and extending the middle finger along the trocar (Fig. 28.1), the trocar should be inserted gently in a twisting motion. This method can prevent excessive insertion of the trocar. Then, the videoscope (either flat or angled) can be inserted through the first trocar (umbilical port), and a brief examination of the abdominal cavity can be made for any organ pathology, adhesions, or trocar-induced injuries.

Two or three additional trocars are then inserted under direct vision. In the four-port method, the second 5- or 10-mm trocar (epigastric port) is inserted into the epigastrium in about the upper 2/3 portion between the umbilicus and the xiphoid process, immediately to the right of the falciform ligament. The third trocar (5 mm, traction port) is inserted into the RUQ abdomen near the midclavicular line, 3–4 cm below the costal margin. The fourth trocar (5 mm, lateral port) is inserted in the anterior axillary 4–5 cm below the costal margin. Because there are personal variations and differences in the anatomical structure, I insert

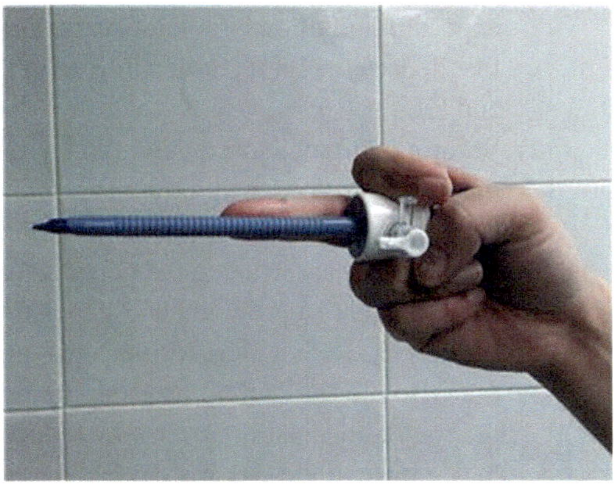

Fig. 28.1 Shape of the hand and fingers grasping a trocar for the umbilical port

the trocar according to the particular anatomical structure. I insert the second trocar 2–3 cm below the liver margin, immediately to the right of the falciform ligament. Every trocar is inserted at an angle of 90° so it can be easily moved in any direction. In the three-port method, the traction port is inserted more laterally than it is in the four-port method, as this is advantageous for an instrument that is opened a lot.

Compared to the four-port method, the three-port method is less invasive, more economical, and has better cosmetic outcomes, but it is difficult to secure a surgical field for this method and to cope with any unforeseen circumstances that arise. Therefore, the three-port method is only recommended after having accumulated enough experience with the four-port method [2]. The basic four-port method usually uses 5 mm trocars in all ports except the umbilical port. Recently, many surgeons have inserted one 5 mm trocar alone as the epigastric port while using 2 or 3 mm trocars for the other ports to reduce the invasiveness and improve the cosmetic outcomes.

3. Cholecystectomy
   (1) A general examination of the abdominal cavity and exposure of the gallbladder (GB): After all trocars have been inserted, the pelvic cavity is first observed by taking a slight reverse Trendelenburg position and then changing the posture to a 10–15° right-side up position; this maneuver achieves full exposure and allows for observation of the ileocecal region, ascending colon, and GB.
   (2) Securing surgical space: The fundus of the GB is grasped with a ratcheted forceps through the lateral port, then the GB and liver are lifted to the upper right of the patient to provide good exposure of the GB. Rather than lifting, pushing the GB with the feeling of propping up the forceps against the liver may reduce the damage to the GB and the liver.
   (3) Exposure and identification of Calot's triangle and the extrahepatic bile duct: The GB infundibulum is grasped with the forceps through the traction port and lifted to the upper right of the patient for full exposure and identification of Calot's triangle and the extrahepatic bile duct. Prior to the dissection of Calot's triangle, correctly identifying the anatomy of Calot's triangle and the extrahepatic duct may reduce bile duct injury. If there is some anatomical distortion, the round ligament and S4 segment of the liver can be good anatomical landmarks, because the confluence of the bile duct is located on the S4 between the GB and round ligament (Fig. 28.2a, b). As a grossly distended GB makes grasping difficult and is more susceptible to rupturing, puncture and aspiration of the GB are recommended.
   (4) Widening Calot's triangle and dissection of the cystic duct and cystic artery: Both aspects of serosa over the presumed junction of the GB and cystic duct should be opened as widely as possible (i.e., widening Calot's triangle) with dissecting forceps or a hook cautery through the epigastric port. The cystic duct and artery are exposed circumferentially with a gentle teasing and spreading motion while checking with the eyes, and the GB infundibulum is also fully dissected and exposed from the liver (i.e., unfolding Calot's triangle) [3]. The dissection is initiated high in the cystic duct or the GB infundibulum, and blunt dissection is preferable in the connective tissue. After identifying the continuous connection between the cystic duct and the GB infundibulum and identifying the liver that is seen posterior to Calot's triangle (i.e., taking a critical view of safety), the cystic duct and artery are clipped and divided to minimize bile duct injury [4].

       If there is a lot of fat or severe edema in Calot's triangle, aspiration of fat or edematous tissue using a suction device will help identify the anatomical struc-

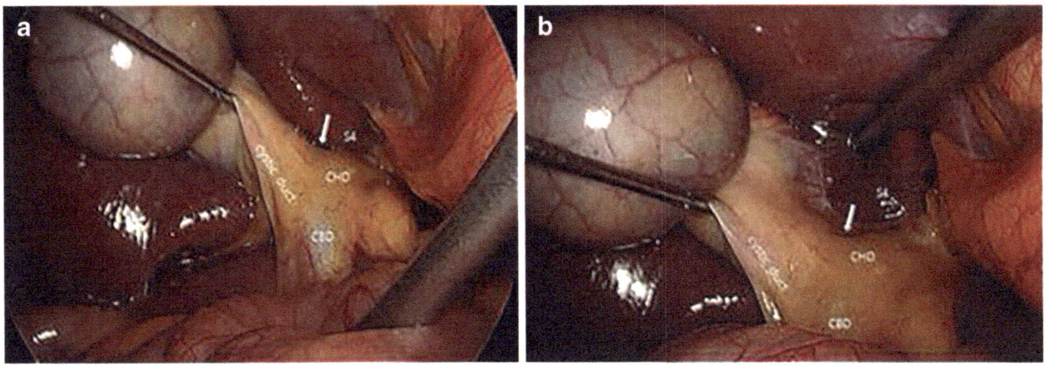

Fig. 28.2 (**a**) Identification of the common duct; (**b**) The groove (white arrow) lateral to the common duct *CBD* common bile duct, *CHD* common hepatic duct

ture. A suction device may be a good blunt dissector as a CUSA. If the cystic duct is clipped near the common duct with too much traction, the bile duct can potentially narrow. Surgical clips should be applied at an angle of 90° without twisting and loosening. If there is a case in which the cystic duct and artery are respectively divided, it is better to cut the artery first, if at all possible. If the cystic duct is divided first, care should be taken not to tear the cystic artery during the GB pull. To prevent thermal injury, the division must be done with scissors rather than electrocautery.

(5) Dissection of the GB from the liver bed: After dividing the cystic duct and the artery, grasp and properly pull the GB with two forceps through the lateral port and the traction port, and open the GB serosa longitudinally about 1 cm away from the liver with a hook cautery (Fig. 28.3). Then, grasp the GB infundibulum with forceps through the traction port, and proceed with the dissection of the GB with electrocautery from the liver bed following from the infundibulum to the fundus of the GB (i.e., retrograde cholecystectomy); in selected cases, antegrade cholecystectomy may be easier. Care should be taken to keep the dissection in the right plane and close to the GB wall, which can prevent

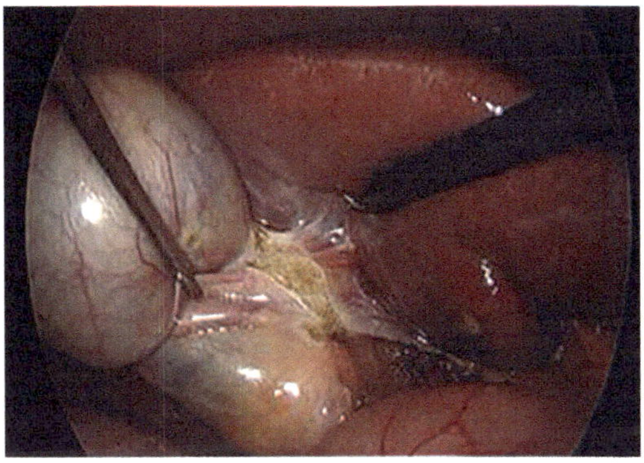

Fig. 28.3 Dissection of the GB from the liver bed

bleeding from the GB bed. The only known prophylactic measure to reduce bile from the bile ducts of Luschka is to dissect as close as possible to the GB wall [5].

(6) Put the resected GB in a retrieval bag: The telescope in the umbilical port is pulled out and an endoscopic removal bag is inserted. After removing the sleeve, only a retrieval bag is left in the abdominal cavity, and after reinsertion of the telescope the bag is unfolded on the liver dome under direct vision using two forceps through the epigastric and traction port. The resected GB is then put in the bag and placed in the pouch between the liver and diaphragm. Some surgeons put in an endoscopic removal bag through the epigastric port using a 10 mm trocar.

(7) Examination of the dissected area: Careful examination of the dissected area is recommended while lifting the liver with forceps and grasping the remaining GB serosa that is still attached to the liver (Fig. 28.4). Bleeding and bile leaks must be checked for and controlled as well. A visual inspection should be made first, after which irrigation and suction are recommended. If either bleeding or bile leaks are suspected, control without hesitation. If there is bleeding that is difficult to control from the exposed portal vein in the liver bed, compression with a retrieval bag filled with the resected GB using sufficient blood clot-inducing materials for a few minutes is safer and more effective than bleeding control with electrocautery or suture.

(8) Perforation of the GB: If perforation of the GB occurs during surgery, measures to minimize any significant spillage should be taken. Putting stones in a preloaded retrieval bag after aspiration of bile may also be needed. Complete removal of spilt stones and sufficient irrigation are likely necessary, and one should not hesitate to insert a drainage catheter.

(9) Intraoperative cholangiogram (IOC): IOC is needed in selected cases. After sufficiently clearing and identifying the cystic duct and artery, the artery is clipped and divided. The cystic duct is clipped as high as possible close to the infundibulum, and an anterolateral ductotomy is made distal to the clip. A cholangiogram catheter is inserted through the ductotomy and secured in place using cholangiogram forceps. Air in the bile duct and the catheter should be removed before cholangiography. It is better to identify the bile leaks through the ductotomy before inserting a cholangiogram catheter, and it is recommended to do so without wasting a lot of time or effort.

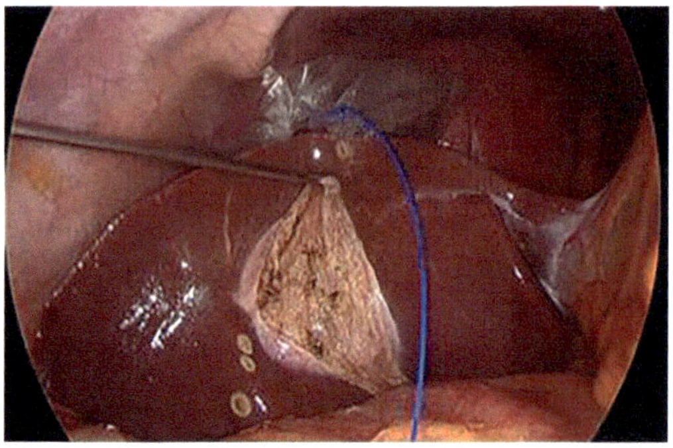

Fig. 28.4 Examination of the dissected area after completion of cholecystectomy

(10) Removal of the trocars and extraction of the resected GB: Before removing the trocars, careful examination of the bleeding and bile leakage in the dissected area and of the upper abdomen should be done, and drains should be installed when necessary without hesitation. The ports are removed under direct vision to evaluate possible bleeding, then the resected GB in the bag is extracted with the umbilical trocar. If the extraction is too difficult because of an excessively thick wall of the GB or exceedingly large stones, you do not need to extend the incision if the GB or the stones are kept in the bag while cutting the GB with scissors or crushing the stones with forceps. All specimens should be placed and removed in a retrieval bag.

(11) Closure of incisions: The fascial defects in the 10 mm port are sutured with absorbable sutures (2–0 size, 3/4 circled and atraumatic needle is preferred). While suturing the defect in the umbilical port, I prefer to perform the suture including the peritoneum and the fascia with my own eyes while lifting the fascia with the clamps. The skin is approximated with absorbable subcutaneous sutures.

28.6 Microlaparoscopic Cholecystectomy

LC may be done to reduce the size and/or number of trocars to minimize invasiveness with improved cosmetic and postoperative outcomes. If LC is performed using 2 or 3 mm ports except for the umbilical port, it is called "microlaparoscopic cholecystectomy" (micro-LC). In micro-LC, the cosmetic effect and the postoperative outcomes are good because of the decreased invasiveness due to the reduce size of the trocars, but there are restrictions on the use of the instruments, which make the operation difficult and the indications narrow [6]. As a result, some surgeons use self-made instruments, and instrument-optimized techniques are needed. I use 2 mm trocars as well as a self-made hook electrocautery and suction-irrigation device. It is difficult to grasp and lift the GB, because 2 mm instruments are small and weak. Therefore, to achieve good exposure, I push rather than pull the GB while keeping the forceps in an open position. When dissecting Calot's triangle, the GB is pulled with the forceps to make a wedge form and remain in an open position between the dissected tissues or between the cystic duct and artery (Fig. 28.5a, b). Another drawback of micro-LC is that a 2 mm telescope placed through the epigastric port shows a dark and low-resolution image when clipping the cystic duct and artery with endoscopic clips through the umbilical port. Therefore, 2 mm telescopes are recommended for use in a temporary and auxiliary manner. Despite the disadvantages of micro-LC, it achieves good postoperative outcomes with high patient satisfaction. It is also easier to learn compared to single port LC, and it can be used in selected patients with acute cholecystitis [6].

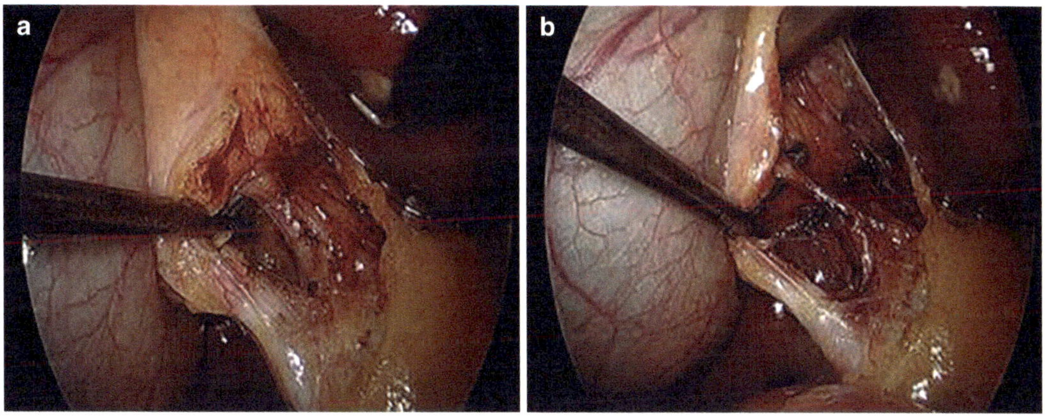

Fig. 28.5 (**a, b**) Traction of the GB with 2 mm forceps through the traction port of the GB, with the forceps making a wedge form and remaining in an open position between the dissected tissues (**a**) or between the cystic duct and the artery (**b**)

References

1. Kim SH, Seo KS. Hepato-biliary-pancreatic surgery. 3rd ed. Euihak Co: Seoul; 2013.
2. Hur SH, Lee SM, Koh SH, et al. The usefulness of three-portal technique for laparoscopic cholecystectomy. JMIS. 1999;2(2):41–8.
3. Ellison EC, Zollinger RM Jr. Zollinger's atlas of surgical operations. 10th ed. Mc Graw Hill; 2016.
4. Strasberg SM, Hertl M, Soper NJ. An analysis of the problem of biliary injury during laparoscopic cholecystectomy. J Am Coll Surg. 1995;180:101–25.
5. Spanos CP, Syrakos T. Bile leaks from the duct of Luschka (subvesical duct): a review. Langenbeck's Arch Surg. 2006;391:441–7.
6. Kwon TS, Lee SM, Park SJ, et al. Clinical application of 2 mm trocar mini-laparoscopic cholecystectomy. JMIS. 2007;10:79–82.

29 Laparoscopic Single-Site Cholecystectomy (Single Port Method)

Dong-Hoon Shin

Abstract

In benign gallbladder disease, laparoscopic cholecystectomy is a standard technique. However, laparoscopic single-incision (single port) cholecystectomy is known to be generally unacceptable for patients with severe acute cholecystitis, chronic cholecystitis, and gall stone-related pancreatitis. In addition, though there is not an official standard, it is known to be difficult to conduct surgery with patients with a high BMI. However, regardless of difficult cases, the range of laparoscopic single-incision cholecystectomy is increasingly expanding by the development of the mechanism and the technique.

Keywords

Single port · Single incision · Single site
Gallbladder · Laparoscopy · Cholecystectomy

29.1 Surgical Procedures

1. Preparing the Operating Room

   The surgeon performs surgery on the left side of the patient and the first assistant helps the puncture for insertion (trocar insertion) on the right side of the patient, and if necessary, moves to the left of the patient to catch a laparoscopic camera next to the surgeon. The patient's left arm is attached next to the patient's body, and the right arm is placed on the armrest slot with open sideways. The monitor is best placed in the position of the patient's right shoulder.

2. Puncture Area

   In the case of three port or four-port surgery, a trocar is inserted a 10 mm or 5 mm around the navel. Laparoscopic single-incision cholecystectomy requires a slightly larger hole than the three-port or four-port method. It is advantageous to make a hole by making a vertical incision in the middle of the navel to insert a single-incision surgical trocar to obtain efficiency with a relatively small skin incision (Fig. 29.1). If the subcutaneous fat is too thick to expose the fascia, piercing the abdominal wall while lifting the bottom of the navel using the Kocher clamp is another way. The single-incision surgical trocar can be used by surgeons using surgical gloves and wound retractors. However, more surgeons use commercially available trocars today. After the incision of the peritoneal membrane is sufficiently made, while retracting the abdominal wall including the peritoneal mem-

Supplementary Information The online version contains supplementary material available at https://doi.org/10.1007/978-981-16-1996-0_29.

D.-H. Shin (✉)
Kosin University Hospital, Busan, South Korea

H. C. Yu (ed.), *Hepato-Biliary-Pancreatic Surgery and Liver Transplantation*,
https://doi.org/10.1007/978-981-16-1996-0_29

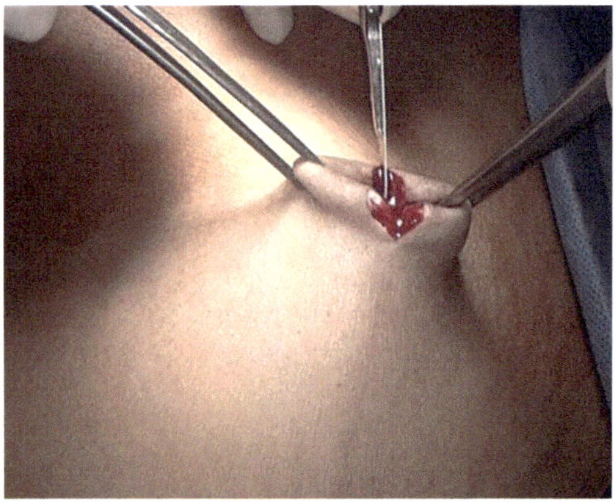

Fig. 29.1 Make a hole by making a vertical incision in the middle of the navel

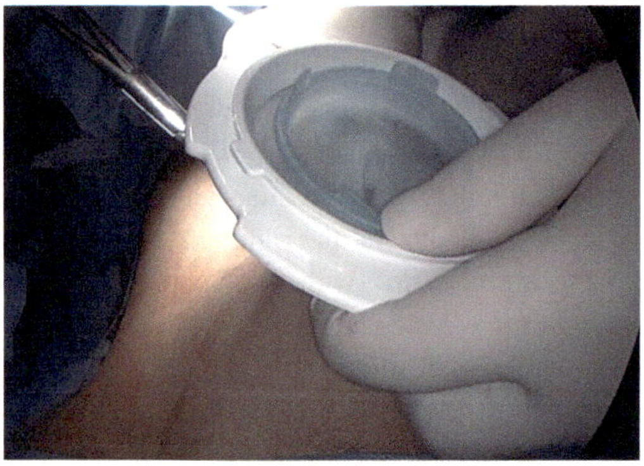

Fig. 29.2 Insert a single-incision surgical trocar

brane, insert a single-incision surgical trocar and make a pneumoperitoneum while maintaining the pressure at 12–14 mmHg (Figs. 29.2 and 29.3).

3. Surgical Techniques

   Use 0–30° telescope or flexible telescope. Check the organs behind the pelvis and abdominal wall, and make sure that there is no damage that occurred when inserting the trocar (Fig. 29.4). In order to expose the gallbladder, make reverse Trendelenburg position by raising the patient's head direction by about 30°. Raising the right side of the operating table also helps to expose the gallbladder. By inserting the endograsper with the left hand, hold the fundus of the gallbladder and expose the surroundings of the cystic duct of the gallbladder (Fig. 29.5). Use the endodissector or right-angled dissector with the right hand to hold the body of the gallbladder, and use the endograsper held with the left hand to help to hold the fundus of the gallbladder in precision. Retract the endo-

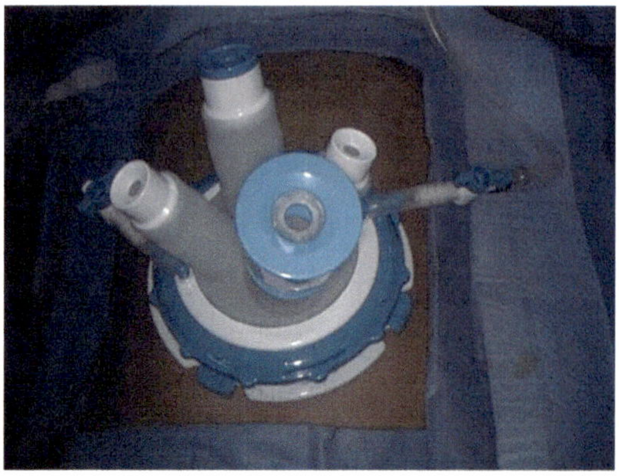

Fig. 29.3 Install a single-incision surgical trocar and make pneumoperitoneum

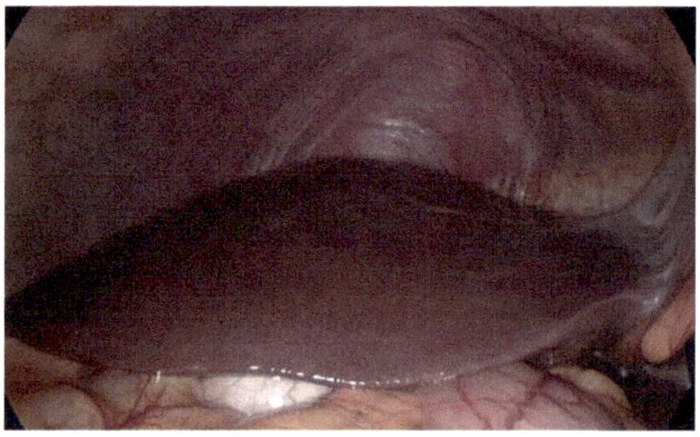

Fig. 29.4 Use a telescope to check intraperitoneal conditions

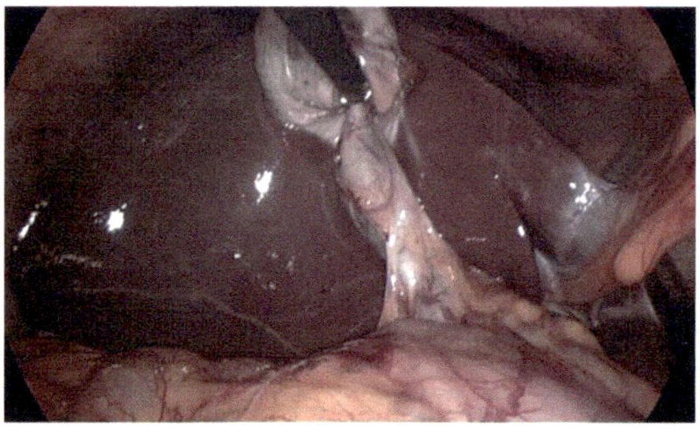

Fig. 29.5 Hold the fundus of the gallbladder with endograsper and expose it around the gallbladder

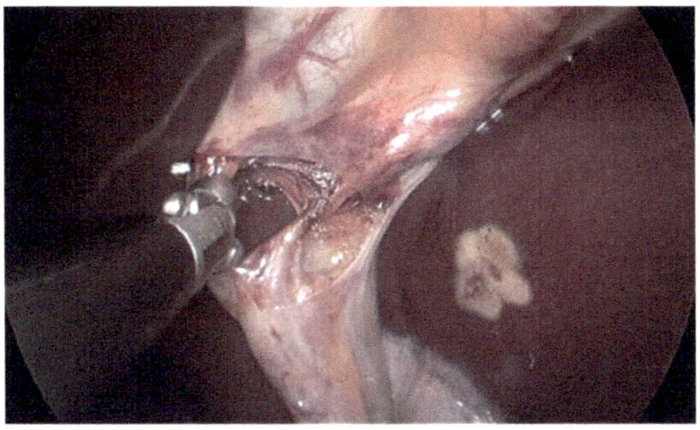

Fig. 29.6 Exposing the triangle of Calot, use endodissector to perform dissection starting with the infundibulum of the gallbladder toward the cystic duct

grasper to the right outer side of the patient to expose the triangle of Callot. Using the endodissector with the right hand, perform dissection from the gallbladder toward the cystic duct. Finding the best angle to retract while moving the endograsper of the left hand properly, it is recommended to perform dissection while ensuring sufficient traction to ensure the surgical view (Fig. 29.6). If the gallbladder ligation is done properly, hold the scissors with your right hand and carefully cut the gallbladder. At this time, it should be careful not to cut the tissue located in the back of the cystic duct because the angle of the scissors enters from the front.

It should be careful not to damage the cystic artery or hepatic artery that passes behind the cystic duct. If the gallbladder is cut off, use endograsper of the left hand to retract the fundus of the gallbladder carefully toward the patient's head, i.e., the liver edge. While doing so, use endodissector or right-angled endodissector of the right hand to dissect the cystic artery (it is also possible to expose both cystic duct and cystic artery through dissection at the same time). If it is confirmed that it is the cystic artery, performs ligation and dissection with the right hand (Fig. 29.7).

In the technique of cholecystectomy, it is crucial to prevent damages of surrounding organs such as common bile duct or hepatic artery, etc. Therefore, the ligation and dissection must be performed after finding the exact cystic duct and cystic artery.

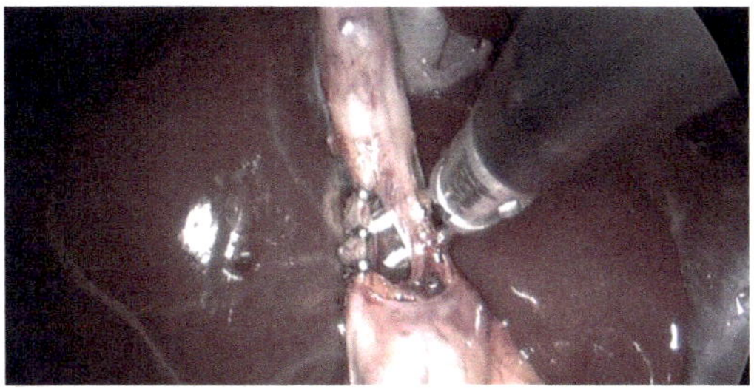

Fig. 29.7 Dissect cystic artery

If the cystic duct and cystic artery are ligated and cut, use endograsper of the left hand to hold the fundus or body of the gallbladder and retract it toward the patient's head or right outer side of the patient. While doing so, perform dissection using suitable endodissector instruments through electrocautery. While performing a dissection, make sure that there is no bleeding site. If there is bleeding, control bleeding through electrocautery and ligation. The dissected gallbladder should be removed through the trocar site located at the navel.

The fascia of the abdominal wall is usually closed with suitable suture materials such as polypropylene sutures, and subcuticular closure should be performed for the dermis of the umbilicus.

29.2 Conclusion

Laparoscopic single-incision cholecystectomy is a safe and efficient surgical method as much as the three-port or four-port laparoscopic cholecystectomy [1–3]. Although the indications of surgery of single-incision laparoscopic cholecystectomy are still limited compared to the three-port or four-port method, especially if the anatomical classification of the gallbladder is difficult for inflammatory diseases or other reasons, the effort to expand the indications continues [4].

References

1. Romanelli JR, Roshek TB 3rd, Lynn DC, et al. Single-port laparoscopic cholecystectomy: initial experience. Surg Endosc. 2010;24:1374–9.
2. Bucher P, Pusin F, Buchs NC, et al. Randomised clinical trial of laparoscopic single-site versus conventional laparoscopic cholecystectomy. Br J Surg. 2011;98:1695–702.
3. Deveci U, Barbaros U, Kapakli MS, Manukyan MN, Şimşek S, Kebudi A, Mercan S. The comparison of single incision laparoscopic cholecystectomy and three port laparoscopic cholecystectomy: prospective randomized study. J Korean Surg Soc. 2013;85:275–82.
4. Kim HS, Han Y, Kang JS, et al. Comparison of single-incision robotic cholecystectomy, single–incision laparoscopic cholecystectomy and 3-port laparoscopic cholecystectomy-postoperative pain, cosmetic outcome and Surgeon's workload. J Minim Invasive Surg. 2018;21(4):168–76.

30 Laparoscopic Surgery for Gallbladder Polyps and Early-Stage Gallbladder Cancer

Woo-Jung Lee and Myung Jae Jung

Abstract

Laparoscopic cholecystectomy is widely performed, to treat such benign gallbladder diseases as gallbladder polyps and cholecystitis. Recently, it is even implemented for early gallbladder cancers in a selective group of patients. However, it must be applied with caution, since lymph node dissection is not always readily performed by laparoscopic surgery. In this chapter, implication of the procedure and principles to be followed during laparoscopic cholecystectomy are discussed.

Keywords

Laparoscopic cholecystectomy · Gallbladder polyp · Early gallbladder cancer · Calot's triangle · Four-port technique · Single-port technique · Radical cholecystectomy Lymphadenectomy

W.-J. Lee (✉)
Yonsei University Severance Hospital, Seoul, South Korea
e-mail: WJLEE@yuhs.ac

M. J. Jung
Myongji Hospital, iGoyand-si, Gyeonggi-do, South Korea

30.1 Gallbladder Polyps and Early-Stage Gallbladder Cancer

30.1.1 Overview

This chapter discusses the laparoscopic surgical technique used to treat gallbladder polyps and early-stage gallbladder cancer. Both diseases are commonly treated with laparoscopic cholecystectomy, and extended cholecystectomy (cholecystectomy + lymphadenectomy) should be considered for early-stage gallbladder cancers (T1b or higher). This chapter will first describe laparoscopic cholecystectomy, then lymphadenectomy. Prior to the surgical techniques, a brief introduction of gallbladder polyps and early-stage gallbladder cancer is presented before the surgical techniques are described.

30.1.2 Gallbladder Polyps

Gallbladder polyps, mostly asymptomatic, are often found incidentally on abdominal ultrasound and computed tomogrhaphy. They are usually finally diagosed as cholesterol polyp or adenoma (Fig. 30.1). Adenomas may be associated with a higher risk of malignant transformation with an increase in the size of the polyps. However,

H. C. Yu (ed.), *Hepato-Biliary-Pancreatic Surgery and Liver Transplantation*,
https://doi.org/10.1007/978-981-16-1996-0_30

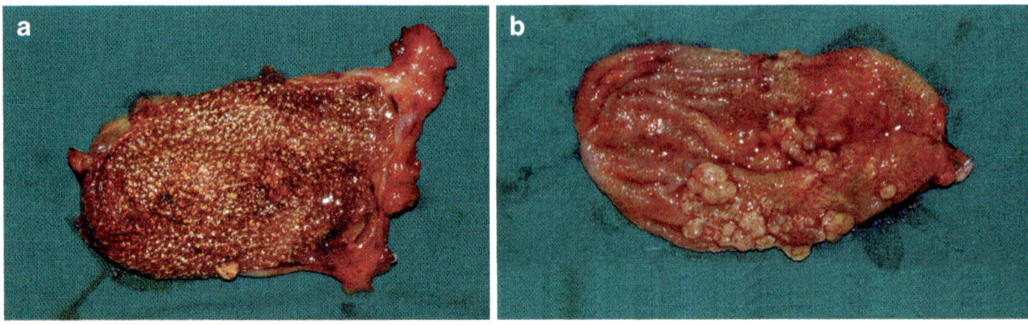

Fig. 30.1 (**a**) Cholesterol polyp, (**b**) gallbladder adenoma

because it is difficult to differentiate between adenoma and cholesterol polyps using the aforementioned method, cholecystectomy is indicated for polyps ≥10 mm.

30.1.3 Early-Stage Gallbladder Cancer

Although there is no clear definition, early-stage gallbladder cancer is considered to be the case when invasion of the cancer cells is restricted to the mucous membrane (T1a) or muscular layer (T1b) of the gallbladder. Current guidelines recommend laparotomy in patients with suspected gallbladder cancer based on preoperative evaluation. However, many recent studies have recommended simple cholecystectomy for T1-stage gallbladder cancer. Further, laparoscopic cholecystectomy has shown outcomes similar or superior to those of open cholecystectomy, and the former procedure has therefore gained popularity in the treatment of early-stage gallbladder cancer [1, 2].

In patients with T1a-stage gallbladder cancer, a five-year survival rate of 95–100%, along with a minor 1% relapse rate, can be achieved with simple cholecystectomy alone, thus avoiding the need for extended cholecystectomy. Lymphadenectomy is not recommended in patients with T1a-stage gallbladder cancer, as the rate of lymph node metastasis has been reported to be <2.5% [3].

There is no reliable evidence indicating that extended cholecystectomy, compared to simple cholecystectomy, would improve the survival rate of patients with T1b stage gallbladder cancer. Moreover, several studies have reported no difference in 5 year survival rates between patients who underwent laparoscopic cholecystectomy and those who underwent open surgery, suggesting that open cholecystectomy may not be necessary. However, a systematic literature review of studies that reported on T1b-stage gallbladder cancer identified a lymph node metastasis rate of approximately 10% and a relapse rate of 9–10%. Thus, lymphadenectomy can be recommended in patients without high operative risk, and this aspect will be discussed further in a later section [4, 5].

30.2 Surgical Techniques

30.2.1 Laparoscopic Cholecystectomy

30.2.1.1 Positioning of Patients

Patients should be placed in the supine position, as in traditional abdominal surgeries. The patient's left arm may be folded toward the body to prevent interference with the surgeon and the first assistant, who both perform the surgery while standing on the left side of the patient. After disinfecting and covering the patient with a surgical drape, the laparoscope is inserted through an incision either at the umbilicus or on the upper or lower side of the umbilicus, depending on the surgeon's preference. Next, the patient's head is turned upward by approximately

30° (in reverse Trendelenburg position), then the patient is turned to the left, which is the ideal position for laparoscopic cholecystectomy.

30.2.1.2 Incision and Trocar Insertion

As explained previously, an incision is made to insert the laparoscope. Different operators have different preferences for insertion, which can largely be divided into the incision method and the closed entry method. A 12-mm camera trocar is inserted either through the umbilicus or through vertical or transverse incisions on the upper or lower side of the umbilicus (Fig. 30.2a). While both methods have their own advantages, the author prefers the open method in which the trocar is inserted through the umbilicus. This technique obtains enhanced cosmetic results and enables the expansion of the incision to remove the gallbladder after the surgery.

After the laparoscope has been inserted through the first trocar, the surgeon should check for intra-abdominal adhesions and anatomical deformities, as well as the degree of inflammation in the gallbladder. Based on this assessment, the decision may be made to perform the surgery laparoscopically, after which the remaining trocars can be inserted.

Laparoscopic cholecystectomy is commonly performed using the four-port technique, wherein one 12-mm camera trocar and three 5-mm trocars are inserted. On the other hand, only two 5-mm trocars are inserted in the three-port technique, which has recently come to be widely adopted. Likewise, single-port cholecystectomy is also gaining popularity. However, the author usually performs laparoscopic cholecystectomy using the four-port technique, and only applies the single-port technique in selected patients (young women, nonobese patients, and those without severe inflammation). Therefore, the four-port technique, which is performed most commonly, will be discussed here.

The camera troca is inserted in umbilical port. And the second trocar is inserted at the upper-third position along the line between the umbilicus and xyphoid process, the third trocar is inserted 2 cm below the intercostal end along the midline of the right axilla, and the fourth trocar is inserted at the point where the lateral line passes the second trocar and the line below the papilla (Fig. 30.2b).

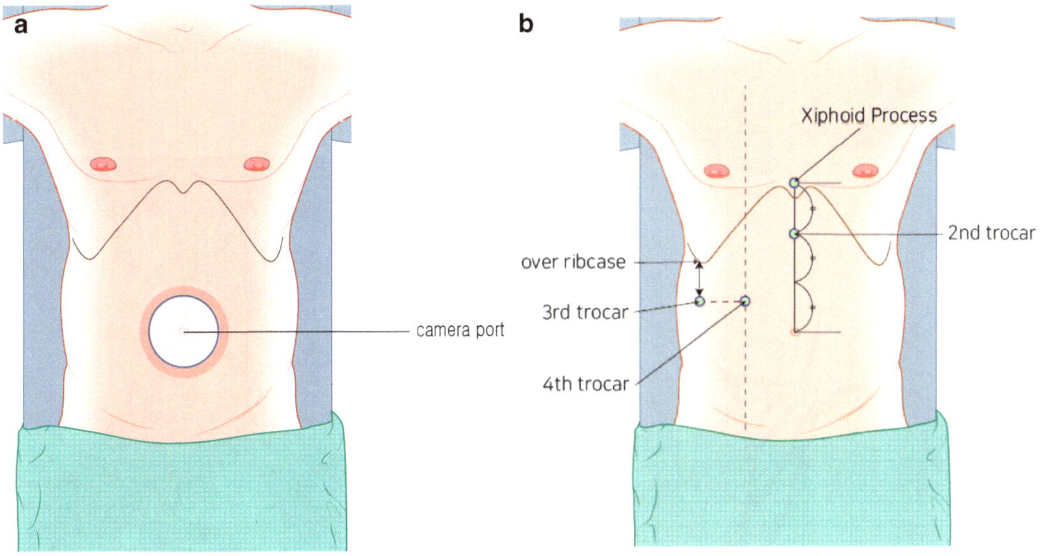

Fig. 30.2 (**a**) Position of the camera port trocar, (**b**) position of the working port trocar

30.2.1.3 Surgical Sequence

First, the surgeon should insert a grasper through the third trocar, then retract the fundus of the gallbladder to the 11-o'clock position of the patient (right side toward the head), and have the second assistant hold or fix it using a tool (Fig. 30.3a). The degree of retraction must be controlled to ensure adequate exposure of Calot's triangle. In some cases, the bottom part of the right liver may be adhered to the transverse colon or to Gerota's fascia, thereby interfering with retraction of the gallbladder. In such cases, the adhesions should first be separated to facilitate retraction of the gallbladder. Then, a hook or dissector attached to a monopolar surgical unit should be inserted through the second trocar, followed by the insertion of the grasper through the third trocar. At this point, it is important to pull the gallbladder toward the surgeon while holding the gallbladder neck with a grasper inserted through the fourth trocar (Fig. 30.3b). Most beginners perform the surgery by pushing the gallbladder backward, which

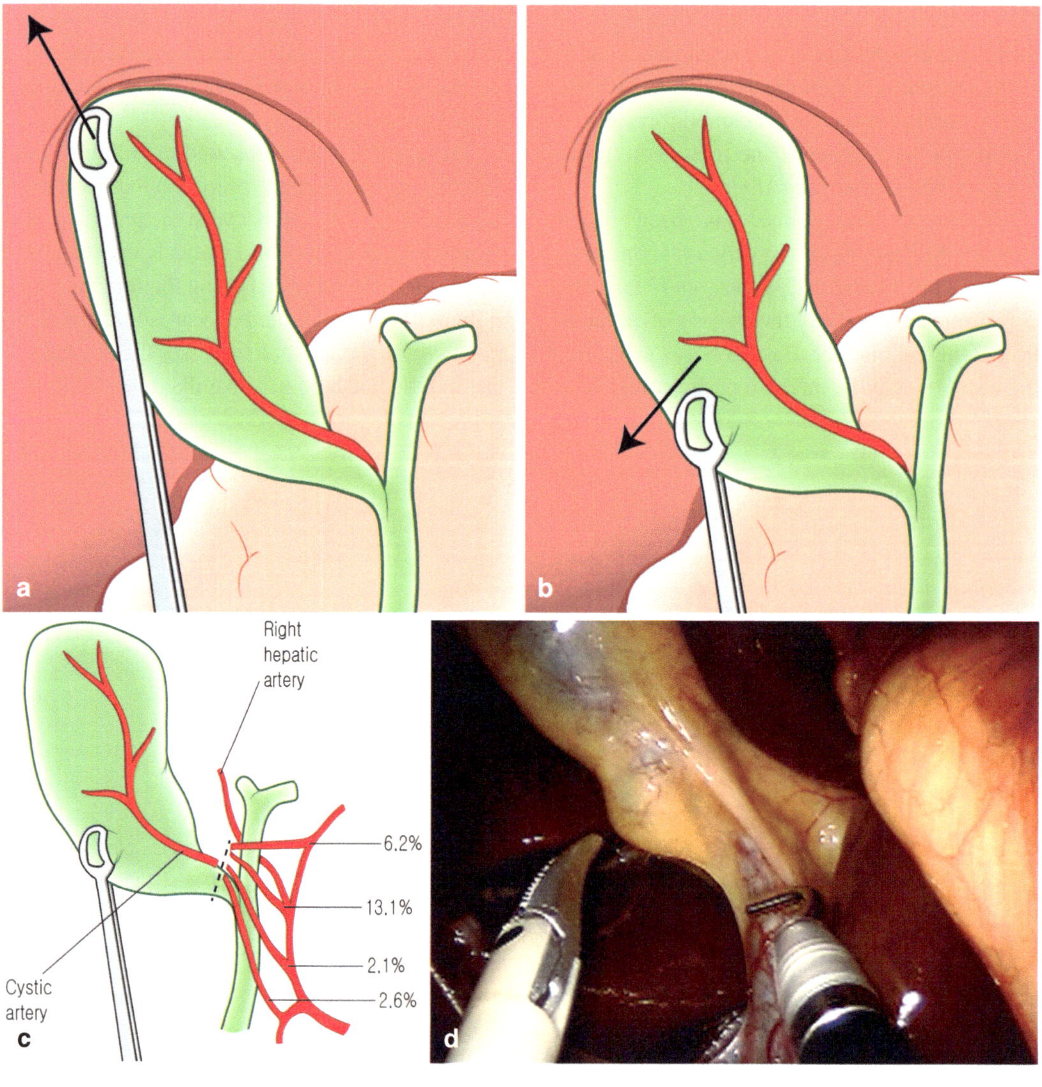

Fig. 30.3 (**a**) Retraction of the fundus of the gallbladder to the 11-o'clock position, (**b**) Pulling the gallbladder neck toward the surgeon to expose the Calot's triangle, (**c**) Resection of the cystic artery, (**d**) Robotic view of cholecystectomy

makes it difficult to expose the cystic duct, thus causing damage to the common bile duct. It is therefore important to assess the course of the common bile duct by examining Calot's triangle while pulling the cystic duct with the grasper. During the identification of the common bile duct, careful sublation of the connective and adipose tissues should begin from the region nearest to the gallbladder. The sublation of adipose tissues proximal to Calot's triangle would expose the cystic duct. The cystic duct is usually exposed from the right side of the patient such that the course of the cystic artery can be identified on the left side. However, in rare cases, the cystic artery may run along the cystic duct or exist on its right side, which should be considered during the surgery.

Following exposure, the cystic duct should be cut after ligation using a laparoscopic clip. The clip should not be placed too close to the common bile duct or while causing excessive retraction of the gallbladder, which could lead to combined ligation of a part of the common bile duct. Although this phenomenon is uncommon in patients with gallbladder polyps, gallstones may move into the cystic duct in some patients, thereby causing severe inflammation of the gallbladder, in turn leading to difficulty in ligating the duct. In such cases, the insertion of a thread or the use of loops enables ligation of the cystic duct. The gallbladder can be moved more easily after cutting the cystic duct, as doing so separates it from the common bile duct, thus facilitating ligation of the cystic artery. However, prior to ligation, it is important to evaluate whether the cystic artery enters the gallbladder. It must be noted that 50% of the patients only have one cystic artery, whereas the remaining 50% often have two or three cystic arteries (Fig. 30.3c).

Upon completion of the procedure in the cystic duct and artery, the gallbladder should be sublated from the liver using a hook with the right hand (the second trocar) while appropriately controlling retraction of the gallbladder with the left hand (the fourth trocar). The gallbladder can be sublated from the liver without any perforation of the gallbladder wall only when the thin membrane between the two structures is exposed though proper retraction with the left hand. Upon complete sublation of the gallbladder from the liver, the operator should insert a plastic bag, place the gallbladder in the bag, and remove it through the camera trocar, indicating completion of the surgery. The excised gallbladder must be dissected and the polyp morphology and mucous membrane of the gallbladder must be examined. In the event of a suspected malignancy, an emergent frozen section procedure must be performed.

30.2.2 Extended Cholecystectomy (Lymphadenectomy)

Here, we discuss lymphadenectomy for patients with early-stage gallbladder cancer (T1b or higher). At present, there is no consensus on the range of lymph node dissection in patients with early-stage gallbladder cancer. The seventh edition of the AJCC defined lymph nodes around hepatoduodenal ligaments, such as cystic duct, common bile duct, hepatic artery, and hepatic portal vein lymph nodes, as group 1 nodes (N1), while those around the pancreaticoduodenal, laparotid artery, mesenteric artery, main artery, and vena cava areas were defined as group 2 nodes (N2). Metastasis in N2 is interpreted as distant lymph node metastasis, leading to a classification of Stage 4 (IVB) cancer according to the TNM staging. As long-term survival cannot be expected in such cases, lymph node dissection is not generally recommended. However, the author includes the lymph nodes around the main artery during dissection in all patients with stage T1b or higher gallbladder cancer. There is no consensus regarding the minimum or appropriate number of lymph nodes that should be dissected to accurately determine the stage of cancer. The sixth edition of the AJCC stated that at least three lymph nodes should be evaluated for metastasis to accurately determine the N stage, but this criterion was removed in the seventh edition.

While lymphadenectomy can be performed using both open and laparoscopic surgery, the author prefers open surgery and employs the right subcostal incision. As lymphadenectomy for hepatoduodenal ligaments has been extensively discussed in the chapters on pancreaticoduodenectomy and hilar cholangiocarcinoma, this chapter does not include a detailed discussion of the same topic.

30.3 Conclusion

Laparoscopic cholecystectomy is a safe and widely used surgical method in patients with gallbladder polyps and early-stage gallbladder cancer, and it is a basic surgical technique for hepatopancreaticobiliary surgeons. Although it is relatively easier than those in the hepatopancreaticobiliary field, laparoscopic cholecystectomy can cause fatal complications if basic principles are not followed; therefore, surgeons should perform the procedure while exercising caution and the utmost safety.

References

1. Blumgart LH. Surgery of the liver, biliary tract and pancreas. 5th ed. Philadelphia: Saunders Elsevier; 2013.
2. Fisher JE. Hepatobiliary and pancreatic surgery. Philadelphia: Lippincott Williams & Wilkins; 2013.
3. Lee SE, Jang JY, Kim SW. The surgical strategy for treating T1 gallbladder cancer. Korean J Hepatobiliary pancreat Surg. 2009;13(2):69–75.
4. Lee SE, Jang JY, Lim CS, et al. Systematic review on the surgical treatment for T1 gallbladder cancer. World J Gastroenterol. 2011;17(2):174–80.
5. Eckel F, Brunner T, Jelic S, et al. ESMO clinical practice guidelines for diagnosis, treatment and follow-up. Ann Oncol. 2011;22(6):40–4.

31 Extended Cholecystectomy (Wedge Resection)

Kim Wan-Joon and Kim Wan-Bae

Abstract

Gallbladder cancer (GBC) is known to have a poor prognosis, and curative radical resection is the gold standard treatment. The factors affecting the prognosis of GBC include depth of tumor invasion and lymph node metastasis, warranting proper hepatic resection and lymphadenectomy.

Several studies have reported that T1 GBC has a good prognosis with simple cholecystectomy alone. Gallbladder cancers T2 and above are still referred to extended cholecystectomy (Kim et al., Cancer Control. 27:2020).

This chapter describes extended cholecystectomy including liver wedge resection and regional lymphadenectomy.

Keywords

Gallbladder cancer · Hepatic resection
Regional lymphadenectomy · Survival rate
Laparoscopic-extended cholecystectomy

Supplementary Information The online version contains supplementary material available at https://doi.org/10.1007/978-981-16-1996-0_31.

K. Wan-Joon (✉) · K. Wan-Bae
Division of Hepato-Biliary-Pancreas Surgery, Department of Surgery, Korea University Guro Hospital, Korea University Medical College, Seoul, South Korea

31.1 Surgical Procedure

The surgical procedure in extended cholecystectomy via open approach is as follows.

31.1.1 Kocherization

In the newly published eighth edition of AJCC TNM staging, the regional lymph nodes harvested during gallbladder cancer surgery were #8, #12a, and #12p. To predict the progression and prognosis of cancer, the author harvested the peri-aortic lymph node #16 after exposure to the aorta via kocherization (Fig. 31.1).

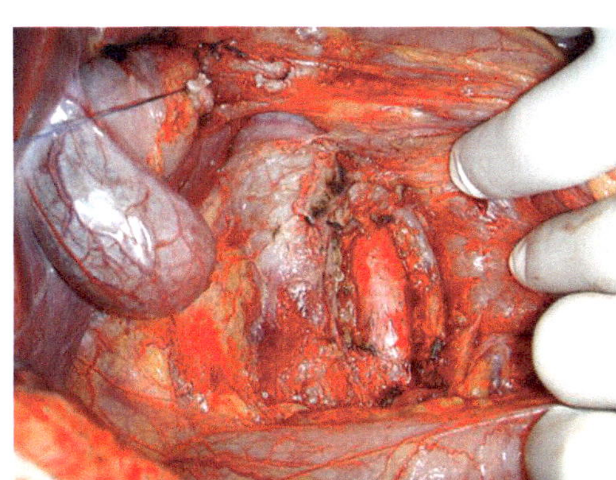

Fig. 31.1 Aortic lymph node dissection

H. C. Yu (ed.), *Hepato-Biliary-Pancreatic Surgery and Liver Transplantation*,
https://doi.org/10.1007/978-981-16-1996-0_31

31.1.2 Dissection of Cystic Duct and Execution of Frozen Biopsy of Cyst Duct Margin

The cystic duct is dissected from the bile duct and divided in order to determine the need for common bile duct (CBD) resection. Frozen biopsy is performed after securing the cystic duct margin from CBD side.

In principle, when cancerous lesion is detected in the cystic duct margin, CBD resection must be performed concomitantly.

After ligation and division of the cystic artery, the gallbladder neck is separated from the surrounding tissue to locate the gallbladder as far away as possible from the hepatoduodenal ligament.

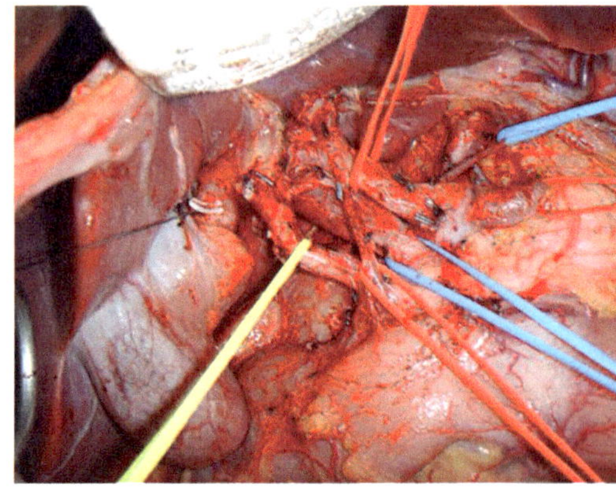

Fig. 31.2 Regional lymphadenectomy (yellow loop: common bile duct, red loop: proper hepatic artery (upper left); right gastric artery (lower left); splenic artery (right), blue loop: portal vein (lower left); left gastric vein (upper right)

31.1.3 Regional Lymphadenectomy

After adequate Kocherization, lymphadenectomy is performed starting with the lymph node #13, located between the common bile duct and the pancreatic head, extending over the liver along the bile duct. The author harvests lymph nodes #8, #12a, #12p, and #13 during lymphadenectomy. Upon completion of lymph node harvesting at the right side of portal vein, the left edge of the hepatoduodenal ligament is opened, and the lymph node is dissected until the left edge of the portal vein is identified.

After confirming the left edge of portal vein, the lymph node that was previously dissected along the right side of portal vein is rotated behind the portal vein to perform lymph node en bloc resection. During lymphadenectomy, the main vessels are tagged with a vessel loop to prevent injury (Fig. 31.2).

31.1.4 Hepatic Resection

Liver mobilization is not always necessary for hepatic wedge resection.

However, if the falciform ligament is cut and a part of the right coronary ligament and the right triangular ligament is incised, the movement of the liver becomes easier and the surgery more convenient. There is no international consensus, but the width of liver resection in wedge resection is generally recommended to be 2–3 cm.

In order to prevent cancer spreading, the gallbladder and liver are excised en bloc. In order to ensure sufficient liver resection, it is important to consider the extent of liver resection when you first start wedge resection.

To ensure adequate width between the gallbladder and the liver resection site, the liver cut surface is made concave shape. To reduce the bleeding level during liver resection, the Pringle technique is used intermittently as needed. The author uses a method of blocking the blood flow for 15 min and reperfusion for 5 min.

Because the terminal end of middle hepatic vein (MHV), V5 vein, and Glissonean pedicle of hepatic segments 4 and 5 appear during liver resection, the above structures are carefully ligated and separated (Fig. 31.3).

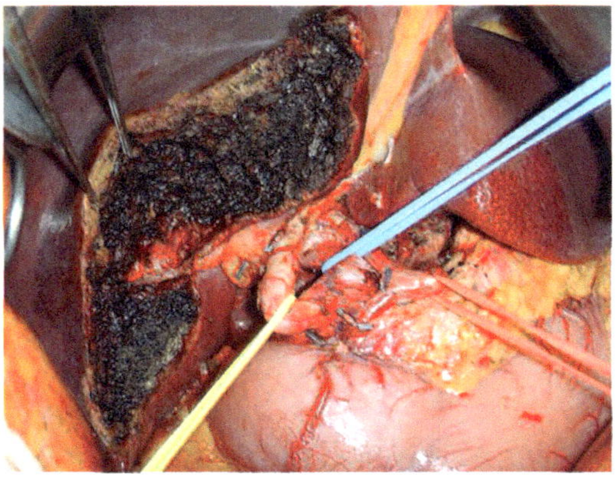

Fig. 31.3 Images after extended cholecystectomy

31.2 Laparoscopic-Extended Cholecystectomy in Gallbladder Cancer

Advances in laparoscopic surgery techniques have led to laparoscopic approaches targeting the biliary system. In the case of GBC, the focus of laparoscopic-extended cholecystectomy is on patients at early-stage GBC (T1 or T2), incidental GBC, and patients with strong suspicion of negative cystic duct margin [1, 2].

The caveats in the laparoscopic approach are that the resection margin cannot be secured due to the unexpected tumor extension and inadequate lymphadenectomy compared to the open approach. There is no consensus on the minimum or appropriate number of harvested lymph nodes required to determine the correct stage. According to the eighth edition of AJCC, at least six lymph node harvests are required to determine the appropriate N stage. Appropriate laparoscopic-extended cholecystectomy can be performed only by improving the proficiency of various techniques such as liver resection, lymph node dissection, and hepaticojejunostomy [3, 4].

References

1. Choi KS, Choi SB, Park P, Kim WB, Choi SY. Clinical characteristics of incidental or unsuspected gallbladder cancers diagnosed during or after cholecystectomy: a systematic review and meta-analysis. World J Gastroenterol. 2015;21(4):1315–23. https://doi.org/10.3748/wjg.v21.i4.1315.
2. Han HS, Yoon YS, Agarwal AK, Belli G, Itano O, Gumbs AA, et al. Laparoscopic surgery for gallbladder cancer: an expert consensus statement. Dig Surg. 2019;36(1):1–6. https://doi.org/10.1159/000486207.
3. Kim HS, Park JW, Kim H, Han Y, Kwon W, Kim SW, et al. Optimal surgical treatment in patients with T1b gallbladder cancer: an international multicenter study. J Hepatobiliary Pancreat Sci. 2018;25(12):533–43. https://doi.org/10.1002/jhbp.593.
4. Kim WJ, Lim TW, Park PJ, Choi SB, Kim WB. Clinicopathological differences in T2 gallbladder cancer according to tumor location. Cancer Control. 2020;27(1):1073274820915514. https://doi.org/10.1177/1073274820915514.

Extended Cholecystectomy (Including Segment IVb and V Resection)

32

Sang-Jae Park

Abstract

Extended cholecystectomy in advanced gallbladder cancer (T2 or higher stage) entails liver resection, although the need for liver resection in T1b GB cancer is disputed. The extent of liver resection is determined by the location, gross type and extent of tumor, and patient's general and liver conditions. Theoretically, extended cholecystectomy including anatomic liver resection with segment IVb and V eliminates potential micrometastasis during venous drainage from gallbladder cancer; however, no randomized controlled studies have demonstrated the potential advantage. Two types of anatomic approach including separate ligation of portal triad (portal vein, hepatic artery, and bile duct) and ligation of Glisson pedicles can be used. I prefer anatomic IVb + V resection via Glisson approach. As the perfect anatomic IVb + V resection is technically complicated, I would like to introduce modified anatomic IVb + V resection, which is simple, safe, and fast.

Keywords

Cholecystectomy · Extended cholecystectomy · Gallbladder cancer · Anatomic resection · Hepatectomy · Lymph node dissection

32.1 Operation

32.1.1 Patient's Position and Diagnostic Laparoscopy (Fig. 32.1)

Supine position is usually recommended.

Diagnostic laparoscopy is recommended for the detection of metastasis missed in the preoperative workup. I applied 2–3 trocars along the midline and evaluated the liver surface, the great omentum, parietal peritoneum, serosa, and pelvic cavity in the counter-clockwise direction and used laparoscopic ultrasound to identify the liver metastasis. The ascites are aspirated; otherwise, 500 mL of normal saline is into the abdominal cavity and aspirated 5 min later for cytology examination.

32.1.2 Incision

Various incisions including inverted L incision, Mercedes-Benz incision (⊥ incision), or midline

S.-J. Park (✉)
Center for Liver and Pancreatobiliary Cancer, National Cancer Center, Goyang-Si, Gyeonggi-Do, South Korea
e-mail: spark@ncc.re.kr

H. C. Yu (ed.), *Hepato-Biliary-Pancreatic Surgery and Liver Transplantation*,
https://doi.org/10.1007/978-981-16-1996-0_32

incision can be used according to the operator's preference. I prefer upper midline incision and occasionally extend to below umbilicus. Next, I used the self-retractors and carefully evaluated possible metastasis.

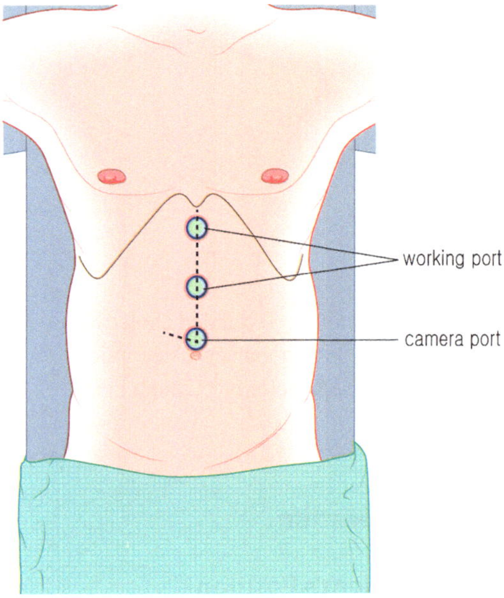

Fig. 32.1 Position of ports in diagnostic laparoscoy

32.1.3 Examination of the Resection Margin of Cystic Duct

First, the frozen biopsy of resection margin of cystic duct is examined, but common bile duct resection is used in case of positive resection margin of cystic duct or lymph node metastasis/perineural invasion in hepatoduodenal ligament. In this chapter, I will explain the case against resection of common bile duct. The cystic artery is resected after confirming the negative resection margin of cystic duct.

32.1.4 Kocher Maneuver and Lymph Node Dissection (Lymph Node Group #13a, 8, 12) (Fig. 32.2)

I do Kocher maneuver for full mobilization of duodenum to remove the LN group #13a from pancreas head, followed by LN dissection upward to hepatoduodenal ligament to remove #13a, 12, 8. Lymph node dissection mostly represents dissection of hepatic artery (common hepatic artery, proper hepatic artery, and right and left hepatic artery) from adjacent soft tissue. For this, I open

Fig. 32.2 Kocher maneuver for lymph node dissection of group #13a, 8, 12

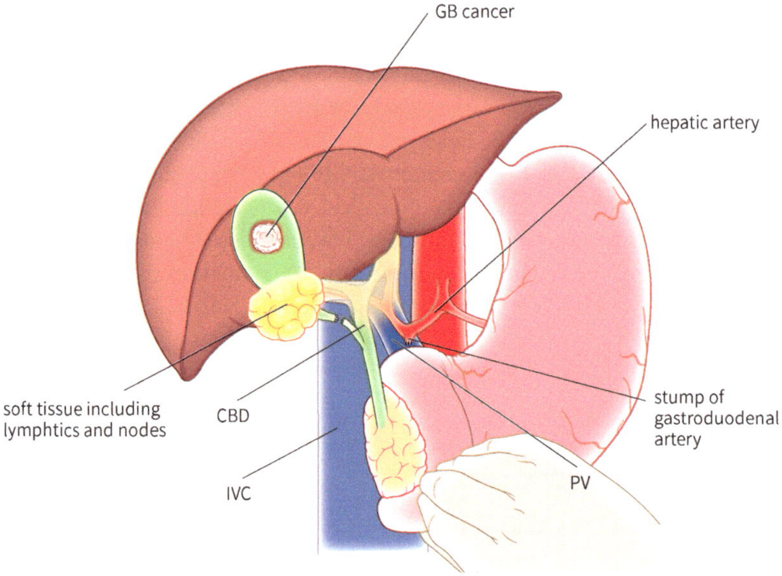

the nerve plexus and incise along the upper part of hepatic artery and mobilize the right- and left-sided soft tissues to the right and the left of hepatic artery. I dissect and cut the right hepatic artery from its origin. I sometimes dissect and cut the gastroduodenal artery (GDA) from its origin for more complete lymph node dissection, which mostly does not harm the blood flow to liver, pancreas, and duodenum. But we should always be very cautious in cutting gastroduodenal artery, which may attenuate hepatic blood flow in very rare cases such as median arcuate ligament syndrome. Therefore, after transient clamping of GDA, you should determine the hepatic blood flow before cutting the GDA. Skeletalization of hepatic artery is followed by skeletalization of portal vein using the same method of incision of the soft tissue along the upper part of portal vein and mobilization of the right-sided soft tissue to the right side and the left-sided soft tissue to the left side of the portal vein. Finally, all the soft tissue around pancreas head, hepatoduodenal ligament, and common hepatic artery are moved from the right to the left side beneath the portal vein, and removed from the right side of the portal vein.

32.1.5 Liver Mobilization

Liver mobilization is not necessary for anatomic IVb + V resection; however, partial mobilization of falciform ligament, coronary ligament, and right triangular ligament can facilitate safe operation. No dissection of the right adrenal gland and IVC ligament is needed.

32.1.6 Dissection of Glisson Pedicle (Right Glisson and Right Anterior Glisson Pedicle) for the Determination of Right Resection Line (Fig. 32.3)

I perform conventional Glisson approach to dissect right Glisson pedicle and right anterior Glisson pedicle. I clamp the right anterior Glisson pedicle and determine the line of the discolored area. Ultrasound examination is performed to evaluate the right and middle hepatic vein without injuring the right hepatic vein during the resection of segment V. The eventual right resection line of segment IVb + V resec-

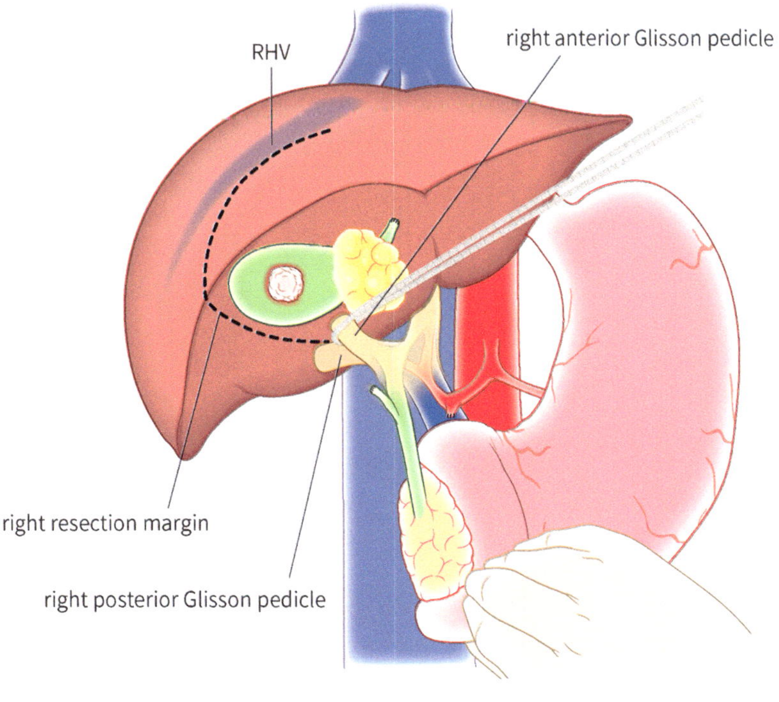

Fig. 32.3 Determination of right resection line

tion is determined by the right side of discolored segment V and also the right side of the right hepatic vein.

32.1.7 Determination of Left and Superior Resection Lines (Fig. 32.4)

Liver resection can be easily initiated along the left resection line (between segment IVb and II/III), which is the left resection line of segment IVb and V resection. IVb Glisson can be dissected and cut from its origin in the left Glisson pedicle. Anatomy of segment IV Glisson is diverse and several Glisson pedicles meet at segments IVa and IVb, and therefore, it is sometimes difficult to discriminate between the two pedicles at these segments. Clamping each pedicle can reveal whether each pedicle is intended for segment IVa or IVb. A transverse line in the middle of segment IV is drawn to demarcate the unclear border between IVa and IV. This line extends to the anterior section as the border of segments V and VIII, which is the superior resection line.

During the resection of liver along the left resection line, caution is needed during the resection of liver along the right resection line to avoid injury to the right hepatic vein. Next, the superior resection line is resected to a depth of 2–3 cm, followed by dissection of the liver toward the lower margin of anterior Glisson pedicle. Multiple resection of right anterior Glisson can be performed without injuring the segment VIII Glisson pedicle, followed by deeper liver resection between segments V and VIII. When the resection is deeper and the resected segment is retracted downward, the border between segments V and VIII is clearer,

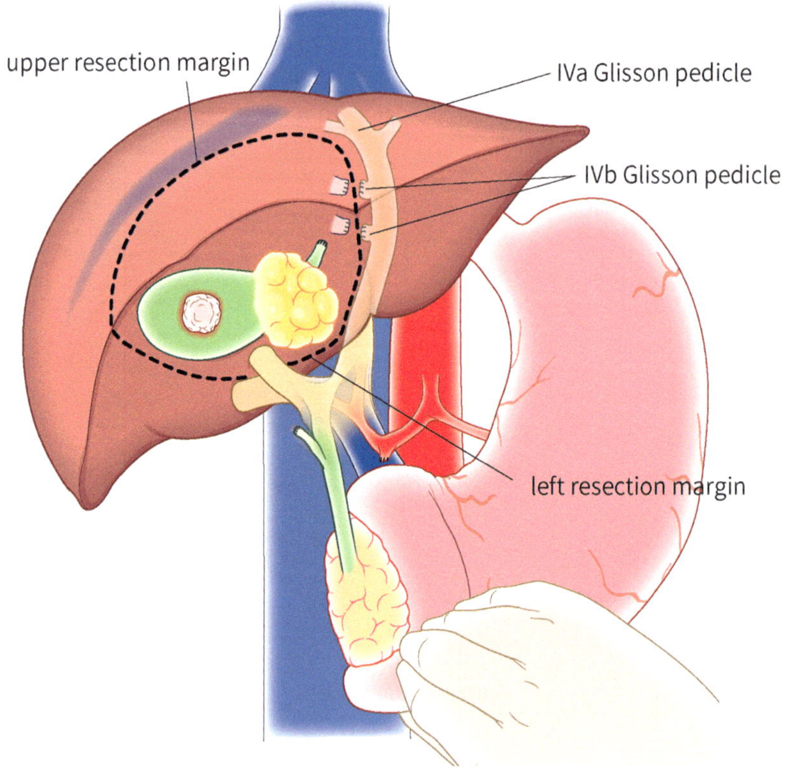

Fig. 32.4 Determination of left and superior resection lines

which enables identification of the remnant Glisson pedicle V for safe ligation. The specimen can be removed.

32.1.8 Management of Liver Cut Surface

Management of liver cut surface is based on the principles of conventional liver resection.

Further Reading

Kim SW, Suh KS. Hepatopancreatobiliary surgery. 3rd ed; 2013.

Korean Society of Surgery. Atlas of Surgery. 2014;156:1278.

Belghiti J, Jarnagin WR, DeMatteo RP, et al. Surgery of the liver, biliary tract and pancreas, 4th ed. 2006.

Part V

Resection of Choledochal Cyst

Open Resection of Chledochal Cyst 33

Kuk Hwan Kwon and Jin Ho Lee

Abstract

Choledochal cyst is a relatively rare disease and is predominantly found in Asian women. The treatment involves complete surgical removal of the cyst, followed by bilioenteric anastomosis. Recent developments in minimally invasive surgery and laparoscopic choledochal cyst excision are gradually increasing. However, open choledochal cyst excision, which has been traditionally performed, is the most basic treatment for choledochal cyst.

Keywords

Adult · Choledochal cyst · Perioperative management · Surgical management

Supplementary Information The online version contains supplementary material available at https://doi.org/10.1007/978-981-16-1996-0_33.

K. H. Kwon (✉)
Department of Surgery, National Health Insurance Service Ilsan Hospital,
Goyang-si, Gyeonggi-do, South Korea

J. H. Lee
Division of HepatoBilioPancreas Surgery,
Department of Surgery, National Health Insurance Service Ilsan Hospital,
Goyang-si, Gyeonggi-do, South Korea
e-mail: jhlee75@nhimc.or.kr

33.1 Introduction

Choledochal cyst is a relatively rare disease constituting approximately 1% of all benign diseases of bile duct. Its incidence, although as high as 1:1000 in the Asian population, is only 1:100000 to 1:150000 in the Western populations. A preponderance of choledochoal cyst disease is observed, especially in Asian women [1]. The etiology and pathogenesis of choledochal cysts are unknown, as the disease is attributed to anomalous pancreaticobiliary duct union (APBDU), but not in all adult cases [2]. The causal relationship between choledochlal cyst and biliary cancer has yet to be clearly identified. However, the causes include recurrent inflammation caused by the reflux of pancreatic enzymes into bile duct or bile stasis, superinfection, repeated cholangitis, or the conversion of bile salt into carcinogens by chronic infections [3]. Clinically, eight types of classification (Fig. 33.1) by Todani are used clinically and the treatment methods vary according to the classification [4]. The surgical approaches used in patients undergoing primary resection include the following: cholecystectomy, cyst excision, and Roux-en-Y hepaticojejunostomy for Todani types I and IVa; cyst excision and duodenal repair for Todani type III; and cholecystectomy and hepatectomy for Todani type V. In the present study, all type V patients carried intrahepatic lesions located in the left liver. In order to preserve liver function

H. C. Yu (ed.), *Hepato-Biliary-Pancreatic Surgery and Liver Transplantation*,
https://doi.org/10.1007/978-981-16-1996-0_33

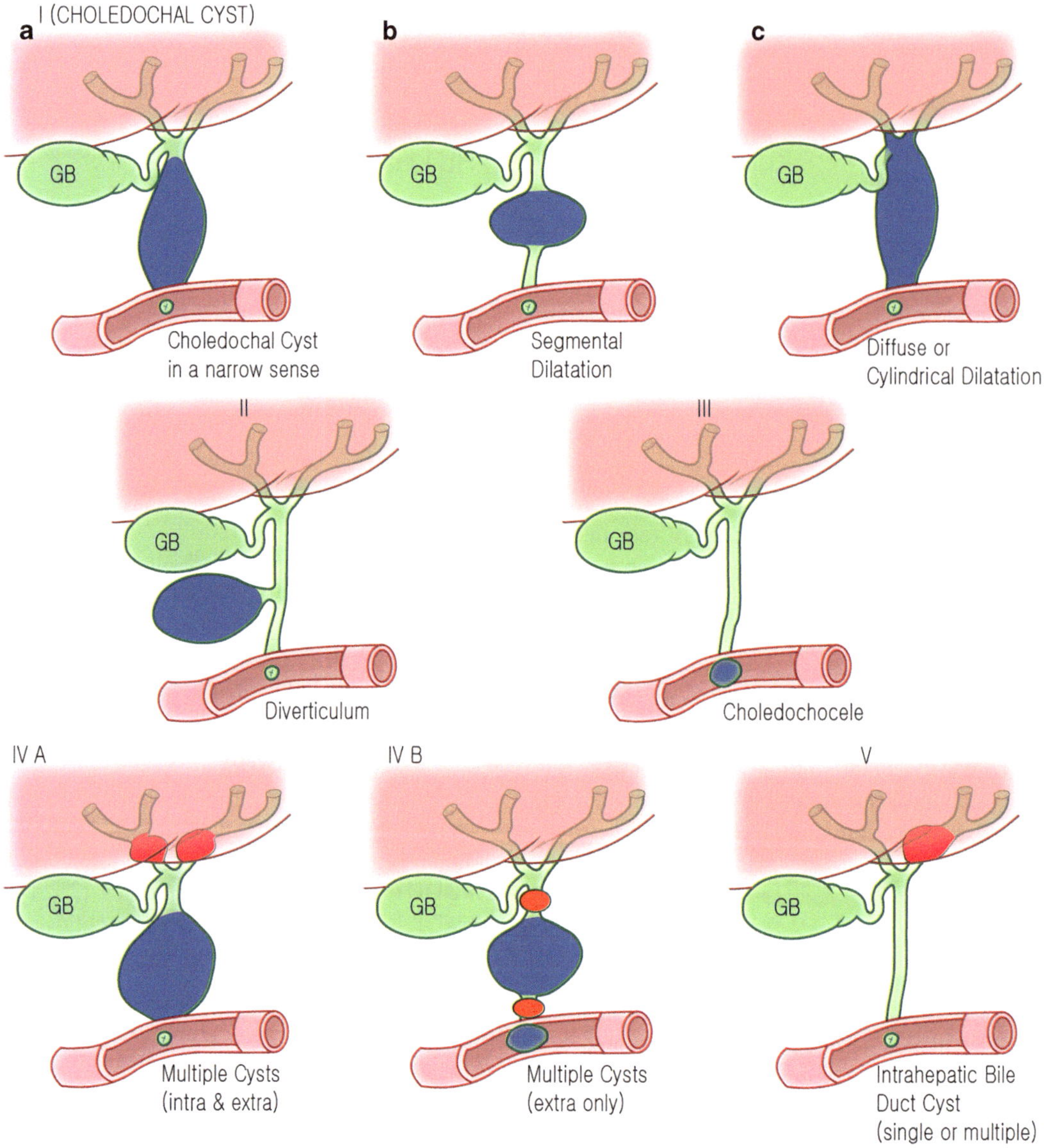

Fig. 33.1 (**a**) Choledochal cyst in a narrow sense (**b**) Segmental dilatation (**c**) Diffuse or cylindrical dilatation

and ensure accurate hepaticojejunostomy, only left hepatectomy was performed [5]. In this section, we will discuss the choledochal cysts in adult cases, mainly seen in the field of hepatobiliary pancreas, and especially focus on the most common disease types (types I and IVb), showing similar clinical manifestations.

33.2 Diagnosis

Most of the choledochal cysts are found in children, but approximately 20% of cases are diagnosed in adults [6]. Choledochal cysts are found in adults incidentally, but during the diagnosis of complications such as cholangitis, pancreatitis, bile duct stones, and malignant changes. It can be diagnosed via imaging tests such as abdominal ultrasound, abdominal computed tomography, magnetic resonance cholangio-pancreatography (MRCP), and endoscopic retrograde cholangio-pancreatography (ERCP) and also confirms the anatomical structure during surgery [7].

33.3 Treatment Before Surgery

The goal of preoperative treatment is to treat inflammation in cholangitis, and to enable precise imaging of the entire choledochal cyst including the pancreaticobiliary duct union or the intrahepatic bile duct, and to determine the bile duct pathology associated with image. Cholangitis accompanied by choledochal cysts warrants conservative treatments such as the usage of effective intravenous antibiotics. However, if the antibiotics are still not effective, percutaneous or endoscopic choledochal cyst drainage is necessary to completely treat sepsis caused by cholangitis before radical surgery. Imaging modalities such as MRCP or ERCP are needed to avoid pancreatic duct damage during surgery, to determine the length of the narrow segment under the choledochal cyst precisely and ascertain the positional relationship between the main pancreatic duct and the choledochal cyst. Also, before surgery, it is necessary to determine whether the intrahepatic bile duct is stenotic or accompanied by choledochal cyst and biliary tract cancer. Stenosis of the intrahepatic bile duct requires excision of the bile duct from the upper stenotic segment. Concurrent choledochal cyst and biliary tract cancer warrant treatment plan similar to cancer treatment. In particular, for patients with repeated symptoms after surgery related to choledochal cyst in the past, it is necessary to determine the presence of strictures at the anastomotic site, bile duct stones, accompanying malignant diseases, liver cirrhosis, and portal hypertension.

33.4 Treatment

Surgical resection is the definitive treatment for choledochal cyst [4]. Surgery is recommended immediately after diagnosis rather than observation because the incidence of biliary cancer increases over time [8]. The surgical management for adults with choledochal cyst is based on the type of choledochal cyst and the presence of associated hepatobiliary pathology. The general principle is to completely excise the choledochal cyst, followed by mucosa-to-mucosa bilioenteric anastomosis. After the resection of the choledochal cyst, bilioenteric anastomosis can be accompanied by Roux-en-Y hepaticojejunostomy or choledochoduodenostomy. However, it is relatively easy in the case of choledochoduodenostomy, but severe complications such as stump syndrome may occur. In general, we follow the standard procedure, which is complete surgical resection of the choledochal cyst and the Roux-en-Y hepaticojejunostomy. If it is not possible to completely resect choledochal cyst, we may consider an alternative surgical option, which is Roux-en-Y cystojejunostomy after maximally excising the choledochal cyst.

However, any stricture in the upper bile ducts warrants excision of the choledochal cyst including the area with stricture, because lack of proper treatment for bile duct stricture may result in complications such as cholangitis, bile duct stone, and cancer. In the past, internal drainage was performed, but the rate of cancer incidence in the case of internal drainage was up to 50% of the rate in surgical patients, which was higher than in those without surgical treatment. In addition, internal drainage induces anastomotic site stenosis, which leads to repeated cholangitis [9]. Accordingly, internal drainage was not performed in recent years. Therefore, with a history of internal drainage warrants radical surgery. Minimally invasive surgeries, such as laparoscopic surgery [10] or robotic surgery [11], have shown remarkable treatment results. In particular, considering the nature of the disease, which is frequent in young women, minimally invasive surgery is expected to become popular in the future. However, additional surgical evaluation is needed to consider minimally invasive surgery as a new standard. Therefore, the first step entails investigation of the role of conventional open surgery for the treatment of choledochal cysts.

33.5 Treatment of Choledochal Cysts Other Than Type I and IVb

In the case of APBDU, bile duct resection is the standard of treatment since the incidence of bile duct cancer increases due to reflux of pancreatic fluid in the bile ducts. In the absence of APBDU, the treatment strategy is to perform surgery to prevent cholestasis. In the absence of conjunctival malformation, surgery to prevent cholestasis is required. In the case of type II, treatment can be performed simply by resecting the diverticulum, which does not require excising the entire extrahepatic duct. In case of type III, treatment in most cases entails endoscopic sphincterectomy except for large cysts warranting surgical resection. In case of type IVa, choledochal cyst excision and hepaticojejunostomy should be widely performed. However, in case of intrahepatic involvement of the cystic lesion with symptoms, such as intrahepatic duct stone, cholangitis, liver cirrhosis, hepatic resection is indicated at the same time as resection for type V. If liver resection is not possible due to extensive intrahepatic involvement of the cystic lesion, liver transplantation should be considered.

33.6 Things to Know before Surgery

According to Lipsett et al., factors to be considered when performing surgery on patients with biliary cystic disease include the following: (1) age, (2) presenting symptoms, (3) cyst type, (4) associated biliary stones, (5) prior biliary surgery, (6) intrahepatic strictures, (7) atrophy/hypertrophy, (8) biliary cirrhosis, (9) portal hypertension, and (10) associated biliary malignancy. In general, regardless of age, presenting symptoms, biliary stones, prior surgery, or other secondary problems, surgery should include cholecystectomy and excision of extrahepatic cyst(s) [12].

1. If cholangitis is accompanied choledochal cyst, conservative treatment using effective intravenous antibiotics should be performed. If there is no improvement in cholangitis with antibiotic treatment alone, percutaneous or endoscopic choledochal cyst drainage should be performed before surgery to completely treat sepsis caused by cholangitis, followed by radical surgery.
2. To avoid injury to the pancreatic ducts in the thinning area of pancreaticobiliary ductal junction, it is particularly important a thorough knowledge of the anatomy between bile duct and ampulla of Vater is essential based on preoperative direct or indirect cholangiography. Before surgery, CT or MRI should be performed to investigate the extent of intrahepatic involvement of choledochal cyst, and simultaneous hepatic resection is indicated if a wide range of choledochal cysts confined to one lobe are identified. Also, the possibility of accompanying malignant lesions should always be borne in mind, and surgical plans should be established if there are cancerous findings such as weight loss, jaundice, tumor marker elevation, mass lesions, or mural nodules in the cyst.
3. If choledochal cyst is found during cholecystectomy, cholangiography should be performed during the surgery to evaluate the structure of the bile ducts.
4. Anatomy of the liver, bile duct, pancreas, and portal vein should be clearly elucidated for safe surgery. In particular, the following anatomical knowledge is important and must be known.
   (a) Hilar bile duct confluence is typically located in front of the right portal vein.
   (b) Hepatic artery is located in the left posterior of the choledochal cyst, and the left and right branches are raised to the liver

in front of the portal vein. The right hepatic artery is located primarily behind the choledochal cyst, where the gallbladder artery is initiated (Calot triangle).

(c) If the right hepatic artery originates from the SMA, it is located behind the choledochal cyst until it enters the Calot triangle and then the liver from the posterior lateral direction along the right side of the common bile duct.

(d) Usually, the portal vein is distorted in the hepatoduodenal ligament by the huge choledochal cyst, suggesting the need for care.

(e) Inflammatory adhesion based on recurrent cholangitis and pancreatitis prior to surgery should be evaluated depending on hepatic artery and portal vein damage due to inflammation around the choledochal cystitis during severe detachment, and it is important to evaluate the portal vein to avoid damage. Lilly et al. suggested that in the case of severe pericystic inflammation, the posterior side of the cyst wall remains intact so as not to damage the portal vein and hepatic artery during efforts such as cyst resection [13].

(f) The distal end of CBD directly enters the pancreatic inferior posterior and forms a short segment before entering the pancreatic parenchyma, or externally on the pancreas in the posterior groove.

(g) In particular, in order to avoid unexpected bleeding and damage to the bile ducts, it is necessary to determine the relationship between the bile duct, the right hepatic artery, and the cystic artery, which show frequent variations.

33.7 Surgical Technique

1. The right subcostal incision method is the most frequently used method for abdominal incision, and when the cyst is large, the midline incision or partial chevron method ensures adequate exposure.
2. Cholecystectomy is performed via top-down method, and the cystic artery is identified in the infundibulum area by gallbladder traction, followed by ligation and resection. If necessary, intraoperative cholangiograms are performed or amylase and lipase concentrations in the choledochal cyst are measured, and bile in the cyst is collected for microbial culture.
3. Duodenal mobilization is performed via Kocher maneuver.
4. The front of the choledochal cyst is evaluated by carefully dissecting the hepatoduodenal ligament along the left side of the bile duct and by incising the upper edge of the duodenum. The circumference of the choledochal cyst is carefully encircled with a vascular loop or umbilical tape, and then, the vascular loop or umbilical tape is pulled to expose the portal vein.
5. During the exfoliation of the portion of pancreatic parenchyma, careful dissection is essential to avoid damage to the pancreatic duct. In addition, small blood vessels must be ligated during surgery to decrease the risk of bleeding in the biliary plexus.
6. When the bile duct suddenly narrows a few mm away from the replaced area of the ductal confluence and the normal diameter of the bile duct is exposed, a 3–0 or 4–0 absorbable suture is used to suture ligation and resection.
7. Then, the bile duct sac is pulled upward and carefully separated from the lower hepatic artery and portal vein before proceeding to the left and the right confluence of the liver. At this time, when the end of the bile duct sac emerges, it is excised from the upper part of the bile duct. In adults, cholangitis is frequent, and repeated internal inflammation is difficult to eliminate from the posterior vessels. In some cases, internal cyst dissection (Lilly surgery) is performed by excising either the anterior or the posterior part alone, with residual posterior wall mucosa. Due to the possibility of cancer, the Lilly surgery is not performed widely.

8. If malignancy is suspected, frozen biopsy is indicated. If malignancy is established, the surgical margin should be excised until negative, followed by radical lymph node dissection.
9. The transverse colon is tracted upward to evaluate the Treitz ligament, and the jejunum is prepared for Roux-en-Y hepaticojejunostomy. The end of the Roux limb is closed in two layers and placed in the hepatic hilum to develop anastomosis by passing a window through the transverse colon and then to the right of the middle colon artery.
10. Hepaticojejunostomy is performed via end-to-side anastomosis. At this time, the bilioenteric anastomosis should be enlarged to prevent anastomotic stenosis. There are several methods to develop anastomosis, which can be adapted to your needs. In general, 4–0 or 5–0 absorbable sutures can be used for anastomosis in a single layer. When the diameter of the bile duct is greater than 1 cm, the posterior wall is continuously sutured, and the anterior wall suture is interrupted. When the diameter of the bile duct is more than 1.5 cm, both walls can be sutured continuously.
11. Subsequently, more than 40 cm Roux limb and jejunojejunostomy are performed to complete the operation.
12. The drain tube is placed around the anastomotic site in hepaticojejunostomy and the abdominal wound is closed to complete the operation.

33.8 Results

Surgery for choledochal cyst has been successfully performed in more than 90%, and postoperative complications are reported to range from 2.5 to 27% and mortality rates from 0 to 6%. Early complications include anastomotic leakage, postoperative bleeding, acute pancreatitis, ileus, gastrointestinal bleeding, and postoperative pancreatic fistula. Late complications include anastomotic stenosis, peptic ulcer, cholangitis, bile duct or intrahepatic duct stones, pancreatitis, liver failure, and cancer. Even though bile duct cancers develop in up to 6% of patients undergoing surgery after choledochal cyst excision, the etiology of bile duct cancer is attributed to remnant choledochal cysts or a history of subclinical malignancy. Therefore, postoperative cancer incidence requires a re-evaluation of the current operation. Due to the possibility of anastomotic stenosis or bile duct cancer, all surgical patients require ultrasound and liver function tests as well as regular follow-up testing for tumor markers such as CA 19–9, CEA, and CA 125.

References

1. Singham J, Schaeffer D, Yoshida E, Scudamore C. Choledochal cysts: analysis of disease pattern and optimal treatment in adult and Paediatric patients. HPB. 2007;9(5):383. https://doi.org/10.1080/13651820701646198.
2. Babbitt DP. Congenital Choledochal cysts: new etiological concept based on anomalous relationships of the common bile duct and pancreatic bulb. Ann Radiol. 1969;12(3):231–40.
3. Funabiki T, Sugiue K, Matsubara T, Amano H, Ochiai M. Bile acids and biliary carcinoma in Pancreaticobiliary Maljunction. Keio J Med. 1991;40(3):118–22. https://doi.org/10.2302/kjm.40.118.
4. Todani T, Watanabe Y, MitsuoNarusue KT, KunioOkajima. Congenital bile duct cysts: classification, operative procedures, and review of thirty-seven cases including cancer arising from Choledochal cyst. Am J Surg. 1977;134(2):263–9. https://doi.org/10.1016/0002-9610(77)90359-2. http://www.sciencedirect.com/science/article/pii/0002961077903592
5. Wu, Xin, Binglu Li, Chaoji Zheng, and Xiaodong He. 2019. Clinical features and surgical Management of Bile Duct Cyst in adults. Gastroenterol Res Pract 2019. https://doi.org/10.1155/2019/2517260.
6. Singham J, Yoshida EM, Scudamore CH. Choledochal cysts: part 1 of 3: classification and pathogenesis. Can J Surg. 2009;52(5):434. http://www.ncbi.nlm.nih.gov.ssl.proxy.medicalinfo.or.kr:8080/pmc/articles/PMC2769090/
7. Lewis VA, Adam SZ, Nikolaidis P, Wood C, Wu JG, Yaghmai V, Miller FH. Imaging of Choledochal cysts. Abdom Imaging. 2015;40(6):1567–80. https://doi.org/10.1007/s00261-015-0381-4.
8. Sastry AV, Abbadessa B, Wayne MG, Steele JG, Cooperman AM. What is the incidence of biliary carcinoma in Choledochal cysts, when do they develop, and how should it affect management? World J Surg. 2015;39(2):487–92. https://doi.org/10.1007/s00268-014-2831-5.

9. Funabiki T, Matsubara T, Ochiai M, Marugami Y, Sakurai Y, Hasegawa S, Imazu H. Surgical strategy for patients with Pancreaticobiliary Maljunction without Choledocal dilatation. Keio J Med. 1997;46(4):169–72. https://doi.org/10.2302/kjm.46.169.
10. Farello GA, Cerofolini A, Rebonato M, Bergamaschi G, Ferrari C, Chiappetta A. Congenital Choledochal cyst: video-guided laparoscopic treatment. Surg Laparosc Endosc. 1995;5(5):354–8.
11. Woo R, Le D, Albanese CT, Kim SS. Robot-assisted laparoscopic resection of a type I Choledochal cyst in a child. J Laparoendosc Adv Surg Tech A. 2006;16(2):179–83. https://doi.org/10.1089/lap.2006.16.179.
12. Lipsett PA, Pitt HA. Surgical treatment of Choledochal cysts. J Hepato-Biliary-Pancreat Surg. 2003;10(5):352–9. https://doi.org/10.1007/s00534-002-0797-4.
13. Lilly JR. Total excision of Choledochal cyst. Surg Gynecol Obstet. 1978;146(2):254–6.

Laparoscopic and Robotic Excision of Choledochal Cyst

34

Jin-Young Jang and Jae Seung Kang

Abstract

Advances in laparoscopic surgery and technique have established laparoscopic excision of the choledochal cyst as a common surgical procedure. It reduces tissue injury, facilitates precise dissection and anastomosis, and leads to better cosmetic outcomes than open surgery. Recently, robotic surgical systems have been introduced for the excision of the choledochal cyst. We introduce the surgical procedures for laparoscopic and robotic excision of the choledochal cyst and provide tips and precautions for preoperative evaluation, surgical skills, and postoperative management.

Keyword

Choledochal cyst · Laparoscopy · Robotic surgical procedure · Minimally invasive surgical procedure

Supplementary Information The online version contains supplementary material available at https://doi.org/10.1007/978-981-16-1996-0_34.

J.-Y. Jang (✉) · J. S. Kang
Department of Surgery and Cancer Research Institute, Seoul National University College of Medicine, Seoul, South Korea
e-mail: jangjy4@snu.ac.kr

34.1 Introduction

Choledochal cysts are rare congenital dilatations of the biliary system and generally affect Asian population [1]. The clinical presentation of a choledochal cyst varies with age [2]. In children, the main symptoms include the presence of a mass, jaundice, and perforation. However, with aging, the manifestations of choledochal cyst can include stones, pancreatitis, and biliary tract cancer. Recently, asymptomatic choledochal cysts have been detected more frequently because of routine health checkups [3]. Although they are known to be benign, they must be surgically resected to prevent the risk of choledocholithiasis, cholangitis, pancreatitis, and biliary malignancy. In the absence of resection, there is a lifetime risk of malignancies such as cholangiocarcinoma and gallbladder cancer [4, 5].

Advances in laparoscopic surgery and instrumentation have resulted in clinical application in a variety of hepato-pancreato-biliary surgeries. Laparoscopic approaches provide magnified surgical views, allowing precise dissection and anastomosis, reduced tissue injury, and better cosmetic outcomes. However, the indications for laparoscopic surgery should be considered carefully, based on patients' safety and the need for complete resection. Recently, robotic surgical systems have been introduced and expanded to a variety of surgeries [6, 7]. Robotic surgeries facilitate wrist movement and three-dimensional

H. C. Yu (ed.), *Hepato-Biliary-Pancreatic Surgery and Liver Transplantation*,
https://doi.org/10.1007/978-981-16-1996-0_34

vision and compensate for hand tremor and therefore can be performed with more precise control than laparoscopic surgery.

Although there are no absolute contraindications, a few relative contraindications for laparoscopic excision of the choledochal cyst include the following: the possibility of combined liver resection, common hepatic duct remnant too small for anastomosis, severe inflammation around the cyst, and suspicion of malignancy.

We elucidate the surgical procedures for minimally invasive excision of a choledochal cyst using a laparoscopic system, followed by the use of robotic system.

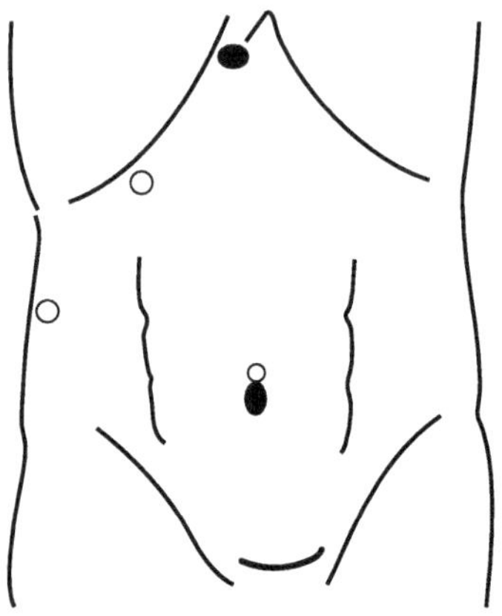

Fig. 34.1 Site and size of the trocars for laparoscopic excision of the choledochal cyst [2]

34.2 Laparoscopic Excision of Choledochal Cyst

34.2.1 Operating Room Setup: Patient Position

The patient is placed in a supine position, in the 15° reverse Trendelenburg position and with a slight right-up rotation. The surgeon and the scopist stand to the left side of the patient, and the first assistant stands on the right side.

34.2.2 Trocar Placement and Exposure

A 12-mm balloon trocar is inserted through an infra-umbilical site using an open access technique, avoiding damage to intra-abdominal organs. A pneumoperitoneum is established, and a laparoscope is inserted through the trocar. The abdominal cavity is explored and the operation site exposed. Another 12-mm trocar is inserted just below the right side of the xiphoid process, a 5-mm trocar at the mid-clavicular subcostal site, and another 5-mm trocar in the axillary line (Fig. 34.1).

34.2.3 Dissection of Calot's Triangle and Exposure of the Distal Margin of the Choledochal Cyst

To expose Calot's triangle, the operator grasps the infundibulum of the gallbladder (GB) and pulls laterally. After dissection of the anterior and posterior peritoneal layers, the cystic duct and artery are exposed and the cystic artery ligated using an endo-clip. From the cystic duct, the hepatoduodenal ligament is dissected along the right choledochal cyst margin, and the dissection extended along the supraduodenal margin. The duodenum is retracted downward using an intestinal grasper. The choledochal cyst is retracted upward, and the retroduodenal and intrapancreatic portion of the choledochal cyst is dissected using a Harmonic Scalpel™ (Ethicon Endo-Surgery, Cincinnati, OH, USA) to ensure hemostasis of the epicholedochal venous plexus (Fig. 34.2).

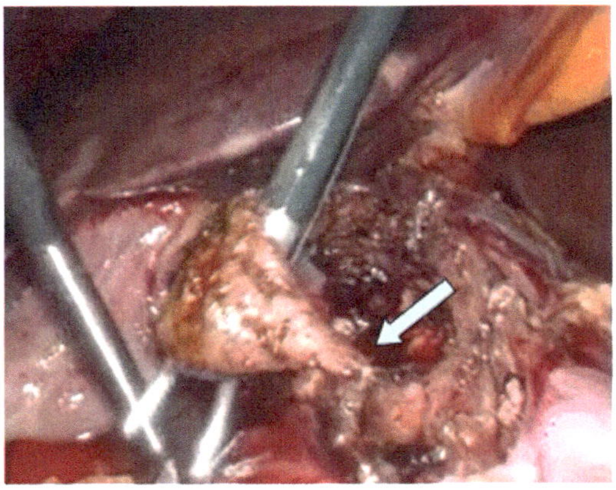

Fig. 34.2 Dissection of intrapancreatic transition point (arrow) of the choledochal cyst

34.2.4 Excision of the Choledochal Cysts

The distal stump is ligated and transected with a 45-mm vascular Endo-GIA once the transection line of the choledochal cyst has been determined (Covidien, Norwalk, CT, USA) (Fig. 34.3). After pulling the distal portion of the choledochal cyst upward, dissection is continued along the medial and posterior margins of the choledochal cyst until the common hepatic duct (CHD) is identified. The choledochal cyst is then transected below the bifurcation with laparoscopic scissors (Fig. 34.4), and the cystic duct is then clipped and divided. The GB is left in its fossa for liver traction during the hepaticojejunostomy (HJ).

34.2.5 Roux-En-Y Reconstruction

After excision of the choledochal cyst, a retrocolic Roux-en-Y HJ is made. A small hole is created in the mesentery of the jejunum 50 cm distal to the ligament of Treitz using the Harmonic scalpel for the passage of the Endo-GIA (Fig. 34.5). After transection of the jejunum using the Endo-GIA, the jejunum mesentery is divided with an endo-clip and LigaSure™ (Medtronic, Minneapolis, MN, USA). A hole is made at the meso-colon lateral to the duodenum, and the Roux limb is brought up to the hepatic hilum behind the colon. LapLoop (Sejong Medical Co., Paju, Korea) facilitates laparoscopic suturing because it carries a premade surgical knot and a

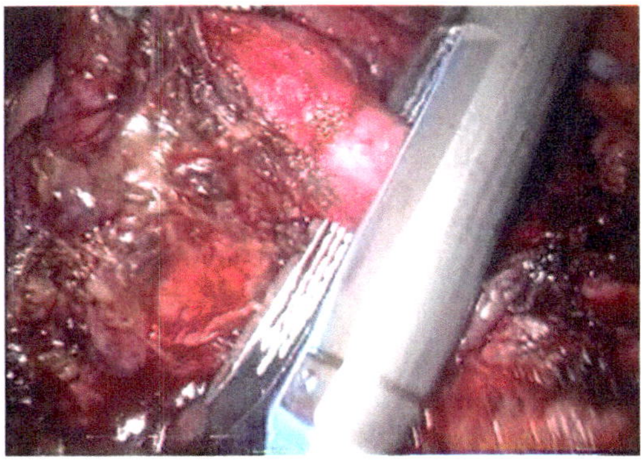

Fig. 34.3 Distal stump ligated using a vascular Endo-GIA

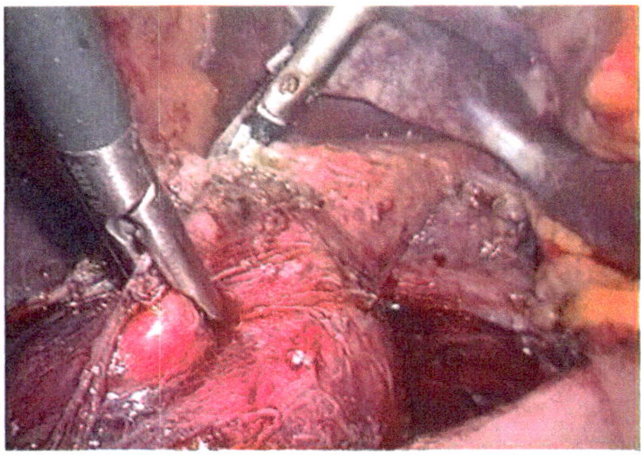

Fig. 34.4 Transection of the choledochal cyst at the hilum level

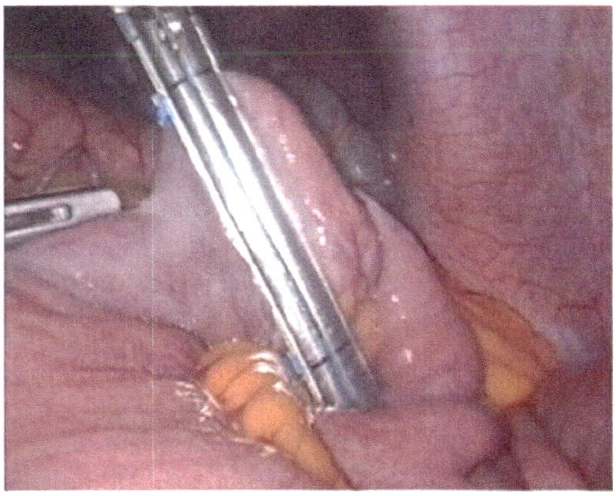

Fig. 34.5 Transection of the jejunum for a Roux-en-Y loop 50 cm distal to the ligament of Treitz

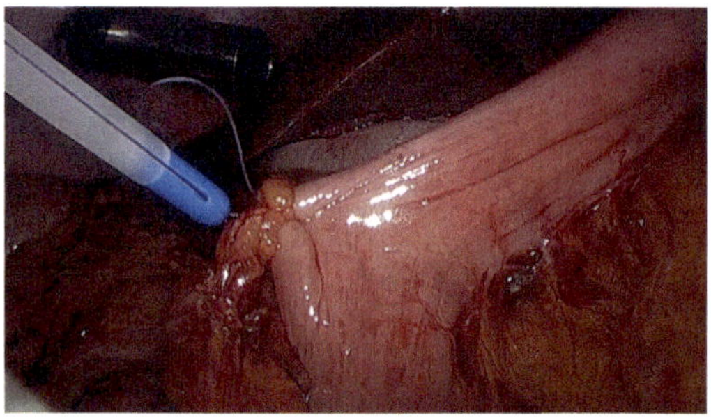

Fig. 34.6 Suture fixation of Roux limb to the meso-colon

knot pusher function. Interrupted sutures are used to fix the Roux limb and fill the meso-colon hole to prevent internal hernia (Fig. 34.6).

34.2.6 Hepaticojejunostomy

After approximation of the jejunum and hepatic duct, a small incision is made in the anti-mesenteric side of the jejunum for an end-to-side HJ. After stay sutures are inserted on both sides of the anastomosis, the posterior aspect of the HJ is secured via interrupted sutures (Fig. 34.7), and the anterior aspect is then sutured similarly. The GB is then dissected free, and a laparoscopic endobag is inserted through the umbilical port trocar, and the specimens are placed in the bag.

34.2.7 Extracorporeal Jejunojejunostomy and Specimen Retrieval

A 1 cm extension of incision to the umbilicus is enough to pull through the jejunum and endobag and perform jejunojejunostomy (JJ). At 60 cm distal to the HJ site, the Roux limb is fixed to the transected upper limb via laparoscopic sutures twice to prevent twisting. After extraction of the endobag, Roux limb and upper limb are pulled through the umbilicus site, followed by side-to-side JJ manually or via Endo-GIA. One Jackson-Pratt drain is inserted through the 5 mm port in the axillary line and located behind the HJ site. The wounds are then closed.

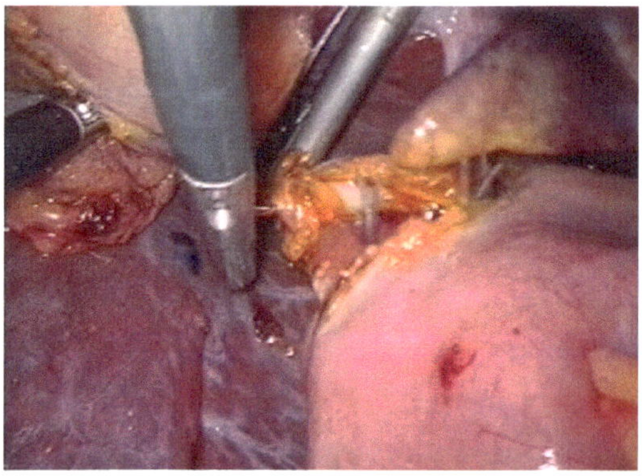

Fig. 34.7 Intracorporeal suture for the posterior aspect of the hepaticojejunostomy

34.2.8 Tips and Comments

Since the bile duct anatomy is complex and may show abnormalities other than the cyst, such as anomalous pancreatic-bile duct union, it is important to evaluate the precise anatomical relationship between the cyst and other important structures such as pancreatic duct, portal vein, and hepatic artery. Because the operator only along the caudal to cephalic direction using the laparoscope, it is difficult to identify accurately the pancreatic duct during dissection near the suprapancreatic part. Therefore, preoperative computed tomography (CT), endoscopic retrograde cholangiopancreatography, or magnetic resonance cholangiopancreatography are needed to determine the extent of surgery and prevent damage to the pancreatic duct, portal vein, or hepatic artery. Intraoperative choledochoscopy facilitates identification and evaluation of the pancreatic and intrahepatic ducts.

To ensure patient's quality of life, it is important to determine the appropriate proximal transection line and perform safe HJ. Dilation of the remnant CHD seldom leads to anastomotic strictures. However, if the diameter of the remnant CHD is very small, surgical complications such as strictures or bile leakage can occur. If the choledochal cyst is not complicated by a malignant lesion, it is better to leave some portion of the proximal cyst for safe and easy anastomosis, rather than perform a radically complete exci-

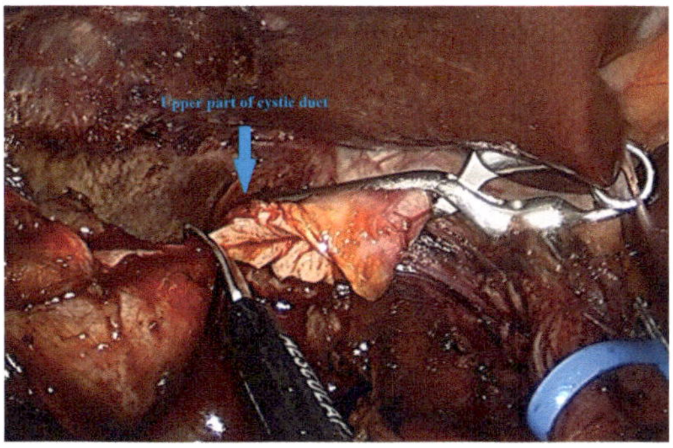

Fig. 34.8 Remnant upper part of the cystic duct for anastomosis

sion. Also, the upper part of the cystic duct can be used like a flap (Fig. 34.8), which along with remnant CHD can be safely and effectively anastomosed to the Roux limb.

34.2.9 Postoperative Management and Follow-Up of Patients

The patient usually starts a liquid diet on postoperative day 1. The closed drain tube is removed if a CT scan on postoperative day 4 shows no abnormal fluid collection. The patient visits the outpatient department 2 weeks after discharge and again at 3 months. In case of no complications, the patient can be followed up every 12–18 months. Appropriate monitoring includes a routine complete blood count, liver function tests, and measurement of tumor markers (including carcinoembryonic antigen and carbohydrate-associated antigen 19–9). CT or MRI is performed to evaluate signs of complications such as pancreatitis, cholangitis, choledocholithiasis, or malignancy.

34.3 Robotic Excision of the Choledochal Cyst

Surgeons can perform dissection using both the laparoscopic and the robotic platforms. Laparoscopic surgery allows quick and easy handling of various instruments, a wider range of motion, a wider surgical field of view during dissection, and tactile sense. Robotic surgery ensures dexterity, precision, and stability of complex techniques, including intracorporeal sutures, which are especially important in HJ after cyst excision [3]. Accordingly, laparoscopic dissection and robotic anastomosis are preferred. However, pure robotic surgery (both dissection and anastomosis) can be selected if surgeons prefer, or if competent surgical assistants are not available.

We introduce below a hybrid technique of laparoscopic excision of the choledochal cyst combined with robotic HJ anastomosis. The da Vinci Surgical System (Intuitive Surgical, Sunnyvale, CA, USA) is used.

34.3.1 Trocar Placement and Excision of the Choledochal Cyst via Laparoscopic Surgery

Trocars are placed in a U-shape in the robotic system (Fig. 34.9). A 12-mm balloon trocar is inserted 3 cm below the umbilicus. Three 8 mm robotic trocars are inserted in the right axilla, right mid-clavicular, and left axillary line. A 12 mm trocar for the assistant is inserted on the mid-clavicular line. A 5 mm trocar is inserted in the epigastrium for traction of the liver during laparoscopic dissection. Dissection and excision

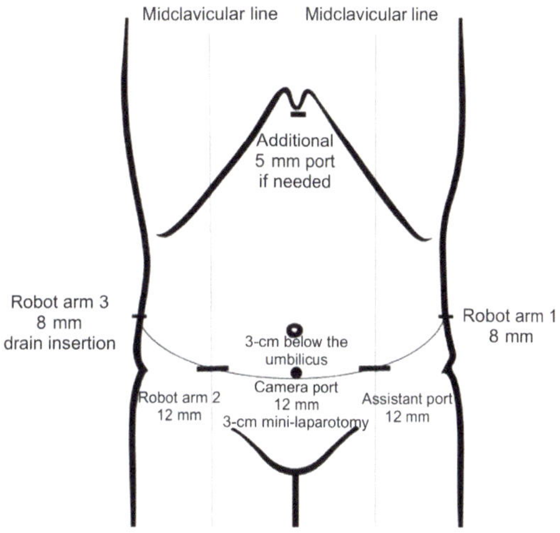

Fig. 34.9 Port placement in robotic choledochal cyst excision [3]

of the choledochal cyst are similar to the laparoscopic procedure. The Harmonic scalpel is used for dissection and hemostasis around the cyst, and the Endo-GIA is used to transect the distal part of the cyst and jejunal limb for a Roux-en-Y reconstruction. The laparoscopic instruments are removed and the robotic surgical system is docked after retrocolic fixation of the Roux limb with premade suture loops (LapLoop) and preparation for extracorporeal performance of a JJ as described in paragraph 34.2.7 above.

34.3.2 Robotic HJ Anastomosis

Vicryl 4–0 interrupted sutures with 1–2 mm spacing are placed at the posterior and anterior walls (Fig. 34.10). If the remnant CHD is large enough, barbed suture material (V-Loc™, Medtronic, MN, USA) is inserted continuously at the posterior wall, and vicryl 4–0 interrupted sutures are inserted in the anterior wall. A Jackson-Pratt drain tube is placed behind the HJ site (Fig. 34.11), and the robotic system is removed from the surgical field. After a 3 cm extension of the umbilical port site, the endobag is extracted and JJ is performed extra-corporeally as described earlier.

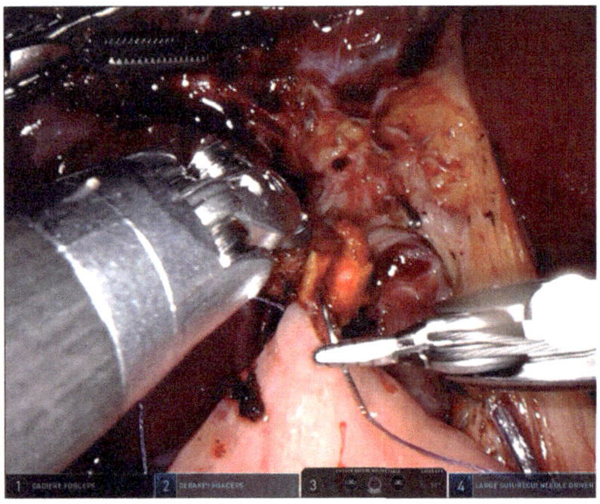

Fig. 34.10 Interrupted suturing with vicryl 4-0 on the posterior wall

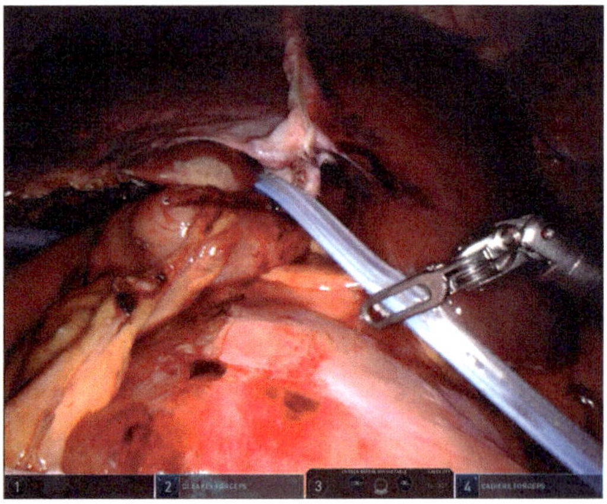

Fig. 34.11 Closed drain placed behind the HJ site

34.4 Short-Term and Long-Term Outcomes

One study reported comparisons of short-term and long-term outcomes between pure-laparoscopic and hybrid robotic groups [3]. The mean operative time was significantly shorter in the laparoscopic group than in the hybrid robotic group (181.31 ± 43.06 min vs. 247.94 ± 54.14 min, $p < 0.05$). The mean estimated blood loss between the two groups was not significantly different (108.71 ± 15.53 mL vs. 172.78 ± 117.46 mL, $p = 0.097$), as was the mean postoperative hospital stay (7.33 ± 2.96 days vs. 6.22 ± 1.06 days, $p = 0.128$). None of the subjects required open conversion.

Short-term surgical complications were defined as complications occurring within 30 days of surgery. Although a total of 11 short-term complications (22.4%) were observed in the laparoscopic group, no complications were observed in the hybrid robotic group (Table 34.1). Long-term surgical complications were observed in seven patients (14.3%) in the pure-laparoscopic group and two patients (11.1%) in the hybrid robotic group. Biliary tract-specific complications occurred more frequently in the pure-laparoscopic group than in the hybrid robotic group (22.4% vs. 0.0%, $p = 0.029$).

Table 34.1 Surgical complications of pure-laparoscopic vs. hybrid robotic group [3]

Complications	Pure-laparoscopic (n = 49)	Hybrid robotic (n = 18)	P value
Short-term	11 (22.4)	0 (0.0)	0.029
Bleeding	1 (2.0)	0 (0.0)	
Fluid collection	1 (2.0)	0 (0.0)	
Bile leakage[a]	7 (14.3)	0 (0.0)	0.176
Wound	1 (2.0)	0 (0.0)	
Ileus	1 (2.0)	0 (0.0)	
Long-term	7 (14.3)	2 (11.1)	0.999
Hepatic duct stone[a]	3 (6.1)	0 (0.0)	0.558
Hepaticojejunostomy stricture[a]	1 (2.0)	0 (0.0)	0.999
Fluid collection	0 (0.0)	1 (5.6)	
Ileus	1 (2.0)	1 (5.6)	
Biliary tract-specific	11 (22.4)	0 (0.0)	0.029

[a] Biliary tract-specific complications. Values are presented as number (%)

34.5 Conclusion

Minimally invasive excision of choledochal cysts yields not only better cosmetic results but also superior functional recovery than open surgery. Therefore, this surgery is more common. Robotic surgery is more precise and stable, and associated with fewer rates of short-term and long-term complications than laparoscopic surgery.

References

1. Wiseman K, Buczkowski AK, Chung SW, Francoeur J, Schaeffer D, Scudamore CH. Epidemiology, presentation, diagnosis, and outcomes of choledochal cysts in adults in an urban environment. Am J Surg. 2005;189(5):527–31.; discussion 31. https://doi.org/10.1016/j.amjsurg.2005.01.025.
2. Jang JY, Kim SW, Han HS, Yoon YS, Han SS, Park YH. Totally laparoscopic management of choledochal cysts using a four-hole method. Surg Endosc. 2006;20(11):1762–5. https://doi.org/10.1007/s00464-005-0565-z.
3. Lee H, Kwon W, Han Y, Kim JR, Kim SW, Jang JY. Comparison of surgical outcomes of intracorporeal hepaticojejunostomy in the excision of choledochal cysts using laparoscopic versus robot techniques. Ann Surg Treat Res. 2018;94(4):190–5. https://doi.org/10.4174/astr.2018.94.4.190.
4. Lee SE, Jang JY, Lee YJ, Choi DW, Lee WJ, Cho BH, et al. Choledochal cyst and associated malignant tumors in adults: a multicenter survey in South Korea. Arch Surg. 2011;146(10):1178–84. https://doi.org/10.1001/archsurg.2011.243.
5. Sastry AV, Abbadessa B, Wayne MG, Steele JG, Cooperman AM. What is the incidence of biliary carcinoma in choledochal cysts, when do they develop, and how should it affect management? World J Surg. 2015;39(2):487–92. https://doi.org/10.1007/s00268-014-2831-5.
6. Jung M, Morel P, Buehler L, Buchs NC, Hagen ME. Robotic general surgery: current practice, evidence, and perspective. Langenbeck's Arch Surg. 2015;400(3):283–92. https://doi.org/10.1007/s00423-015-1278-y.
7. Stefanidis D, Wang F, Korndorffer JR Jr, Dunne JB, Scott DJ. Robotic assistance improves intracorporeal suturing performance and safety in the operating room while decreasing operator workload. Surg Endosc. 2010;24(2):377–82. https://doi.org/10.1007/s00464-009-0578-0.

Part VI

Hilar Cholangiocarcinoma

35 Extended Right Hepatectomy and Caudate Lobectomy

Shin Hwang

Abstract

Perihilar cholangiocarcinoma is defined as adenocarcinoma occurring at the hepatic hilum. This tumor grows longitudinally along the bile duct and penetrates the bile duct wall. It invades the connective tissue along the bile duct. Therefore, curative resection requires en bloc resection of the bile duct and surrounding connective tissues, and concurrent resection of the invaded vessels if needed.

Keywords

Perihilar bile duct cancer · Gallbladder cancer Hepatectomy · Post-hepatectomy hepatic failure · Postoperative pancreatic leak Complication · Abdominal drain

Supplementary Information The online version contains supplementary material available at https://doi.org/10.1007/978-981-16-1996-0_35.

S. Hwang (✉)
Division of Hepatobiliary Surgery and Liver Transplantation, Department of Surgery, Asan Medical Center, University of Ulsan College of Medicine, Seoul, South Korea
e-mail: shwang@amc.seoul.kr

35.1 Indications

- Bismuth–Corlette IIIA cholangiocarcinoma invading the right hepatic duct.
- Complete resection of the right lobe and caudate lobe is recommended to increase surgical curability even in Bismuth–Corlette II type bile duct cancer, where the tumor is limited to the hepatic duct without spreading to either side of the left or right hepatic duct.
- Although the perihilar bile duct cancer is Bismuth-Corlette IV type, which infiltrates both left and right sides of the hepatic duct, it is also applicable to tumor-negative resection of the left bile duct.

35.2 The Concept of Extended Right Hepatectomy

The relationship between the bile ducts and the surrounding blood vessels in the hepatic hilum exhibits the following characteristics (Fig. 35.1).

1. Because the bile duct runs in an inclined direction to the right side of the hepatoduodenal ligament, the branches of the left and the right hepatic duct are located on the right side of the hepatic hilum. The left hepatic duct is longer, and thus, it can be resected with a longer stump.

H. C. Yu (ed.), *Hepato-Biliary-Pancreatic Surgery and Liver Transplantation*,
https://doi.org/10.1007/978-981-16-1996-0_35

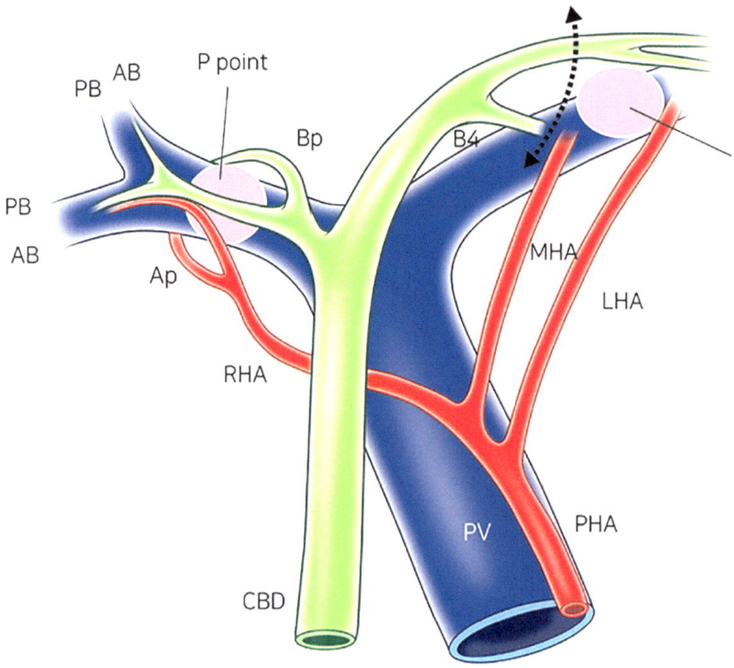

Fig. 35.1 Standard vasculature of the portal vein. *PHA* = proper hepatic artery, *LHA* = left hepatic artery, *MHA* = middle hepatic artery, *RHA* = right hepatic artery, *Ap* = right posterior hepatic artery, *CBD* = common bile duct, *B2* = segment II bile duct, *B3* = segment III bile duct, *B4* = segment IV bile duct, *Bp* = right posterior duct, *PV* = main portal vein, *UP* = umbilical portion of the portal vein

2. The left hepatic artery is located on the left side of the hepatoduodenal ligament and away from the bile duct infiltrated with tumor. In contrast, in most cases, the right hepatic artery reaches the right side of the common hepatic duct while traversing the dorsal side of the common bile duct, and thus easily infiltrated with cancer. In addition, even if there is no invasion, the right hepatic artery must be carefully separated from the adjacent bile ducts invaded by the tumor, and thus, the tumor is inevitably over-manipulated in this process, which can lead to the dissemination of cancer cells.
3. Since most of the caudate lobe bile ducts are infiltrated with cancer, resection of the caudate lobe is essential for radical resection.
4. When portal vein resection is required, the long transverse portion of the left portal vein easily ensures sufficient distance during resection and reconstruction compared to the right portal vein. For these reasons, except when the occupied site of hepatic bile duct cancer is clearly dominant in the left hepatic duct (Bismuth-Corlette IIIB type bile duct cancer), (extended) right lobectomy and caudal lobectomy are the preferred forms of radical surgery. In this procedure, since the volume of the liver that is normally resected is more than two-third of the volume of the total liver, it is essential to ensure adequate volume of the remaining liver before surgery to prevent liver failure. Therefore, if the right lobe is not already atrophied sufficiently, preoperative right portal vein embolization is performed to induce hypertrophy of the left lobe.

35.3 Preoperative Evaluation and Management

Preoperative evaluation is defined as evaluation of the degree of cancer progression (the extent of bile duct invasion, the presence or absence of vascular invasion and its site), liver function, and rate of hepatic parenchymal resection. Preoperative management is a biliary decompression procedure and portal vein embolization.

1. Preoperative evaluation

   For curative surgery for cancer, the achievement of tumor-negative resection margins is the most important goal. Magnetic resonance cholangio-pancreatography (MRCP), which was performed before decompression of the obstructed bile duct, provides important information by accurately revealing the extent of dilated bile ducts. Cholangiography according to endoscopic retrograde cholangiography (ERC) or percutaneous transhepatic biliary drainage (PTBD) also shows the extent of tumor. The extent of tumor invasion outside the wall of the bile duct, such as invasion of the surrounding blood vessels, is evaluated via dynamic computed tomography (CT) and contrast MRI, and the extent of invasion can be more accurately identified in the 3-dimensional images of reconstruction.

2. Since the right lobe occupies more than two-third of the total volume of the liver, including the caudate lobe, preoperative volumetry via dynamic CT is used to calculate the parenchymal resection rate. In general, since obstructive jaundice is accompanied by perihilar bile duct cancer, the reliability of the indocyanine green retention test for evaluating hepatic functional reserve is low. Based on the decompression degree of obstructive jaundice, patient's age, chronic hepatitis, combined pancreatoduodenectomy, and the patient's general condition, it is important to ensure that the estimated future remnant liver volume is 40% or more of the total liver volume.
3. Biliary decompression procedures

   If there is jaundice before surgery, sufficient biliary decompression is necessary to improve liver function and prevent cholangitis. When massive hepatic resection, including right hepatectomy, is scheduled, the target reduction in total bilirubin is less than 2 mg/dL. Biliary decompression via endoscopic naso-biliary drainage (ENBD) is attempted first, and PTBD can be used concurrently in cases with a slow rate of biliary decompression and uncontrolled cholangitis. ENBD can be performed on one or both sides. In perihilar bile duct cancer where the left and right bile ducts are separated, bilateral biliary drainage is recommended to control cholangitis if possible. Although a few cases of cancer cell spread at the PTBD tract have been reported, it is reasonable to perform PTBD without hesitation if indicated. In some cases, endoscopic retrograde biliary drainage (ERBD) is performed to ensure patient comfort before surgery. However, it increases the risk of ascending cholangitis, and thus, it should be avoided in patients scheduled for surgery.
4. Portal vein embolization

   In perihilar bile duct cancer, the decrease of hepatic functional reserve is accompanied by prior obstructive jaundice. Therefore, the future remnant liver volume should remain at least 40% of the total liver volume. In cases of severe preoperative jaundice or deteriorated liver function, and when minor future remnant liver volume is expected, it is important to increase the safety of the operation by inducing hypertrophy of the future remnant liver via portal vein embolization. Within a few days after performing the percutaneous right portal vein embolization, a dynamic CT is used to evaluate the status of portal vein embolization. In order to prevent rapid deterioration in liver function after the portal vein embolization, right portal vein embolization is recommended when the total bilirubin level is decreased to about 5–8 mg/dL. Doppler ultrasonography may be performed to establish the absence of residual blood flow in the right portal vein several days after the portal vein embolization procedure, but dynamic CT yields more accurate information. Dynamic CT is performed at 1-week intervals to determine the degree of right liver atrophy and left liver hypertrophy. Surgery is indicated when the estimated future remnant liver is more than 40% of the total liver volume and the total bilirubin value is less than 2 mg/dL. If the patient has to wait for a long time because of inadequate biliary decompression, the tumor progresses slowly even during the waiting period, so surgery is recommended within 4 weeks after portal vein embolization if possible.

5. Hepatic vein embolization

   If it is difficult to expect adequate levels of right hepatic atrophy and left hepatic hypertrophy only with right portal vein embolization, additional hepatic vein embolization can be performed to block the right hepatic vein and the inferior hepatic vein. When both the portal vein and hepatic venous blood flow of the right liver are blocked, the amount of blood flowing to the right posterior region is decreased significantly, resulting in effective induction of parenchymal atrophy of the right liver and efficient hypertrophy of the left liver.

35.4 Intraoperative Management of Biliary Decompression Tubes

A bile drainage tube (PTBD or ENBD) is inserted because most of the patients with perihilar bile duct cancer show accompanying obstructive jaundice. Aggressive curative surgery is a time-consuming operation, and inappropriate bile drainage during surgery adversely affects the postoperative course, so management of the drainage tube is important. Before starting the surgery, the PTBD drainage tube should be disconnected, and the end of the PTBD tube should be wrapped with surgical gloves, for use as a temporary drainage bag during surgery. The ENBD tube remains intact until the common bile duct is transected.

35.5 Operative Procedures

After dissecting the common bile duct within the hepatoduodenal ligament and transecting it at the upper edge of the pancreas, the bile duct and surrounding connective tissues, lymph nodes are resected, followed by transection of the right hepatic artery and the right portal vein. By skeletonizing the main portal vein and hepatic arteries, all connective tissues that may carry cancer cells are removed leading to the planned site of the left hepatic duct transection in the liver. The parenchymal transection leads to this site, and the bile duct and surrounding connective tissues and the right lobe and caudate lobe are excised together.

The actual surgical procedures are as follows: (1) dissection of the bile duct and surrounding connective tissue in the hepatoduodenal ligament;(2) skeletonization of the left and middle arteries and the left portal vein to the intended site of the left hepatic duct transection; (3) mobilization and dissection of the right lobe and caudal lobes; (4) hepatic parenchymal transection; and (6) transection of the left hepatic duct and bile duct reconstruction (Fig. 35.2).

The hepatic parenchymal transection plane differs depending on the extent of hepatic resection. Extended right lobectomy can be performed to completely remove the middle hepatic vein if the left liver is large enough and carries a fissural vein between the middle and left hepatic veins. If the left liver is not large enough or the risk of surgery is high, the ventral half of the middle hepatic vein is removed and the dorsal half of the middle hepatic vein is preserved in order to conserve some of the segment IV parenchyma. Such extensive surgical resection is preferred to ensure high surgical safety.

1. Incision and surgical field of view

   The surgical field of view is secured via a mirrored-L-shaped, right horizontal incision

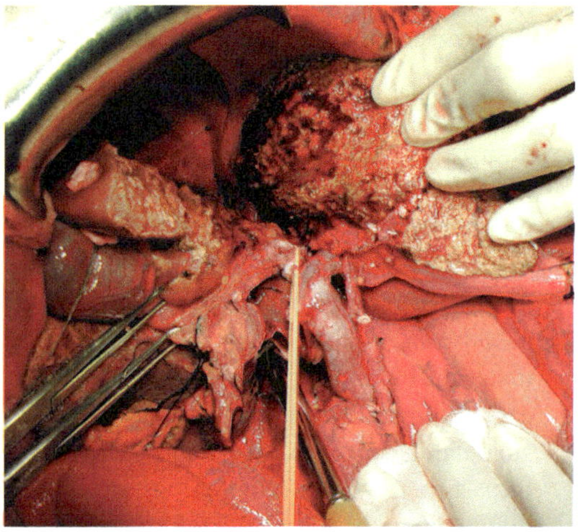

Fig. 35.2 Extent of hepatic resection and skeletonization of the hepatoduodenal ligament

after exploring for ascites, peritoneal dissemination, and liver metastasis by opening an upper median incision from the xyphoid process to the upper part of the umbilicus. A horizontal incision on the left side is usually not required although the extent of incision varies depending on the type of retractors. A better surgical field of view can be secured by resecting the xiphoid process. The PTBD tube on the left side is released by cutting the fixation suture, thereby pushing the tube into the abdominal cavity and reconnecting the surgical rubber gloves, to continuously drain the bile into the glove during surgery. If the reconstruction of the biliary tract is incomplete or there is a risk of post-hepatectomy liver failure, the PTBD tube on the left side is left uncut because PTBD can be maintained after surgery. The lesser omentum is opened to observe whether the cancer has infiltrated the peritoneum and observe the status of lymph node metastasis. The falciform ligament is cut to expose the inferior vena cava inlet of the major hepatic veins. After ligating the round ligament to secure the visual field of view of the liver, the suture material is pulled and fixed with a towel clamp over the retractor.

2. Cholecystectomy and dissection and transection of the extrahepatic bile duct

   If cholecystectomy is not performed first, it is difficult to secure the field of view. Therefore, unless there is extensive tumor infiltration in the cystic duct, retrograde cholecystectomy is performed first. Subsequently, while touching the right hepatic artery, the connective tissue of the hepatoduodenal ligament is removed bit by bit to expose the right hepatic artery and the portal vein. The dissection is continued towards the pancreas after grasping the common bile duct.

   The duodenum is mobilized by Kocher's maneuver, and the pancreatic capsule and surrounding tissues are dissected to expose the pancreatic parenchyma in the posterior part of the pancreas, and the lymph node No. 13 is then removed. The posterior-superior pancreaticoduodenal artery and vein is exposed and dissection continues cephalad along the pancreatic parenchyma until it reaches the pancreatic upper margin. The posterior-superior pancreaticoduodenal artery is proximal to the branch of the gastroduodenal artery from the common hepatic artery, and the posterior-superior pancreaticoduodenal vein enters the portal vein from the dorsal side. While hooking and pulling the lower common bile duct with a vascular rubber loop, the common bile duct is transected at the upper edge of the pancreas warranting intraoperative frozen-section biopsy with the end of the bile duct resection margin (Fig. 35.3). It is essential to ensure the absence of free tumor mass or blood clots in the residual bile duct by strongly injecting normal saline using a ball-tip syringe into the residual bile duct in the pancreas. It is safer to suture the end of the bile duct in the pancreas continuously with a 5–0 non-absorbable monofilament rather than suture ligation.

   If the end of the bile duct is tumor-positive, the distal bile duct is further excavated into the pancreas by 1–3 cm to secure the maximum marginal distance. It is transected, and a frozen-section biopsy is repeated. Excavation of the pancreatic parenchyma increases the risk of pancreatic leakage after surgery, so the detached pancreatic tissues must be carefully sutured (Fig. 35.4).

3. Skeletonization of blood vessels in the hepatoduodenal ligament

   Once the common bile duct is cut and pulled cephalad, the portal vein and the hepatic artery are well exposed, and the surgical field of view is secured. The periportal lymph nodes are dissected to simplify the vascular structures of the hepatic hilum, followed by the skeletonization of the hepatic arteries in the hepatoduodenal ligament. Starting from the right hepatic artery or gastroduodenal artery, the periarterial neural plexus is carefully dissected to expose the entire length of the hepatic artery leading to the right hepatic artery, middle artery, left hepatic artery, proper hepatic artery, common hepatic artery, and gastroduodenal artery. At this time, if any of the lymph nodes around the hepatic artery are enlarged, a

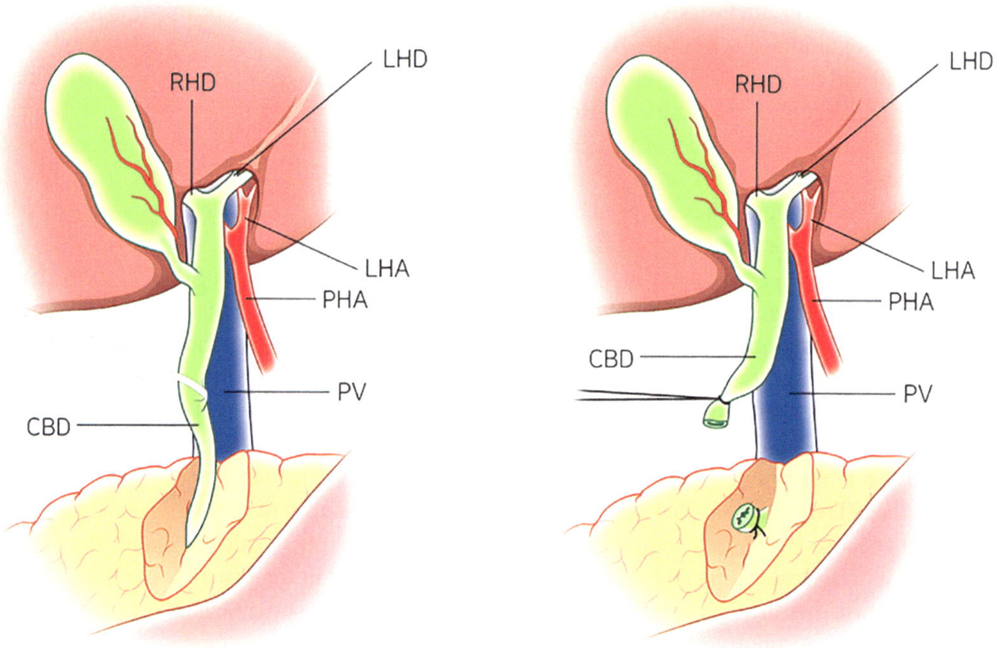

Fig. 35.3 Transection of the distal bile duct within the pancreas. *CBD* = common bile duct, *RHD* = right hepatic duct, *LHD* = left hepatic duct, *PV* = portal vein, *PHA* = proper hepatic artery, *LHA* = left hepatic artery

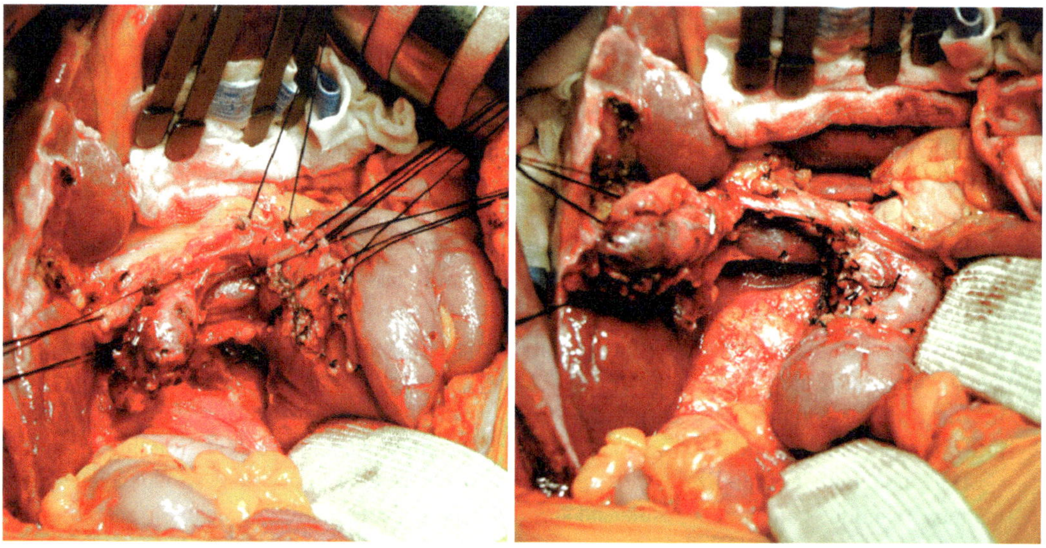

Fig. 35.4 Extended bile duct resection performed by deep excavation into the pancreas

frozen-section biopsy is performed. In case of a positive tumor, the periarterial neural plexus is removed thoroughly, without damaging the adventitia of the hepatic artery, since there is a risk of developing pseudoaneurysm in the future if the periarterial neural plexus is removed excessively. Excessive use of electrosurgery around the hepatic artery may induce blood vessel damage, suggesting the need for meticulous mechanical dissection. Although it is convenient to hang with a vascular rubber loop to traction the isolated artery, care should be taken because excessive traction can cause vascular damage.

4. Transection of the right hepatic artery and exposure of the portal system

The right hepatic artery is cut and ligated, and the surrounding connective tissues including lymph nodes and the common bile duct are lifted to the right and pulled. The main portal vein is pulled with a vascular rubber loop to the right and the proper hepatic artery to the left, followed by dissection of the hepatic artery and the connective tissues around the portal vein along the longitudinal axis to expose the left and right portal branches (Fig. 35.5).

The transverse portion of the left portal vein is dissected to sufficiently expose the left portal vein branch. At this time, since the dilated bile duct often adheres to the left portal vein wall due to cholangitis, no portal infiltration should occur, which is confirmed by dissecting only to the easily exposed area. The

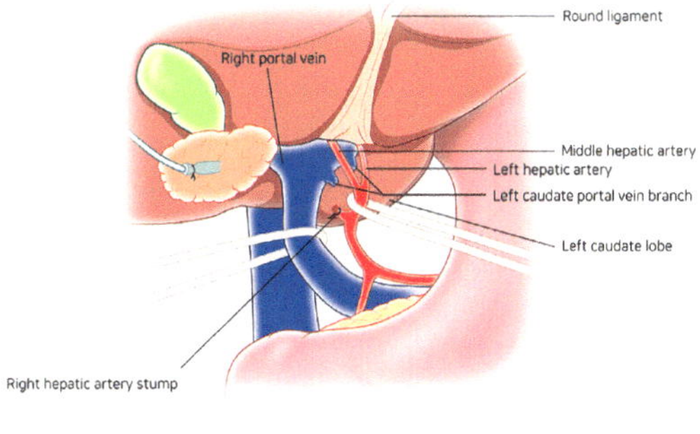

Fig. 35.5 Dissection of the portal vein branches at the hepatic hilum

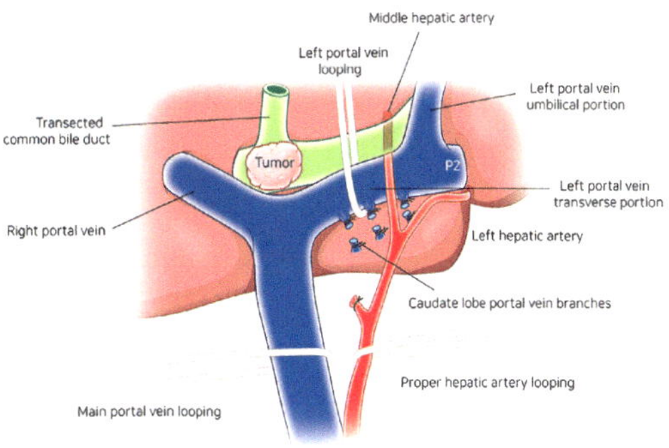

Fig. 35.6 Dissection of the left portal vein

2–3 caudate portal vein branches attached to the left portal vein are cut and ligated (Fig. 35.6).

5. Mobilization of the right lobe and caudate lobe

If the right portal vein is well exposed and easily cut, it must be transected immediately. If its detachment is difficult due to adhesion, the right portal blood flow is blocked with bulldog clamps, and the right liver is mobilized. At this stage, both the arterial and portal blood flow to the right liver are blocked, so the surface of the right liver exhibits ischemic color change. The right coronary ligament, right triangular ligament, and hepatorenal ligament are cut via electrosurgery and the inferior vena cava is exposed by releasing the liver and the right adrenal gland. More than 10 short hepatic veins that drain the caudate lobe between the liver and the inferior vena cava are exposed and cut one by one from the caudal side. The vein stumps at the inferior vena cava side are ligated with sutures and those on the liver side are ligated with metal clips. If the diameter of the short hepatic vein is more than 3 mm, it is safe to suture continuously with 5–0 Prolene. Inferior vena cava dissection proceeds to the left side, and the right inferior vena cava ligament that exists outside the inferior vena cava near the inlet of the right hepatic vein can be seen. When this is cut, the proximal part of the right hepatic vein is exposed. At this stage, a tonsil forceps is inserted between the right hepatic vein and the middle vein, followed by

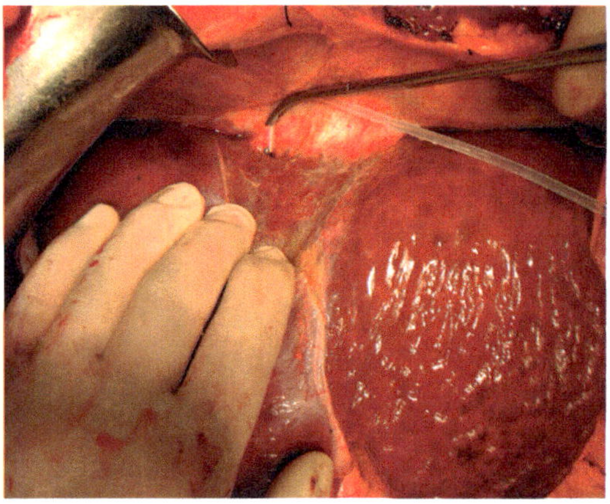

Fig. 35.7 Hanging the lifting string between the right hepatic vein and the middle vein

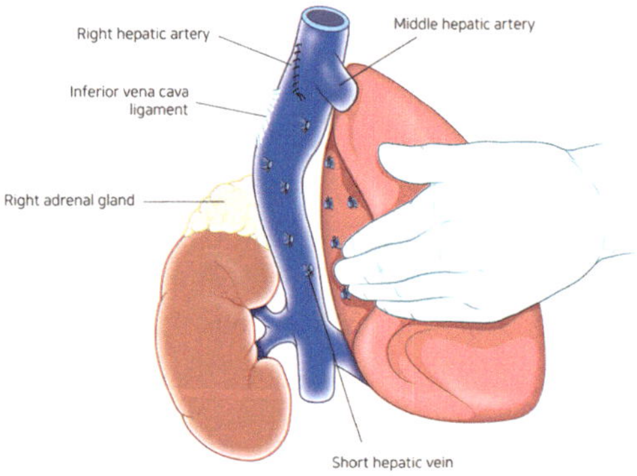

Fig. 35.8 Mobilization of the left liver

insertion of a vascular rubber loop, nylon string, or Penrose drain (Fig. 35.7).

If all the short hepatic veins on the left caudal lobe (Spiegel lobe) are cut, the entire caudal lobe can be completely mobilized. Since the left inferior vena cava ligament is still attached, the caudate lobe is not completely mobilized, and the surgical field of view is not good, so there is no need to forcefully cut the left inferior vena cava ligament. The right lobe and caudate lobe after liver mobilization are firmly brought into the operator's left hand (Fig. 35.8). The right hepatic vein can be cut at this stage, but it is convenient not to cut it during a hanging maneuver.

6. Transection of the hepatic parenchyma.

   After cutting the right hepatic artery and right portal vein, the hepatic parenchyma is transected along the Cantlie line, which demarcates the discolored right lobe from the left lobe (Fig. 35.9).

   The transection plane of the liver differs depending on the location of cut and uncut ventral portions of the segment IV. The main features of the hepatic parenchymal transection are as follows: (1) preservation of the middle hepatic vein and exposure of its right wall, (2) total resection of the right lobe and

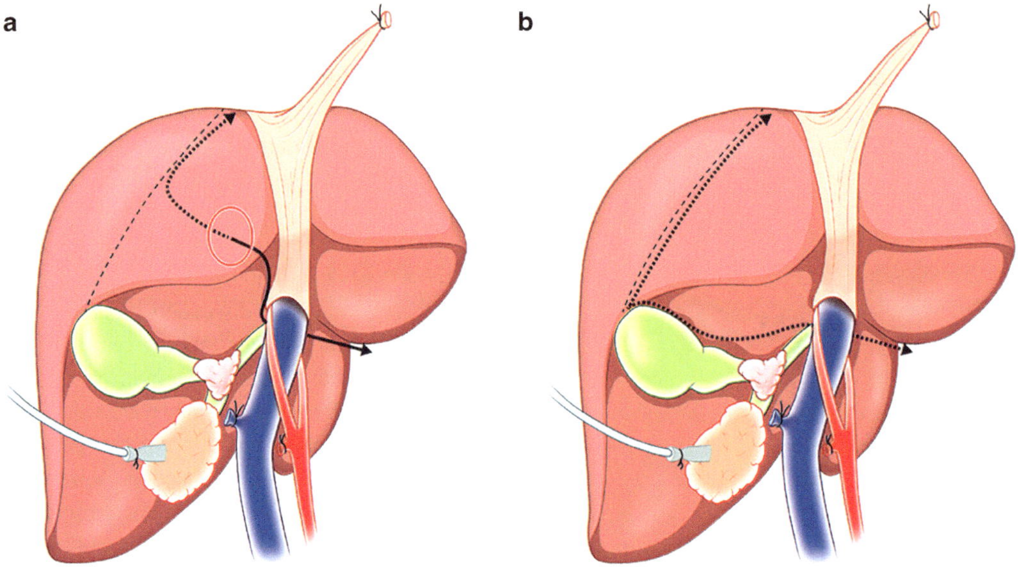

Fig. 35.9 Determination of the hepatic transection plane with (**a**) or without (**b**) concurrent resection of the ventral segment IV parenchyma

caudate lobe, (3) excision of the left hepatic duct as far as possible at the location when the hepatic transection is almost complete, and at this time, the caudal lobe duct is completely within the extent of resection. (4) Since the left hepatic duct enters the back side of the portal vein, a concurrent resection of the ventral part of the segment IV ensures better visibility for biliary reconstruction.

If the size of the segment IV is larger or comparable to that of the left lateral section in preoperative volumetry CT, additional resection of the ventral segment IV parenchyma may trigger post-hepatectomy hepatic failure due to insufficient volume of the remnant liver, so a careful approach is required. For further resection of ventral segment IV, a few small portal branches from the portal vein to the ventral segment IV should be cut to expose the right wall of the umbilical portion of the left portal vein. At this time, it is important to preserve the portal vein branches into the dorsal segment IV (Fig. 35.9a). When the ventral segment IV is not excised, the hepatic transection proceeds upwards and backward along the Cantlie line, but in the vicinity of the hepatic hilum, it is safe to prevent cancer infiltration into the hepatic parenchyma about 10 mm away from the hepatic hilar plate (Fig. 35.9b). Therefore, only a small part of ventral segment IV parenchyma is excised together with the right lobe, and the actual transection plane of ventral segment IV differs in each case according to the degree of bile duct infiltration. There is no need to completely remove the ventral segment IV parenchyma in all cases.

The hepatic parenchymal transection is performed by holding the left hepatic artery and the left portal vein with bulldog clamps; thus, the blood inflow to the liver is blocked (Pringle maneuver). The blood flow is repeatedly blocked by 15 min of blockade and 5 min of release. Bleeding hemorrhage during the parenchymal transection usually involves the branches of middle hepatic vein. Therefore, a vein branch from the beginning of the hepatic parenchymal transection near the gallbladder draining segment V is located and cut to guide along the path to reach the main trunk of the middle hepatic vein. Exposing the right wall of the middle hepatic vein at the hepatic transection plane reduces bleeding during surgery. In case of middle hepatic vein injury, the bleeding point is gently pressed to stop bleeding, and accurately identify the origin of bleeding, for hemostasis with a 6–0 Prolene suture if it is uncontrolled.

While exposing the middle hepatic vein longitudinally, along the inferior vena cava inlet cephalad, the left caudate lobe can be found to the right when the Arantius canal is cut at the site where the Arantius canal is connected near the junction of the inferior vena cava and the left hepatic vein (Fig. 35.10).

The hanging method for hepatic transection not only reduces bleeding from the hepatic veins, but also prevents the risk of misdirection of the hepatic parenchymal transection (Fig. 35.11). In the deeper part of the

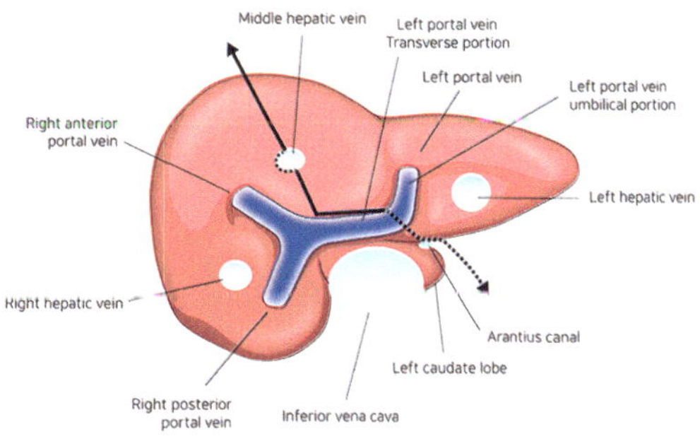

Fig. 35.10 Hepatic transection plane

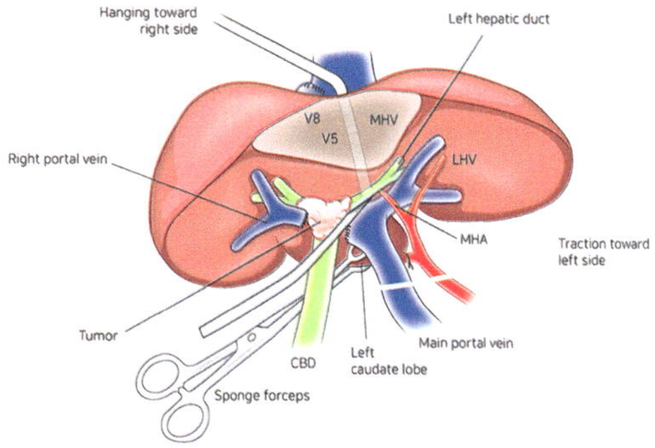

Fig. 35.11 Hanging method via loop lifting

hepatic transection plane after the main trunk of the middle hepatic vein is exposed, upward lifting of the hanging string opens the hepatic transection plane wide and improves the view of the transection to easily control the bleeding from the hepatic transection plane. The left caudate lobe is pulled to the right, which is also useful in locating the direction of transection.

7. Transection of the left hepatic duct and biliary reconstruction.

   The last step of bile duct transection involves transection of the left hepatic duct on the right side of the umbilical portion of the left portal vein. The left caudal lobe Glisson branches should be resected at the left hepatic duct. Therefore, the right hepatic duct is pulled to the right and the bile duct is gently cut with sharp surgical scissors to ensure a safe distance of 5–10 mm without tumor invasion (Fig. 35.12).

Since the end of the transected left hepatic duct is shorter than before cutting, it is recommended to leave 2–3 mm of bile duct resection margin on the remaining side to facilitate biliary reconstruction. A frozen-section biopsy with the end of the bile duct can be used to confirm whether the tumor is negative, and the bleeding at the end of the left hepatic duct is sutured with 6–0 Prolene. If the left hepatic duct resection margin is tumor-positive, if possible, the end of the left hepatic duct is cut a little further and a frozen-section biopsy is repeated. The resected left hepatic duct is exposed via 2 to 3 openings (Fig. 35.13). Usually, the most ventral side is segment II duct (B2) and the most ventral side is segment IV duct (B4), and most of them are cut into two openings, B4 and segment II + III duct (B2 + 3) (Fig. 35.14).

When a single Glissonean sheath carries 2–3 bile duct openings and are connected by fibrous connective tissues, each opening drains into a

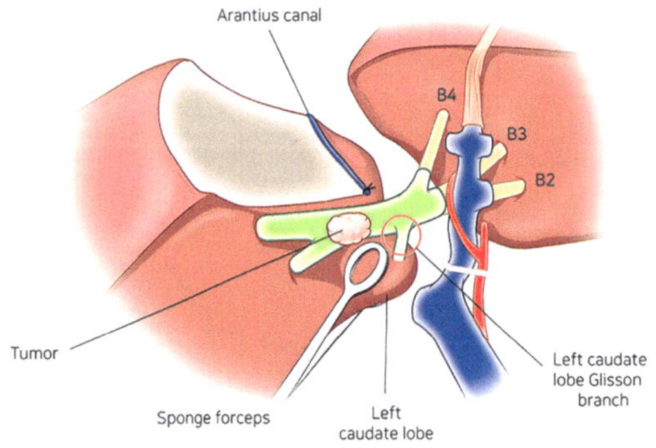

Fig. 35.12 Transection of the left bile duct

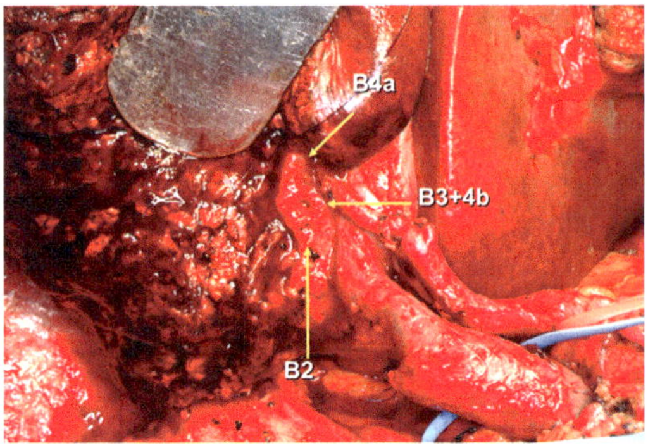

Fig. 35.13 Three left hepatic duct openings within a single connective tissue sheath

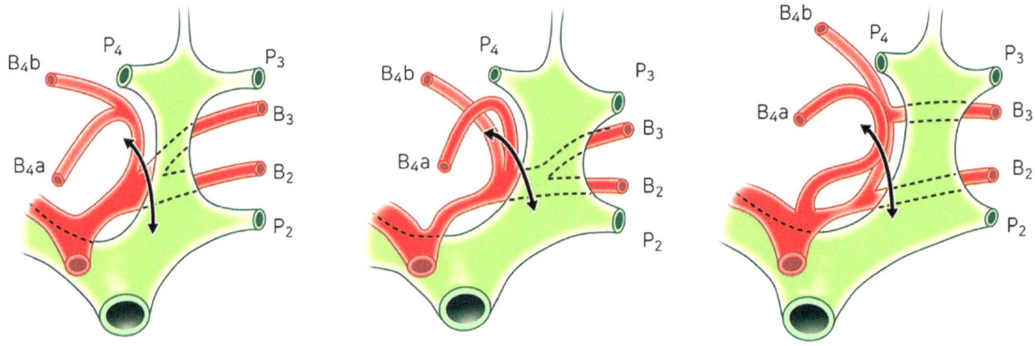

Fig. 35.14 Types of left hepatic duct opening that are cut according to anatomical variations

single bile duct with 6–0 Prolene or absorbable material, to facilitate bile duct-enteric anastomosis (Fig. 35.15).

Prior to biliary reconstruction, a number of traction sutures are placed on the ventral wall of each opening at 1.5-mm intervals; thus, the lumen of each bile duct can is clearly visible. A 50-cm-long jejunum loop is made for biliary-enteric anastomosis. In case of independent anastomoses of two bile duct openings, the distance between the anastomotic openings at the jejunum should be more than threefold the distance between the bile duct openings to create a natural anastomosis (Fig. 35.16).

Sutures are made of 5-0 to 6-0 Prolene or absorbable material. Continuous or intermittent sutures are used on the dorsal wall of the anastomosis, and intermittent sutures ventrally. A short stent over the anastomosis is inserted and secured with an absorbable suture to allow escape later. A residual left PTBD tube can be used to insert an external drainage tube using the PTBD tract (Fig. 35.17).

The PTBD insertion site on the right side of the abdominal wall is electrocauterized or coagulated with an Argon laser to remove buried cancer cells. When the PTBD tube is removed from the left side of the abdominal wall, the side of the abdominal wall is partially excised electrosurgically. The remaining liver-side hepatic parenchyma is burned with Argon coagulation to reduce the risk of local recurrence following the spread of cancer cells.

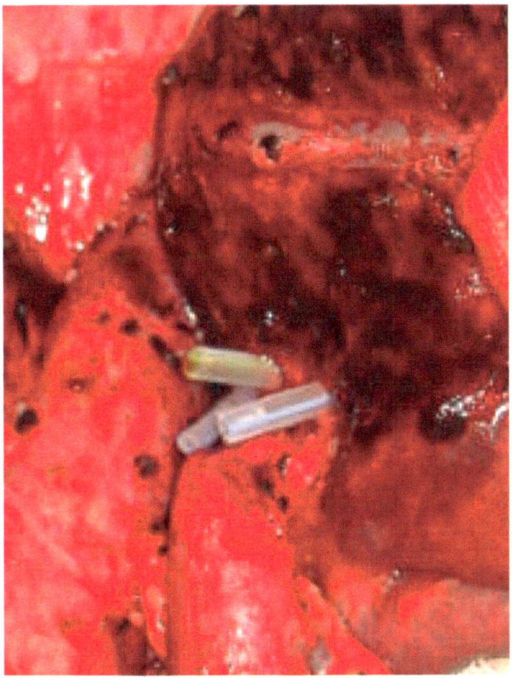

Fig. 35.15 Three bile duct openings molded to enable single bile duct-enteric anastomosis

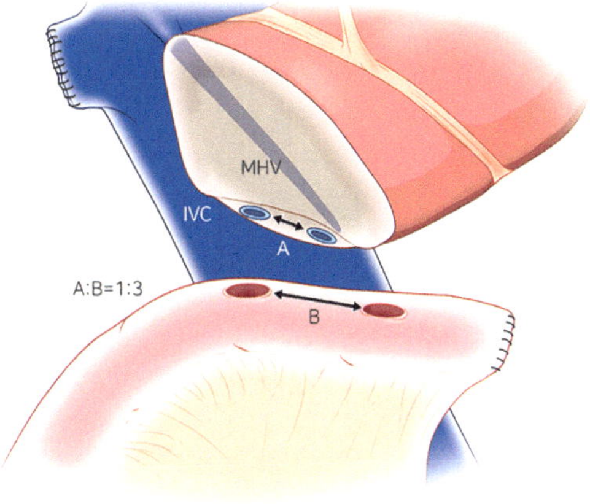

Fig. 35.16 Separate reconstruction of two bile duct openings

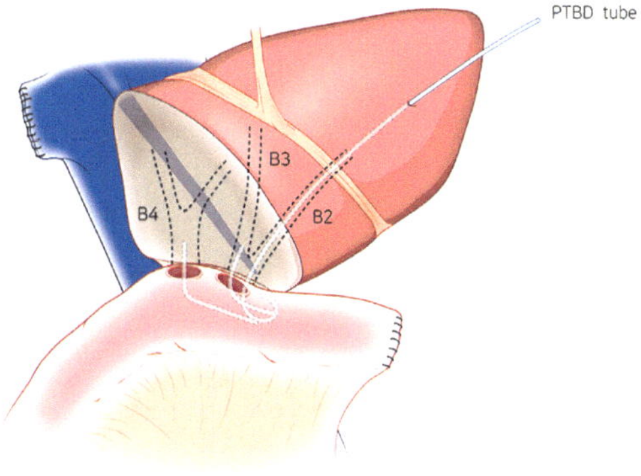

Fig. 35.17 Insertion of the internal and external biliary drainage tubes. B2–4 denotes segment II–IV ducts

Part VII

Extrahepatic Bile Duct Cancer

Bile Duct Resection

36

Joo Seop Kim

Abstract

Segmental bile duct resection (BDR) is not a routine procedure. This operation is mainly indicated for middle bile duct cancer and rarely for Bismuth type I and II hilar bile duct cancer with papillary tumor or lesions less than T2 stage. Segmental BDR is less invasive than pancreatoduodenectomy or major hepatic resection. This procedure should be performed when the resection margin is more than 10 mm for R0 resection.

Keywords

Segmental bile duct resection

36.1 Introduction

Neoplasms of extrahepatic carcinoma are divided into hilar (49%), middle (25%), distal (19%), and diffuse types (7%), according to location and corresponding surgical treatment modalities [1]. Pancreatoduodenectomy is a standard surgical option for distal bile duct cancer, and bile duct resection with combined hepatic resection is indicated for patients with proximal bile duct cancer. Segmental BDR is mainly indicated for mid-bile duct cancer. However, most cancers show longitudinal growth along the duct [2–4], and securing safe proximal margin of 10 mm for the R0 resection is impossible [5]. The method is indicated basically for the middle bile duct cancer, and the Bismuth type I and II hilar cholangiocarcinoma with papillary tumor and lesions less than T2.

36.2 Preoperative Management and Evaluation

Most patients present with jaundice following biliary obstruction. The necessity of preoperative biliary decompression is controversial and not recommended universally for all jaundiced patients. The procedures of decompression are determined according to the severity of icterus and concomitant cholangitis. The decompression methods are performed via transhepatic route: percutaneous transhepatic biliary drainage (PTBD) or endoscopic route; endoscopic nasobiliary drainage (ENBD); or endoscopic retrograde biliary drainage (ERBD). The timing of operation does not depend entirely on the level of total bilirubin. The author has performed operation when the level of total bilirubin is decreased to 5 mg/dL.

J. S. Kim (✉)
Department of Surgery, Hallym University Kangdong Sacred Heart Hospital, Hallym University School of Medicine, Seoul, South Korea
e-mail: jskim324@naver.com

H. C. Yu (ed.), *Hepato-Biliary-Pancreatic Surgery and Liver Transplantation*,
https://doi.org/10.1007/978-981-16-1996-0_36

36.3 Operative Method

Author recommends an upper midline incision with or without extension below the umbilicus for rapid and extensive results. As the upper abdomen is opened, resectability is first determined via palpation of the hepatoduodenal ligament. The absence of hepatic, peritoneal, or bulky nodal metastasis is confirmed. The need for aspiration cytology is determined by the presence of ascites in the abdominal cavity. The incision is extended below the umbilicus when the resection is decided. Using a Kent-type retractor, the bilateral costal arches are elevated. A self-retractor can be used in the low parts of incision for a stable and wide surgical view (Fig. 36.1).

The lesser sac is opened and the dissection of lymph nodes is initiated from the celiac axis. The coronary vein is dissected and divided. The common hepatic artery is exposed along the upper border of the pancreas and nodal dissection is continued to the right side. At the duodenal pylorus, the periduodenal arteries and veins are ligated and divided. After dissection of vessels, a bilateral ligation is performed. Ligation of the duodenal side using hemostats should be avoided to prevent injury to the duodenal wall. Wide devascularization of the duodenum results in discolorization. Although the risk of ischemia is not high, delayed gastric emptying occurs when the vagal nerve is cut. The nasogastric tube facilitates the management. Dissection around the common hepatic artery is continued and the tributaries of right gastric artery are exposed. Each artery is encircled and lifted with a vessel loop to enable the dissection and to avoid vascular injury. The distal portion of the bile duct is identified and dissected. When the distance is greater than 10 mm between the upper border of pancreas and the main tumor, the bile duct is transected (Fig. 36.2). Distal resection margin is sent to the pathology laboratory for frozen examination. When the frozen examination is positive for carcinoma, the distal bile duct is dissected from the surrounding pancreatic tissue similar to the surgery for congenital choledochal cyst. The tumor shows an infiltrative growth within and outside the bile duct lumen, prompting suggestions for excavation type resection of pancreas parenchyma to avoid pancreatoduodenectomy [6]. This operation is less invasive than classical pancreatoduodenectomy and is indicated for elderly patients or patients with major comorbidities. However, atypical resection of pancreas is not easy because CUSA or forceps fracture method is not practical like in hepatic resection. Also, the procedure is time-consuming. Hence, conversion to pancreatoduodenectomy is rather safe for low-risk patients with positive resection margins. The duodenum is fully mobilized by Kocher maneuver and lymph node # 13 is dissected. The anterior border of hepatoduodenal ligament is incised. The dissection of common hepatic artery is carried upward and the origin of right gastric artery is identified and divided. The portal vein is then exposed. Lymph nodes #12a are dissected to the left side, and lymph nodes #12b, 12p are cleared to the right side with bile duct. The bifurcation of right hepatic artery is met and encircled in a vessel loop. Concomitant cholangitis complicates the identification of the bifurcation of left and right hepatic artery. In such cases, the level of cystic duct is useful to identify the bifurcation point, because both levels are approximately similar in anatomic location. The middle hepatic artery generally originates from the left hepatic arteries. The division of middle hepatic artery is sometimes carried out to facilitate nodal dissection. After the skeletonization of hepatic arteries,

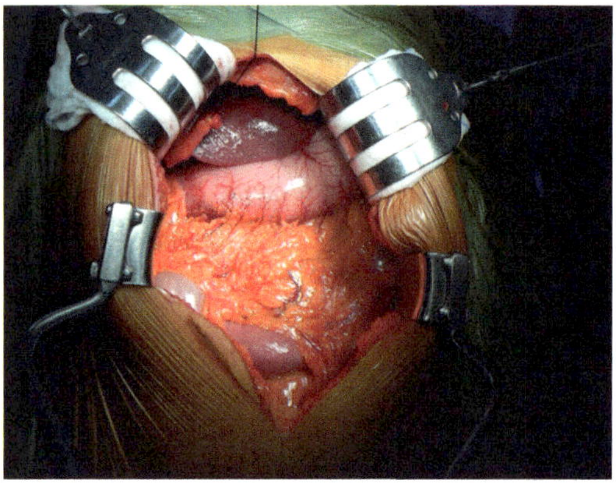

Fig. 36.1 Author prefers an upper midline incision with extension below the umbilicus. Using the Kent-type retractor and the self-retractor, the costal arch is elevated and the optimal area of operation is exposed

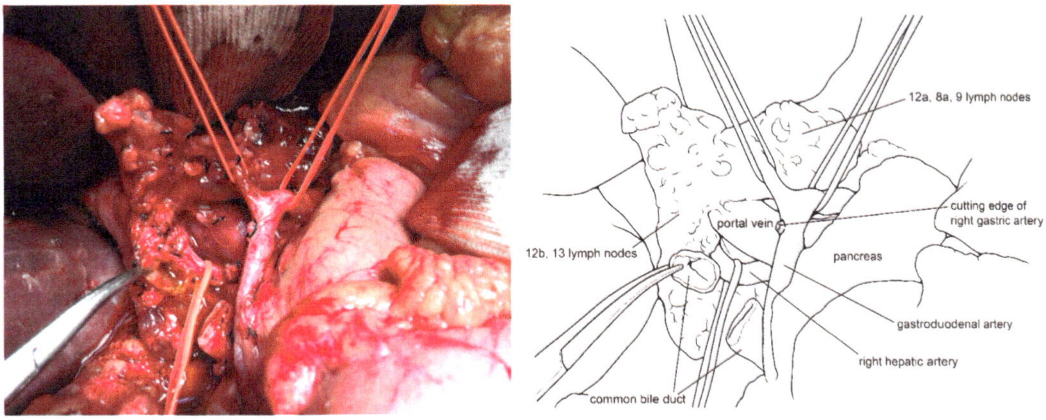

Fig. 36.2 Dissection of lymph nodes is started at the celiac axis and continued to the right side. The distal part of common bile duct is transected. Skeletonized portal vein and hepatic artery are obtained

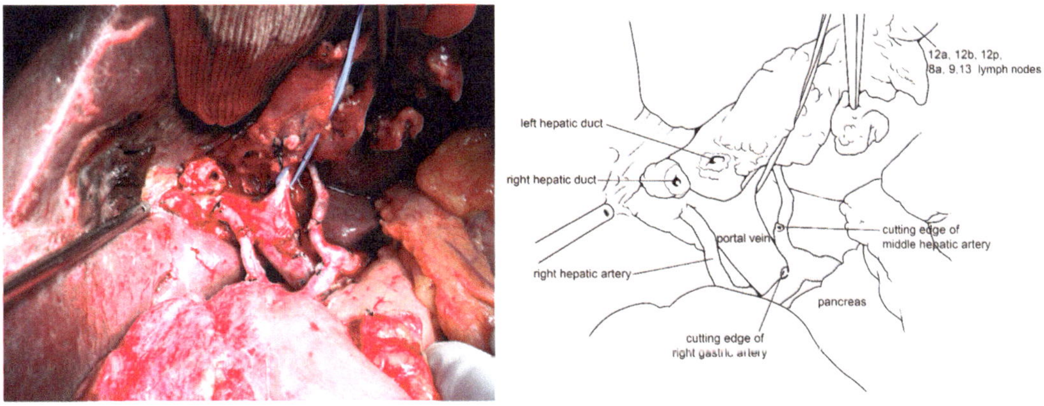

Fig. 36.3 Right and left hepatic ducts are separately transected. The middle hepatic artery is ligated and cut to facilitate the dissection of lymph nodes

the gallbladder is removed from fundus to neck. The cystic duct is not divided and should be included in the resected specimen. The uppermost border of the hepatoduodenal ligament is dissected from the hepatic hilum. The bile duct is cut from 10 mm of the tumor and resected margin is sent for pathology examination (Fig. 36.3). When the pathology is positive for the proximal margin, additional resection of 5 mm is done and right and left bile ducts are separately obtained. If the pathology is positive again in this step, liver resection is the next choice of procedure. As the right hepatic artery is generally invaded by the tumor in hilar cholangiocarcinoma, hepatic resection of right lobe is considered first if the volume of remaining lobe is greater than 35%. Finally, the resected bile duct and lymph nodes are removed as a whole. The distal margin of bile duct is closed continuously with 4-0 or 5-0 prolene. The jejunum is cut below the Treitz ligament. Choledocho- or hepatojejunostomy is performed in Roux-en-Y fashion. When left and right bile ducts are separated, choledochoplasty is conducted to generate an orifice (Fig. 36.4). The use of internal or external stent depends on the surgeon's preference. Author prefers 5-0 polydioxanone (PDS) as a suture material for choledochoenteric anastomosis. Author uses two PDS sutures with needles on both sides. Each side is anchored with 5-0 PDS. The anterior and posterior walls of anastomosis are sutured continuously. If the lumen of anastomosis is less than

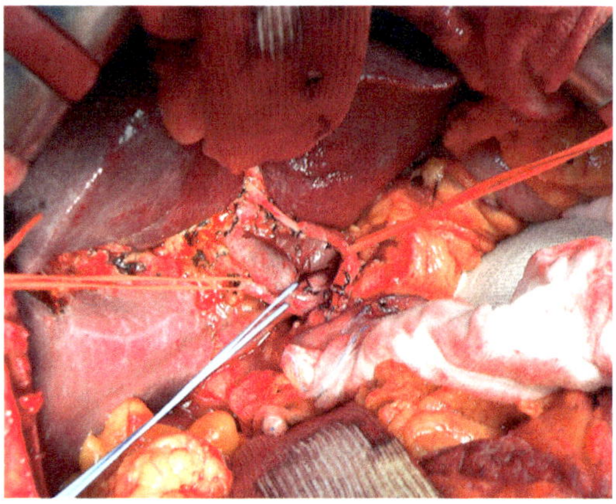

Fig. 36.4 Segmental bile duct resection is completed. The separate hepatic ducts (arrows) are converted to a single orifice after ductoplasty in this patient

7 mm, an interrupted suture is used to avoid anastomotic strictures after operation. Careful hemostasis is done. One or two drainage tubes are placed and the abdomen is closed layer by layer.

References

1. Kondo S, Takada T, Miyazaki M, et al. Guidelines for the management of biliary tract and ampullary carcinoma: surgical treatment. J Hepatobiliary Pancreat Surg. 2008;15:41–54.
2. Kim N, Lee H, Min SK, et al. Bile duct segmental resection versus pancreatoduodenectomy for middle and distal bile duct cancer. Ann Surg Treatment Res. 2018;94:240–6.
3. Chen RX, Li CX, Luo CH et al. Surgical strategies for the treatment of bismuth type I and II hilar bile duct cholangiocarcinoma: bile duct resection with or without hepatectomy? Ann Surg Oncol 2020.
4. Ikeyama T, Nagina M, Odda K, et al. Surgical approach to bismuth type I and II hilar cholangiocarcinomas: audit of 54 consecutive cases. Ann Surg. 2007;246:1052–7.
5. Ebata T, Watanabe H, Ajioka Y, et al. Pathologic appraisal of lines of resection for bile duct carcinoma. Br J Surg. 2002;89:1260–7.
6. Hwang S, Lee SG, Kim KH, et al. Extended extrahepatic bile duct resection to avoid performing pancreatoduodenectomy in patients with mid bile duct cancer. Dig Surg. 2008;25:74–9.

37 Pancreatico-duodenectomy

Sang Geol Kim and Hyung Jun Kwon

Abstract

Extrahepatic bile duct cancer is defined as the presence of a malignant tumor arising at the biliary tree distal to second-order branches. Extrahepatic bile duct cancer can be further divided into hilar and distal bile duct cancers. The site of an extrahepatic bile duct cancer has clinical importance because it affects the selection of the appropriate type of surgical resection and outcomes after the surgery. Compared to hilar bile duct cancer, which requires concomitant bile duct and liver resection, surgical resection for a distal bile duct cancer requires pancreaticoduodenectomy with regional lymph node dissection and subsequent reconstruction with a hepaticojejunostomy, pancreaticojejunostomy, and duodenojejunostomy.

The first pancreatoduodenectomy was described by Kausch in 1909. The procedure traditionally involves en bloc removal of the gastric antrum, duodenum, pancreatic head, gallbladder, and bile duct. Since its first introduction in 1978 by Traverso and Longmire, the pylorus-preserving technique is now performed for most distal bile duct cancers.

Keywords

Extrahepatic bile duct · Distal bile duct
Common bile duct · Cholangiocarcinoma
Surgery · Pancreaticoduodenectomy

37.1 Position

The patient is placed supine on the table with 90 degrees abduction of the right arm.

37.2 Incision and Exposure

While various types of incision such as oblique or curved incision below right costal margin are employed, the authors usually prefer the midline incision extending below umbilicus. The xiphoid process can be excised if it is too long and xiphicostal angle is narrow hindering adequate exposure. After opening the abdomen, the round ligament is ligated and divided leaving the 2–0 silk clamped with a hemostat at the end, which is used to expose the liver by pulling the silk. The incision can be extended to lower the abdomen or via additional transverse incision above umbilicus if required to ensure adequate exposure. The fal-

Supplementary Information The online version contains supplementary material available at https://doi.org/10.1007/978-981-16-1996-0_37.

S. G. Kim (✉) · H. J. Kwon
Department of Surgery, Kyungpook National University School of Medicine, Daegu, South Korea
e-mail: ksg@knu.ac.kr

H. C. Yu (ed.), *Hepato-Biliary-Pancreatic Surgery and Liver Transplantation*,
https://doi.org/10.1007/978-981-16-1996-0_37

ciform ligament is divided cranially via electrosurgery until the triangular ligament, followed by the application of abdominal retractors to fully expose the upper abdomen.

To determine the resectability, the degree of invasion of the primary tumor, gross features of the lymph nodes, the presence of peritoneal seeding, and distant metastasis need to be analyzed systemically.

First, hepatoduodenal ligament, hepatic hilum, tissues around celiac artery, and the pancreas head are examined by inspection and palpation to determine the invasiveness of the primary tumor and the probability of lymph node metastasis. Then, the surface of the liver is evaluated for possible metastasis. Lastly, peritoneal seeding is examined by tracing the intestine from the Treitz ligament to the rectovesical pouch including mesentery, mesocolon, and para-aortic area.

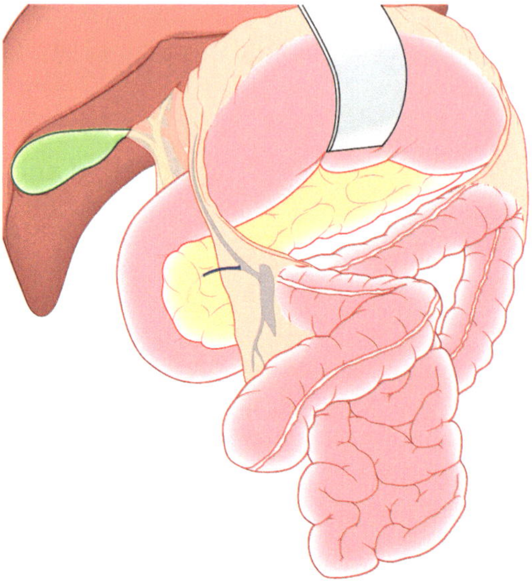

Fig. 37.1 Dissection between great omentum and transverse colon continued to hepatic flexure of ascending colon to facilitate the mobilization of duodenum via Kocher maneuver

37.3 Mobilization of Pancreas Head and Duodenum

The avascular plane between the great omentum and the transverse colon is dissected by pulling the omentum cranially and the transverse colon caudally. The dissection is continued to expose the second and third portions of the duodenum, the anterior surface of pancreas head, the right side of superior mesenteric vein, and the inferior margin of pancreas body. During this procedure, the hepatic flexure of ascending colon can be dissected downward from the third portion of duodenum to facilitate the mobilization of duodenum by Kocher maneuver (Fig. 37.1). Mobilization of the duodenum requires ligation and division of supraduodenal vessel and right gastric artery followed by the Kocher maneuver. The Kocher maneuver, dissecting the duodenum off the retroperitoneum over right kidney, exposes the inferior vena cava, left renal vein, and right side of aorta retracting the C-loop of duodenum and pancreas head (Fig. 37.2). During this procedure, great care is needed to avoid injury to the ureter and annoying bleeding from mesocolic artery and gastrocolic trunk.

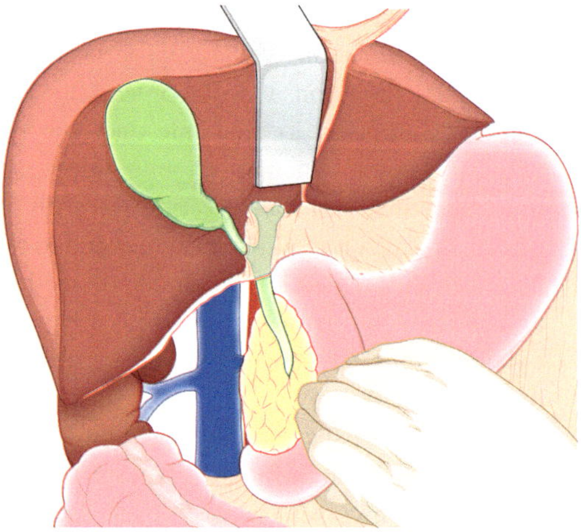

Fig. 37.2 Kocher maneuver, retracting the C-loop of duodenum and pancreas head, exposes the inferior vena cava, left renal vein, and right side of aorta

37.4 Tunneling of Pancreatic Neck

When duodenum is completely mobilized and the gastrocolic trunk is exposed, the veins from gastrocolic trunk draining into superior mesenteric vein need to be ligated and divided early to prevent tearing and bleeding. The division of these veins from gastrocolic trunk mobilizes the upper part of superior mesenteric vein. The dissection between SMV and inferior part of pancreatic neck proceeds to adjacent inferior margin of pancreas body to facilitate tunneling along the SMV under the neck of pancreas. The peripancreatic tissues of both superior and inferior margins are dissected and the transfixed bilaterally with 3–0 Prolene tagging sutures on remnants of pancreatic body. These tagging sutures enable tunneling procedure and control the bleeding (Fig. 37.3). The space between SMV and pancreatic neck is usually in the avascular plane; thus, blunt dissection by Kelly or right-angle clamp easily results in the tunnel between SMV and posterior surface of pancreatic neck.

37.5 Division of Duodenum

The right gastroepiploic artery supplying pylorus and duodenum is ligated and divided at its origin in the gastroduodenal artery. In this area, we included the subpyloric lymph node (no. 6) in the tissue for removal by dividing the right gastroepiploic artery far distally from the origin of gastroepiploic artery (Fig. 37.4).

As described in the procedure for Kocher maneuver, the supraduodenal vessel and the right gastric artery are divided near the gastroduodenal wall to dissect suprapyloric lymphatic tissue completely (no. 5) (Fig. 37.5). Although the right gastric artery may be preserved to ensure blood supply, the authors usually divide the right gastric artery at its origin.

After dissection between pancreatic head and duodenal c-loop to obtain adequate length of duodenum, the duodenum is divided more than 2–3 cm below the pylorus using a GIA stapler.

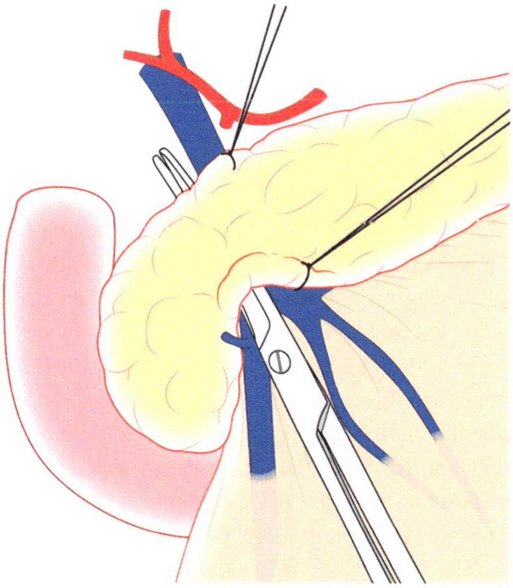

Fig. 37.3 After the division gastrocolic trunk from SMV, transfixing tagging sutures of 3-0 Prolene are placed on both sides of remnant pancreatic body to facilitate the tunneling procedure

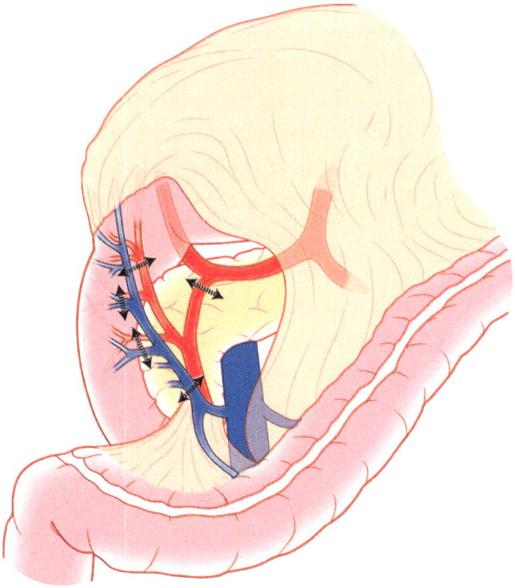

Fig. 37.4 Right gastroepiploic artery is ligated and divided near the division line of duodenum

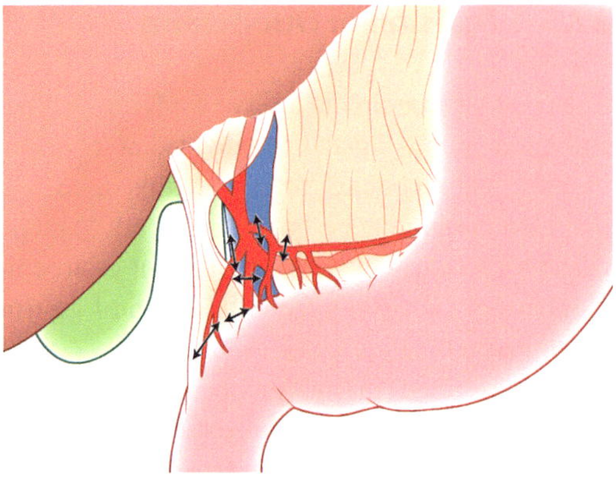

Fig. 37.5 Supraduodenal vessels are divided near gastroduodenal wall and the right gastric artery is divided at its origin. The dissection is continued to obtain adequate length of duodenum and the duodenum is divided more than 2–3 cm below the pylorus

37.6 Division of Pancreatic Neck

Pancreatic neck is divided usually just above the SMV-portal vein but the division line may extend beyond the left margin of SMV according to the left margin of the primary tumor.

The proximal portion of the neck to be removed is ligated with a 2–0 black silk before the division. The tagging sutures with 3–0 Prolene placed on the superior and inferior border of the distal portion of pancreatic neck enable the elevation of the neck during tunneling. The authors prefer to divide the pancreatic neck with a knife because it provides clear resection surface and easy identification of bleeding vessels. The pulsating arterial bleeding is ligated with sutures and the non-pulsating minor bleeding is controlled via electrosurgery.

37.7 Division of Bile Duct and Regional Lymphadenectomy

The regional lymphadenectomy around hepatoduodenal ligament starts with longitudinal dissection of the hepatoduodenal ligament and opening of the lesser sac. The isolation of bile duct is followed by cholecystectomy. By pulling the fundus of gallbladder via clamp, dissection is used to remove the gallbladder off the bed of liver without division of the cystic duct. Further dissection from right to left side of hepatoduodenal ligament opens the serosa connected to hilar plate and exposes the anterior surface of bile duct. The dissection proceeds caudally along the left side of the hepatoduodenal ligament to identify hepatic artery, and further along the hepatic artery proper and common hepatic artery. The origin of right gastric artery is ligated and divided to dissect the lymph nodes # 5, 12a, and 8. After exposing hepatic artery proper and common hepatic artery, the right hepatic artery is traced to skeletonize via dissection of the lymphatic tissue leaving only vascular structures behind.

The gastroduodenal artery is exposed. Before the ligation and division of the artery, the anomalous origin of the hepatic artery from GDA is confirmed utilizing a Bulldog clamp. The gastroduodenal artery is the largest artery among the arteries ligated and divided during the entire surgery. Because the location of the gastroduodenal artery stump is located near the site of future pancreatic jejunostomy, a significant pancreatic fistula is strongly associated with pseudoaneurysm and lethal bleeding from gastroduodenal artery. The gastroduodenal artery needs to be double ligated securely.

The dissection of the bile duct may be substantially facilitated by the skeletonization of the vessel. Using a right-angle dissector, the bile duct is dissected from the portal vein and isolated by a vessel loop. By pulling the vessel loop around the bile duct, the bile duct can be further mobilized to identify the right hepatic artery behind the duct. The division line of the bile duct differs depending on the extension of the primary tumor and the usual division line is on the level of hepatic bifurcation.

The distal bile duct is ligated. The lymph nodes around portal vein (12b, 12p) are dissected after the bile duct is divided and dissected off the portal vein. Proximal resection margin should be examined by frozen biopsy to determine the need to resect the bile duct further.

37.8 Division of Jejunum

Jejunum is divided about 15-cm distal from Treitz ligament. The vascular pattern of the jejunal mesentery is identified by transilluminating the mesentery to determine the line of mesenteric division. In order to dissect the first jejunal branch of SMA, the division of mesentery occurs near the mesenteric border of proximal jejunum. Because the proximal jejunum is actively involved in the absorption of nutrients, it is better to leave behind as much as possible avoiding excessive tension and ischemia of the intestine. The first jejunal branch of SMA is ligated and divided after rotating the divided proximal jejunum under superior mesenteric vessels, followed by the dissection of SMA nerve plexus and lymph nodes (Fig. 37.6).

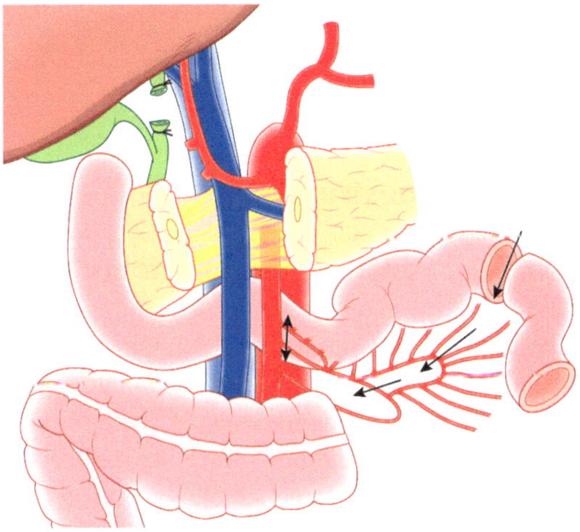

Fig. 37.6 After the division of pancreatic neck just above the SMV, the divided proximal jejunum is rotated under superior mesenteric vessels, followed by ligation of the first jejunal branch of SMA and division of the right side of SMA

37.9 Dissection of Uncinate Process, Retroperitoneal Tissues, and Nerve Plexus

37.9.1 Dissection of Uncinate Process

Uncinate process of pancreas is located behind SMV usually extending to immediate right of superior mesenteric artery, rarely extending to the left beyond SMA. The nerve plexus is divided and the arteries between SMA and uncinate process are ligated and divided by retracting the portal vein to the left using a vein retractor and pulling the uncinated process to the right side.

37.9.2 Retroperitoneal Tissues

Pulling the pancreatic head to the right side and retracting portomesenteric trunk to the left side with a vein retractor, the retro-pancreatic connective tissues adjacent to pancreatic head containing vessels are ligated and divided. Great caution should be taken to avoid troublesome bleeding from the arterial branches from SMA (Fig. 37.7).

37.9.3 Dissection of Lymph Nodes and Nerve Plexus around SMA

Primary tumor and metastatic lymph nodes around SMA often invade the nerve plexus; thus, we prefer dissection of lymph nodes in a lump with nerve plexus around SMA. When the pancreatic head is pulled to the right after dividing the pancreatic neck, the nerve plexuses can be

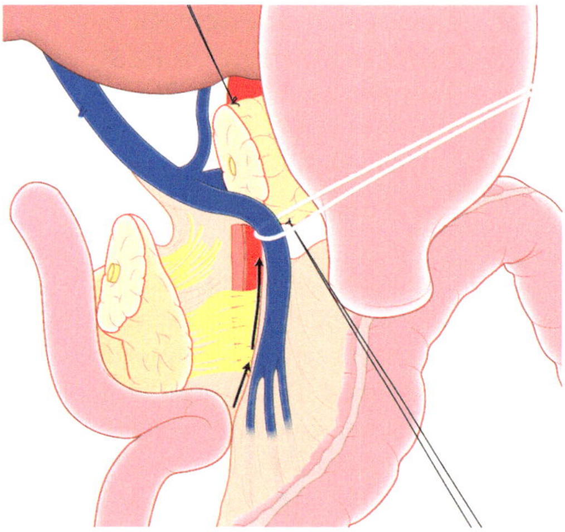

Fig. 37.7 Retracting portomesenteric trunk to the left side, uncinated process, nerve plexus, and vessels such as inferior pancreaticoduodenal artery are ligated and divided

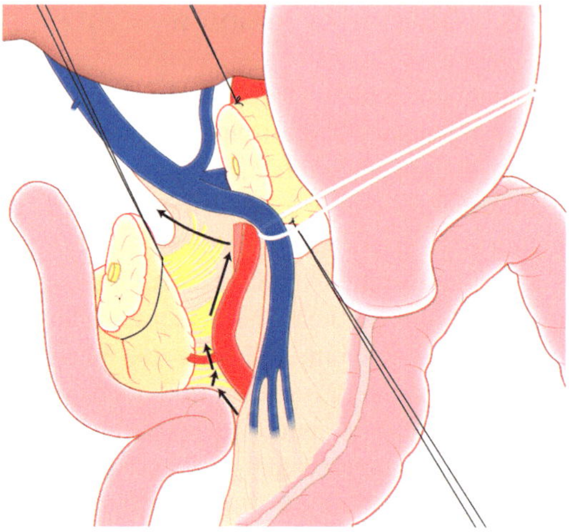

Fig. 37.8 Retracting portomesenteric trunk to the left side using a vein retractor, the nerve plexus to the right of SMA and celiac trunk is dissected in a lump containing the lymph nodes and retroperitoneal tissues and resected combined with pancreas head

identified from the uncinated process along SMA, common hepatic artery, and celiac trunk.

Pulling the divided jejunum to the right side of SMA after dividing the first jejunal branch of SMA, the nerve plexus near uncinated process is dissected longitudinally upward. The dissection of nerve plexus is continued upward retracting the SMV to the left with a vein retractor. Finally, the nerve plexus is dissected off the SMA in a lump containing the lymph nodes and retroperitoneal tissues.

Several vessels including inferior pancreaticoduodenal artery branching from SMA should be carefully ligated. The occasional right hepatic artery from SMA should be carefully handled to avoid injury. The remaining tissue during the dissection of lymph nodes and nerve plexus is ligated to prevent lymphorrhea. Following the dissection of nerve plexus around SMA, the pancreatic head is connected to the root of celiac axis by the retro-pancreatic tissues carrying the SMA nerve plexus. Finally, the nerve plexus on the right side of celiac axis is dissected and resected combined with pancreatic head (Fig. 37.8).

37.10 Reconstruction

37.10.1 Pancreaticojejunostomy

The blind end of the divided jejunum is pulled through the opening of mesocolon along the retro-colic route and placed near the proximal end of remnant pancreas. Since we utilize the inverted mattress pancreaticojejunostomy, a kind of invagination technique, the superior and inferior margins of the remnant pancreas are mobilized for easy insertion inside the jejunum. Every active bleeding point of pancreatic cut surface is securely controlled with a 4–0 Prolene to prevent postoperative intraluminal bleeding. The size of external stent is determined after identification of pancreatic duct.

The inverted mattress pancreaticojejunostomy is an invagination technique, in which the proximal remnant pancreas is inserted through the opening created in antimesenteric side wall of jejunum. The jejunum and inserted proximal jejunum are secured by four U-shaped mattresses and one suture at each corner; thus, a total of 5–6 sutures are placed between jejunum and the remnant pancreatic body. This suture technique is easy and reduces tangential shear force with a reduced risk of significant pancreatic fistula. Since the cut surface of pancreas is exposed inside the jejunal lumen without contacting tissues, the pulsating bleeding from cut surface of pancreas is securely sutured with a non-absorbable monofilament.

The inverted mattress technique for pancreatojejunostomy is described below.

1. Antimesenteric border of the proximal jejunum is longitudinally opened with the same-sized pancreatic cut surface via electrosurgery.
2. External stent is inserted through a small opening of jejunum into pancreatic duct.
3. Based on the location of the pancreatic duct and the size of the cut surface, the number of sutures is determined. If the duct is located at the center of pancreatic cut surface, four U-shaped mattress sutures are placed, and if it is located on the periphery of cut surface, three U-shaped mattress sutures are placed. The U-shaped mattress sutures (4–0 Prolene) are made starting at the mucosa of posterior jejunal wall using one arm of non-absorbable 4–0 monofilament, going in-out through the full thickness of jejunum (Fig. 37.9). The other arm is also used similarly going in-out through the full thickness of jejunum.
4. Both arms of 4–0 monofilament penetrate the proximal end of remnant pancreatic body straight constituting a unit of U-shaped mattress suture. Totally, 3–4 U-shaped mattress sutures are completed between the posterior wall of jejunum and the proximal pancreatic body.
5. The sero-muscular layer of anterior jejunal wall is inverted by the transpancreatic U-shaped sutures going out-in followed by a full-thickness stitch of anterior jejunal wall going in-out, thereby invaginating the proximal pancreatic body into the lumen of jejunum.
6. Finally, the U-sutures were placed in both corners of jejunum. The needle is placed on one side of jejunal corner inverting the seromuscular layer followed by penetration of a corner of pancreatic body. The needle is passed through the other side of jejunal corner out-in followed by a full-thickness stitch, invaginating the corner of proximal pancreatic body into the lumen of jejunum.
7. All five to six stitches are tied carefully at the anterior wall and both corners of the jejunum enclosing the jejunal opening around the pancreas remnant (Fig. 37.10).

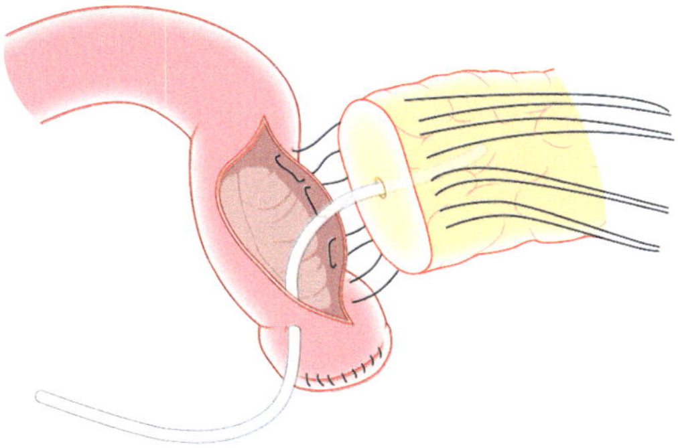

Fig. 37.9 Three to four U-shaped mattress sutures (4-0 Prolene) are made starting at the mucosa of posterior jejunal wall using a double-arm non-absorbable 4-0 monofilament. The tagging sutures of 3–0 Prolene placed at both superior and inferior border of pancreas body used for traction after penetrating the jejunum from inside to outside of the jejunal wall

37.10.2 Hepaticojejunostomy

Since the bile duct is usually dilatated in cases of extrahepatic bile duct cancer, the authors prefer continuous hepaticojejunostomy. According to the size of the bile duct, a smaller jejunal opening than the bile duct is created via electrosurgery. The 4–0 absorbable monofilament (PDS) sutures are placed between the bile duct and the jejunal wall at both right and left corners. Continuous intraluminal running sutures of posterior walls

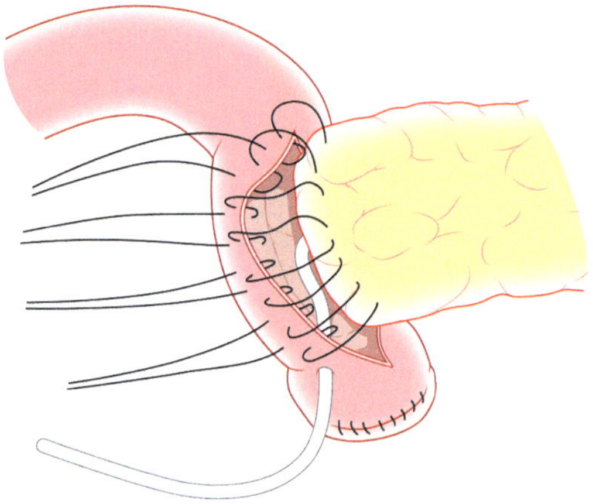

Fig. 37.10 Anterior wall of jejunum is sutured with the transpancreatic U-shaped sutures. The sero-muscular layer of anterior jejunal wall was inverted going out-in, followed by a full-thickness stitch of anterior jejunal wall going in-out. The traction of 3-0 prolene tagging sutures facilitates invagination of proximal pancreatic body into the lumen of jejunum and all four U-shaped sutures are tied at the anterior wall jejunum

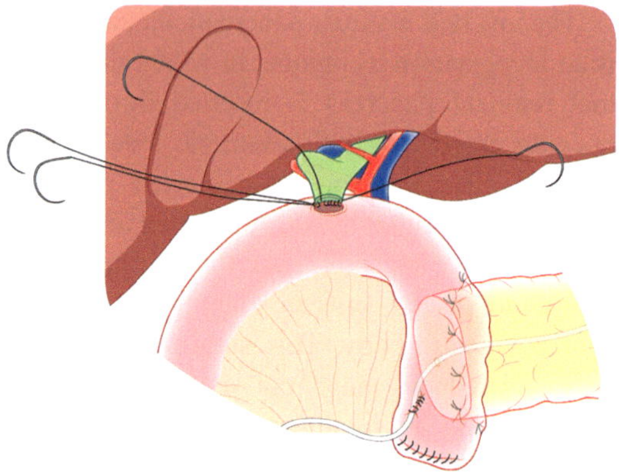

Fig. 37.11 In case of dilated bile duct, continuous hepaticojejunostomy is performed

are performed from the left to the right corner. Once the posterior wall sutures are completed, the anterior wall sutures are performed from the left to the other side. Hepaticojejunostomy is completed after tying both posterior and anterior running sutures after completing the anterior wall (Fig. 37.11).

37.10.3 Duodenojejunostomy

The authors anastomose duodenum and jejunum at least about 40 cm apart from the opening of mesocolon anterior to the T-colon via continuous sutures using 4–0 absorbable monofilament (4–0 PDS). According to the size of opening in the divided duodenum, an appropriate opening is created at the antimesenteric border of jejunum. Two double-arm PDS are placed through the full thickness of duodenal and jejunal walls at both right and left corners with all the needles inside the lumen. After tying at the right corner intraluminally, one single arm is passed through duodenal wall in-out and left outside the duodenal wall to be utilized in anterior continuous running. The other single arm is utilized to perform intraluminal continuous running from right corner to left corner suturing posterior walls. Once the running suture of posterior wall reaches the other end, all three arms are tied. At the left corner, a single arm is passed through duodenal wall in-out and through jejunal wall out-in in extramucosal anastomosis. The stitches run a quarter of anterior wall leftward in the same manner. The remaining single arm on the right side is utilized in continuous extramucosal running sutures for anterior walls. After running 3 quarters of anterior wall, the suture is completed tying with the other single arm from left corner. If it is required, several reinforcement stitches are made to secure the anastomosis. (Fig. 37.12).

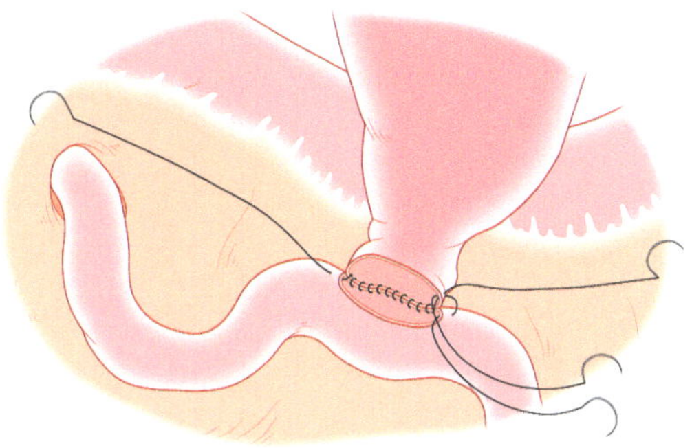

Fig. 37.12 Continuous duodenojejunostomy: Two double-arm PDS are placed at both right and left corners with the all needles inside of the lumen. After tying at the right corner intraluminally, a single arm was run to suture the posterior wall and tied with the other double arm at the left corner, where a single arm passes through the duodenal wall in-out and through jejunal wall out-in as in extramucosal anastomosis in addition to a quarter of anterior wall leftward in the same manner. The remaining single arm in the right suture anterior wall was run leftward in the method of extramucosal anastomosis. Finally, the suture is completed by tying with the other single arm from the left corner

37.11 Insertion of Drain and Closure

Openings at mesocolon and Treitz ligament are closed to prevent internal hernia. Drainages are placed near hepaticojejunostomy and pancreaticojejunostomy. The abdomen is closed layer by layer after confirming the absence of bleeding and other complications.

38 Hepatopancreatoduodenectomy

Shin Hwang

Abstract

Hepatopancreatoduodenectomy (HPD) is a combination of hepatectomy and pancreaticoduodenectomy. Its primary indications are diffuse bile duct cancer and advanced gallbladder cancer involving the peripancreatic lymph nodes. Since each phase of surgery is associated with high operative risk, it is important to lower the risk by reasonably adjusting the extent of hepatectomy, obviating the need for excessive and unnecessary dissection of the neural plexus around the hepatic arteries, and insertion of multiple abdominal drains.

Keywords

Diffuse bile duct cancer · Gallbladder cancer
Hepatectomy · Pancreaticoduodenectomy
Post-hepatectomy hepatic failure
Postoperative pancreatic leak · Complication
Lymph node metastasis · abdominal drain

S. Hwang (✉)
Division of Hepatobiliary Surgery and Liver Transplantation, Department of Surgery, Asan Medical Center, University of Ulsan College of Medicine, Seoul, South Korea
e-mail: shwang@amc.seoul.kr

38.1 Indications and Contraindications

The primary indications for HPD are diffuse bile duct cancer and advanced gallbladder cancer involving the peripancreatic lymph nodes [1–4].

Localized extrahepatic bile duct cancer, which is not diagnosed with diffuse bile duct cancer, is an indication for hepatic resection if the hepatic bile duct resection margin is tumor-positive on intraoperative frozen-section biopsy during bile duct resection. Another indication for pancreaticoduodenectomy is tumor-positive distal bile duct resection margin following intraoperative frozen-section biopsy during extended bile duct resection excavating the intrapancreatic bile duct. Consequently, if both proximal and distal bile duct resection margins are tumor-positive, HPD is indicated [1, 2]. In contrast, since HPD is considered a high-risk surgery for non-curative resection leading to microscopic tumor-positive resection margins, it is selectively performed to achieve curative resection with a high probability [4].

In case of advanced gallbladder cancer, pancreaticoduodenectomy is indicated if hepatectomy and bile duct resection cannot ensure complete removal of the tumor including the regional lymph nodes due to extensive involvement of the peripancreatic lymph nodes [3]. However, the outcome of HPD in advanced gallbladder cancers with deep involvement of the

H. C. Yu (ed.), *Hepato-Biliary-Pancreatic Surgery and Liver Transplantation*,
https://doi.org/10.1007/978-981-16-1996-0_38

hepatic parenchyma or suspected involvement of the para-aortic lymph nodes is associated with a high risk of early tumor recurrence leading to futile surgery [5, 6].

38.2 Preoperative Evaluation and Design for Surgical Resection

HPD can be divided into pre-planned and intra-operative categories for more aggressive surgery. In the case of pre-planned operation, if the hepatic parenchymal resection rate is more than 60% for right hepatectomy, preoperative right portal vein embolization is recommended to prevent liver failure after surgery. In surgically confirmed cases, it is safe to perform hepatectomy only when the rate of hepatic parenchymal resection is less than 60%. Not only does massive hepatic resection cause hepatic insufficiency, but the decrease in hepatic function due to massive hepatic resection significantly delays recovery and incidence of infection at the site of pancreaticoduodenectomy [7].

If the reason for hepatic resection in biliary tract cancer is to secure tumor-free hepatic duct resection margins, the hepatic parenchymal resection rate can be decreased via left hepatectomy or central parenchyma-preserving hepatectomy. If the reason for hepatic resection is removal of the hepatic infiltrating tumor in the gallbladder cancer, the prognosis is not significantly affected even if only a 2-cm-deep hepatic resection margin is secured via extended cholecystectomy or central partial hepatectomy. In gallbladder cancer, unlike perihilar bile duct cancer, the caudate bile duct is rarely infiltrated; thus, it is usually unnecessary to remove the caudal lobe concurrently.

When the pancreatic duct is not enlarged and the pancreatic parenchyma is normal, the risk of postoperative pancreatic leak after HPD is elevated. Thus, special attention is needed during hepatic artery resection due to hepatic artery invasion because of the high risk of rupture or pseudoaneurysm at the arterial anastomosis [8].

Portal vein invasion can be treated with end-to-end anastomosis after segmental resection up to 3 cm. If excessive tension is applied to the site of portal vein anastomosis due to forceful pulling after portal vein resection, the risk of anastomotic stenosis increases. Therefore, for resection of a long segment of the portal vein, interposition can be performed using a homologous or autologous vascular conduit.

The risk of postoperative pancreatic leak in pancreaticoduodenectomy is largely determined by the condition of the pancreatic parenchyma. In case of chronic pancreatitis or dilated pancreatic duct, aggressive periarterial plexus dissection is allowed because the risk of pancreatic leak is relatively low. However, in the case of normal pancreas, it is better to avoid complete peeling of the neural plexus around the hepatic artery over the entire length.

38.3 Surgical Techniques

Except for cases in which the gallbladder cancer is widely infiltrated and there is a risk of tumor cells spreading during transection of the tumor in the mid-portion of the common bile duct, HPD does not require resection of the liver–biliary tract–pancreas–duodenum in a single mass. In the case of diffuse biliary cancer, since the extrahepatic biliary tract is transected to confirm the bile duct resection margins, surgical resection is performed on the hepatic and the pancreatic sides.

Hepatic resection depends on the patterns of hepatic duct invasion. Since the left hepatic duct is relatively long, it is easy to obtain a tumor-negative resection margin, so HPD including right hepatectomy is generally performed (Fig. 38.1). However, it is advisable to avoid right hepatectomy with a hepatic parenchymal resection rate of 60% or more unless previously planned before surgery. The caudate lobe should be excised altogether given the tumor progression in diffuse bile duct cancer. Therefore, left hepatectomy combined with caudate lobectomy is one of the preferred methods.

As for hepatic parenchyma-preserving resection, the conventional approach is resection of the left medial section (segment IV) via caudate lobectomy (Fig. 38.2). Although this extent of surgery is technically difficult and requires reconstruction of both left and right hepatic ducts (Fig. 38.3), the hepatic parenchymal resection rate is as low as 15%. Because it is low enough, it has the advantage of virtually no risk of liver failure and can be performed in almost all cases without invading the major blood vessels in the hepatic hilum.

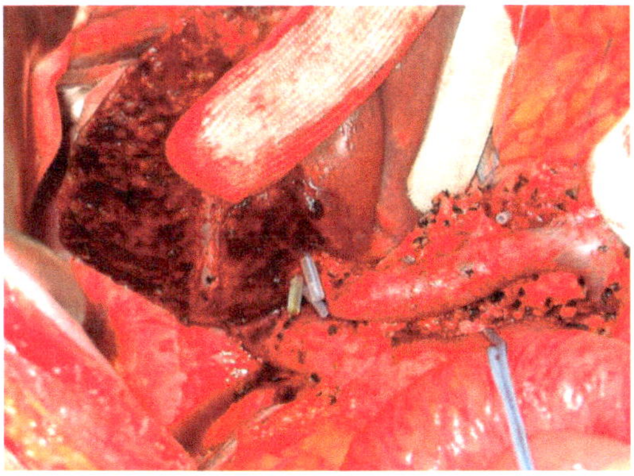

Fig. 38.1 Resection in a patient with diffuse bile duct cancer treated with right hepatopancreatoduodenectomy. The right lobe and caudal lobe were excised, and the remaining left lobe with three bile ducts exposed. Right portal vein embolization was performed before surgery; thus, the left liver is significantly enlarged. The left renal vein was encircled with a vascular loop for para-aortic lymph node resection

In diffuse biliary cancer, conventional pancreaticoduodenectomy is performed since the depth of bile duct wall infiltration within the pancreas is not severe. In the case of normal pancreas, a pan-

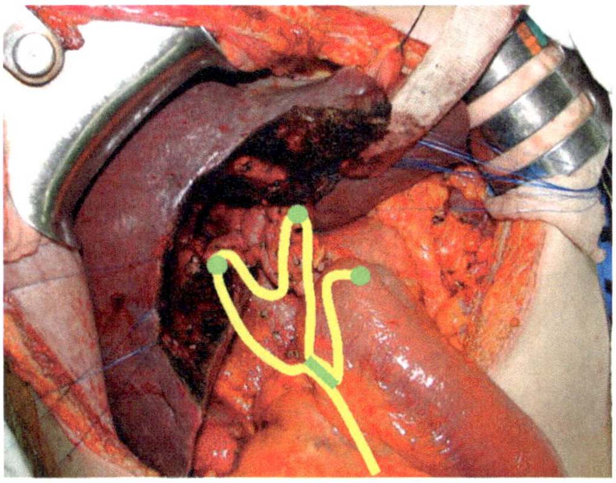

Fig. 38.3 Extent of resection in hepatopancreatoduodenectomy performed in a patient with diffuse bile duct cancer. The ventral portions of the segment IV, segment V, and caudate lobe were resected, and pylorus-preserving pancreaticoduodenectomy was performed. The photograph shows the preparation for biliary reconstruction after pancreato-enteric anastomosis. As shown in the illustration, a wide gap is made between the anastomoses at the jejunal limb side to anastomose the left and right bile ducts easily. Braun jejunojejunostomy was performed in the middle portion in order to prevent the pancreatic fluid flowing into the jejunum through the pancreatic-jejunal anastomosis from entering the biliary-enteric anastomosis

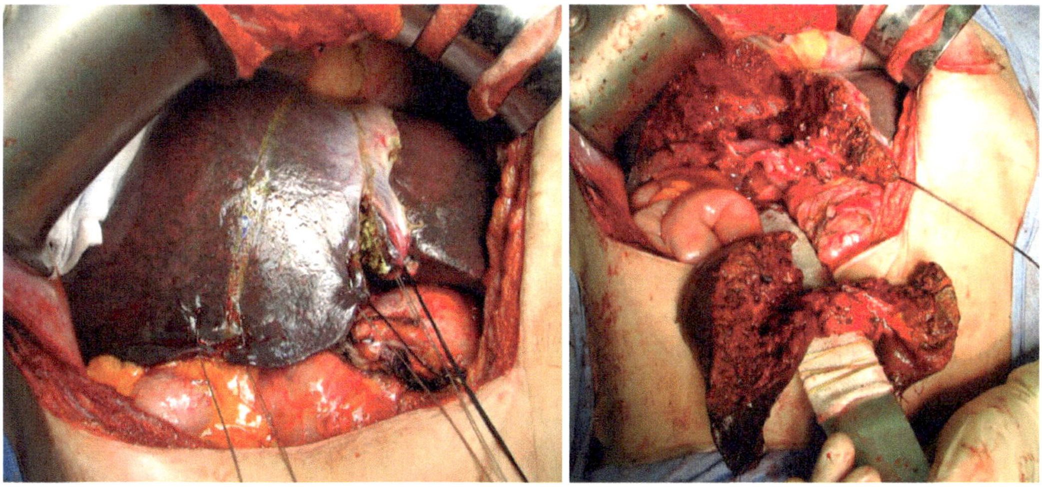

Fig. 38.2 Extent of hepatic parenchyma-preserving resection performed in a patient with diffuse bile duct cancer. The entire segment IV and caudate lobe were excised

creatic anastomosis at the pancreatic body after resecting the pancreas more than 2–3 cm to the left of the portal vein completely exposes the superior mesenteric and splenic vein confluence and reduces the risk of pancreatic leakage (extended pancreaticoduodenectomy).

In patients with advanced gallbladder cancer, if metastatic lymph nodes do not directly infiltrate the pancreatic parenchyma, only lymph node dissection is usually performed. Because the surgical field of view is relatively well secured via bile duct resection alone, it is possible to extensively dissect lymph nodes around the pancreatic head. When the metastatic lymph nodes locally infiltrate the pancreatic parenchyma, a small amount of pancreatic parenchyma can be removed at the lymph node level. Considering the poor prognosis after surgery due to extensive peripancreatic lymph node metastasis, it is rare to perform combined pancreatoduodenectomy only for extensive lymph node dissection.

Pancreatoduodenectomy is contraindicated if direct infiltration of the duodenum and gastric pyloric area is not clearly visible on the preoperative imaging studies, because it is usually locally resectable. Extensive invasion of the common bile duct along the cystic duct may be an indication for pancreaticoduodenectomy.

In cases where the gallbladder carcinoma is not associated with severe lymph node metastasis but involves extensive invasion of the surrounding tissues, pancreaticoduodenectomy may be performed for complete tumor resection. A large gallbladder mass is not uncommon in cases where the gallbladder cancer is associated with xanthogranulomatous cholecystitis. In advanced gallbladder cancer, hepatic parenchyma-preserving resection, such as central hepatectomy, is more commonly performed than major hepatic resection. Resection of the right lobe requires accurate evaluation of the extent of hepatic parenchymal resection because it entails extended right hepatectomy due to the location of the gallbladder.

38.4 Risks and Pitfalls During Surgery

Liver failure and pancreatic leak are the major surgical complications associated with HPD, resulting in severe outcomes. Therefore, special care should be taken to prevent such major complications.

Hepatic insufficiency is primarily due to excessive hepatic resection and rarely occurs unless right hepatectomy is performed. If right hepatectomy with a parenchymal resection rate of more than 60% is required, portal vein embolization before surgery is recommended to reduce the parenchymal resection rate [7].

The incidence of pancreatic leak following pancreaticoduodenectomy is quite high in normal pancreas. If there is such a risk, it is better to avoid excessive periarterial neural plexus dissection so that the arteries can partially withstand exposure to pancreatic fluid.

Fibrin glue can be applied to the hepatic artery dissection sites to form a protective film. The greater omentum can be separated to form an omental flap, which can be placed between the common hepatic artery and the pancreatic anastomosis to prevent pancreatic anastomotic leakage [9]. However, these protective measures are not effective once an anastomotic leakage occurs, so efficient intraperitoneal drainage tubes must be inserted in advance. The Jackson-Pratt type drainage tube has a relatively poor drainage effect on abscess fluid induced by pancreatic leak due to its structural limitation. Therefore, it is effective to insert a number of reliable Penrose or Cigarette drainage tubes [8, 10].

If the drainage tube is inserted from the right side around the pancreatic anastomosis, it is difficult to discharge the stuff that accumulates in the resection site of the pancreatic head and uncinate process. Thus, it is necessary to insert at least one drainage tube from the left upper abdomen toward the hepatic hilum along the path from which the duodenum was removed [10, 11].

Appropriate selection of patients is the most important criterion in HPD. Additional hepatic resection or pancreaticoduodenectomy is required to improve the prognosis via complete resection. The surgical risk is decreased if the extent of hepatic resection is reduced or accompanied by chronic pancreatitis, and the indications for operation can be expanded. Conversely, the risk of operation increases and the operation indication should be prudently selected if massive hepatic resection is required or in case of normal pancreas.

38.5 Conclusion

HPD is performed in combination with standard or pylorus-preserving pancreaticoduodenectomy as well as variable hepatectomy including right hepatectomy. The indications for this aggressive surgery are very limited and are associated with a relatively high risk of complications. The extent of resection is usually fixed in pancreaticoduodenectomy, but the extent of hepatic resection varies depending on the extent of tumor. It can be performed when the surgical risk is acceptable in patients who can expect to improve their prognosis following extended aggressive resection. Precise evaluation before surgery and delicate surgical intervention to prevent complications are required in order to decrease the risk of surgery.

References

1. Ebata T, Yokoyama Y, Igami T, Sugawara G, Mizuno T, Nagino M. Review of hepatopancreatoduodenectomy for biliary cancer: an extended radical approach of Japanese origin. J Hepatobiliary Pancreat Sci. 2014;21:550–5.
2. Lim CS, Jang JY, Lee SE, Kang MJ, Kim SW. Reappraisal of hepatopancreatoduodenectomy as a treatment modality for bile duct and gallbladder cancer. J Gastrointest Surg. 2012;16:1012–8.
3. Kaneoka Y, Yamaguchi A, Isogai M. Hepatopancreatoduodenectomy: its suitability for bile duct cancer versus gallbladder cancer. J Hepato-Biliary-Pancreat Surg. 2007;14:142–8.
4. Ebata T, Nagino M, Nishio H, Arai T, Nimura Y. Right hepatopancreatoduodenectomy: improvements over 23 years to attain acceptability. J Hepato-Biliary-Pancreat Surg. 2007;14:131–5.
5. Kaneoka Y, Yamaguchi A, Isogai M, Kumada T. Survival benefit of hepatopancreatoduodenectomy for cholangiocarcinoma in comparison to hepatectomy or pancreatoduodenectomy. World J Surg. 2010;34:2662–70.
6. Seyama Y, Kokudo N, Makuuchi M. Radical resection of biliary tract cancers and the role of extended lymphadenectomy. Surg Oncol Clin N Am. 2009;18:339–59.
7. Hwang S, Lee SG, Lee YJ, Park KM, Jeon HB, Min PC. Liver regeneration following extended liver resection combined with pancreatoduodenectomy. Korean J Hepatobiliary Pancreat Surg. 1998;2:73–8.
8. Jwa EK, Hwang S. Extended pancreatic transection for secure pancreatic reconstruction during pancreaticoduodenectomy. Ann Hepatobiliary Pancreat Surg. 2017;21:138–45.
9. Seyama Y, Kubota K, Kobayashi T, Hirata Y, Itoh A, Makuuchi M. Two-staged pancreatoduodenectomy with external drainage of pancreatic juice and omental graft technique. J Am Coll Surg. 1998;187:103–5.
10. Hwang S, Jung DH, Ha TY. Application of suction-type cigarette drain in leak-prone hepatopancreatobiliary surgery. Ann Hepatobiliary Pancreat Surg. 2020;24:305–8.
11. Yoon YI, Hwang S, Cho YJ, Ha TY, Song GW, Jung DH. Therapeutic effect of trans-drain administration of antibiotics in patients showing intractable pancreatic leak-associated pus drainage after pancreaticoduodenectomy. Korean J Hepatobiliary Pancreat Surg. 2015;19:17–24.

Part VIII

Operative Technique of Pancreatectomy

39 Pylorus-Preserving Pancreaticoduodenectomy

Dong Sup Yoon and Joon Seong Park

Abstract

Pancreaticoduodenectomy (PD) is the standard surgical treatment for tumors of the pancreatic head, proximal bile duct, duodenum, and ampulla. Since its initial description by Whipple et al. in the 1930s, it has evolved and undergone several modifications. The development of specialist units has contributed to a marked reduction in postoperative mortality from approximately 30% to 5–6% or less.

Keywords

Pancreatic resection · Pancreatoduodenectomy

Since its introduction in 1978 by Traverso and Long-mire, pylorus-preserving pancreaticoduodenectomy (PPPD) has become the standard of treatment in periampullary disease [1]. Current mortality rates are 3% or less at high-volume centers because of advances in intraoperative and postoperative care, as well as technical refinements [2].

39.1 Surgical Techniques

39.1.1 Patient Position and Skin Incision

Adequate exposure is mandatory for safe PPPD. The patient is positioned supine and a midline incision is performed (Fig. 39.1). An abdominal retractor is used for secure retraction. A thorough abdominal exploration is used to investigate peritoneal or hepatic metastases, focused on the pelvis for unexpected metastases.

39.1.2 Kocher Maneuver

Occasionally, the hepatic flexure of the colon is released inferiorly, and a Kocher maneuver is performed to elevate the duodenum and the head of pancreas. Kocher maneuver should be performed to the left of the abdominal aorta. The dissection is conducted cephalad above the retrocholedochal lymph node, inferior to the transverse duodenum, and medially to the aorta (Fig. 39.2).

Supplementary Information The online version contains supplementary material available at https://doi.org/10.1007/978-981-16-1996-0_39.

D. S. Yoon (✉) · J. S. Park
Pancreatobiliary Cancer Clinic, Department of Surgery, Gangnam Severance Hospital, Seoul, South Korea
e-mail: yds6110@yuhs.ac; JSPARK330@yuhs.ac

H. C. Yu (ed.), *Hepato-Biliary-Pancreatic Surgery and Liver Transplantation*,
https://doi.org/10.1007/978-981-16-1996-0_39

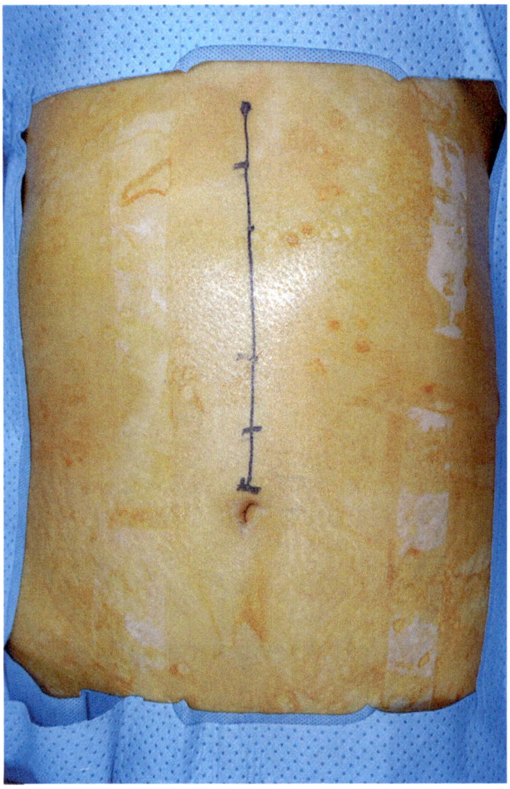

Fig. 39.1 Midline incision

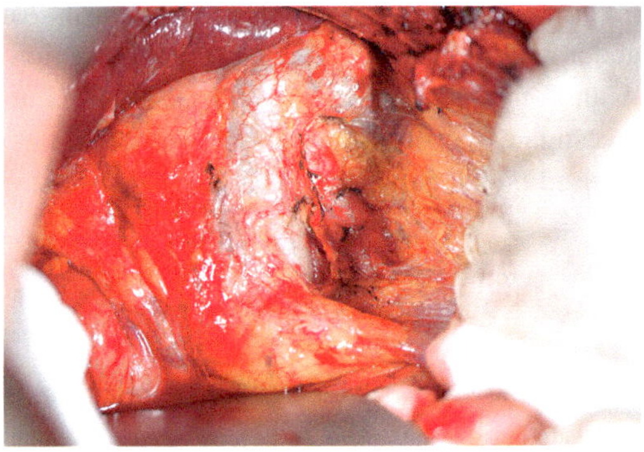

Fig. 39.2 Kocher Maneuver

39.1.3 Pancreatic Approach

The omentum is freed from the transverse colon in an avascular manner. The omental dissection is carried out from the right to the left, to complete separate the omentum from the right transverse mesocolon. The lesser sac is entered, and the entire anterior aspect of the pancreas is explored (Fig. 39.3a, b).

39.1.4 Duodenal Surgery

The right half of the omentum is mobilized and the proximal pancreas exposed, followed by the identification of middle colic vein down to its junction with the SMV. Exposing the lateral aspect of the SMV, the right lateral SMV is followed in a cephalad direction to the gastrocolic venous trunk. The gastrocolic trunk is ligated with fine sutures and divided (Fig. 39.4a, b). The right gastroepiploic artery and vein are divided and the stomach is retraced directly anteriorly, followed by duodenal traction. (Fig. 39.5) The duodenum can be severed at this time with GIA 2–3 cm distal to the pylorus (Fig. 39.6a, b).

39.1.5 Dissection of Lesser Sac

The gastrohepatic omentum beneath the left lobe of liver incised in an avascular manner carefully protects the nerves of Latarjet. Tissues anterior to the hepatoduodenal ligament are carefully incised and the right gastric artery divided. The common hepatic artery is identified and retraced (Fig. 39.7). The plane between the superior border of the pancreas and the common hepatic artery is dissected superiorly, and PV is identified. GB is mobilized from GB bed above downward. The cystic artery is ligated and divided. The common bile duct is palpated posteriorly to determine the presence of the accessory or the right hepatic artery arising from the SMA is replaced. The bile duct is then mobilized along the plane between the PV and the common hepatic duct, and clamped and severed (Fig. 39.8).

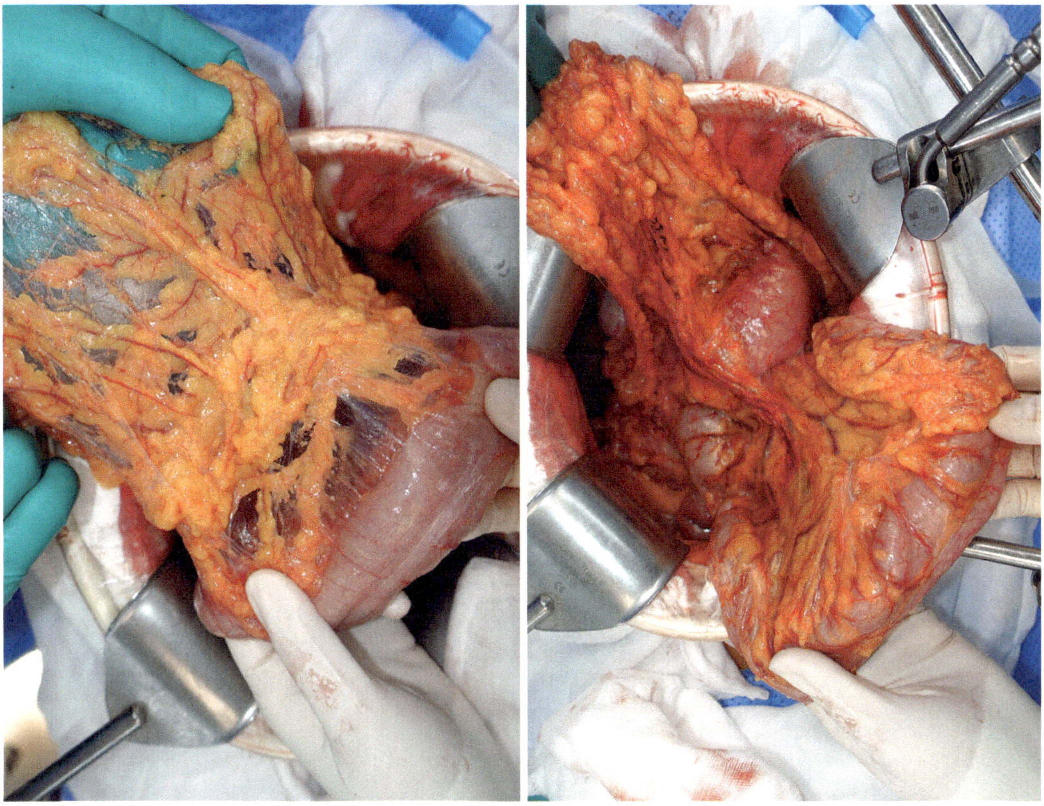

Fig. 39.3 Omentectomy

39.1.6 Division of the Pancreas

The space under the pancreatic neck anterior to superior mesenteric vein is suitable for dissection. Using a blunt clamp alternately advancing and spreading, a plane is then developed between the pancreatic neck anteriorly and the SMV-PV confluence posteriorly. A blunt clamp is then placed behind the pancreatic neck and slightly elevated. The pancreatic neck is divided carefully. The consistency of the pancreas and the size of the pancreatic duct is noted, and a specimen from the neck of the pancreas is removed and submitted as margin. Bleeding from the transected pancreas is controlled with sutures and ligated as needed.

Hemostasis is completed. The superior and inferior longitudinal pancreatic arteries are secured by suture ligatures. The end of the pancreas must be freed up for about 2 cm before the anastomosis is attempted, and any bleeding must be controlled via electrocoagulation or interrupted sutures (Fig. 39.9a, b).

Intraoperative assessment of the flow through the hepatic artery is performed before GDA ligation.

If median arcuate ligament syndrome is diagnosed during procedure, the median arcuate ligament must be divided before GDA ligation. GDA is identified and double-ligated after confirming the flow in the hepatic artery (Fig. 39.10a, b).

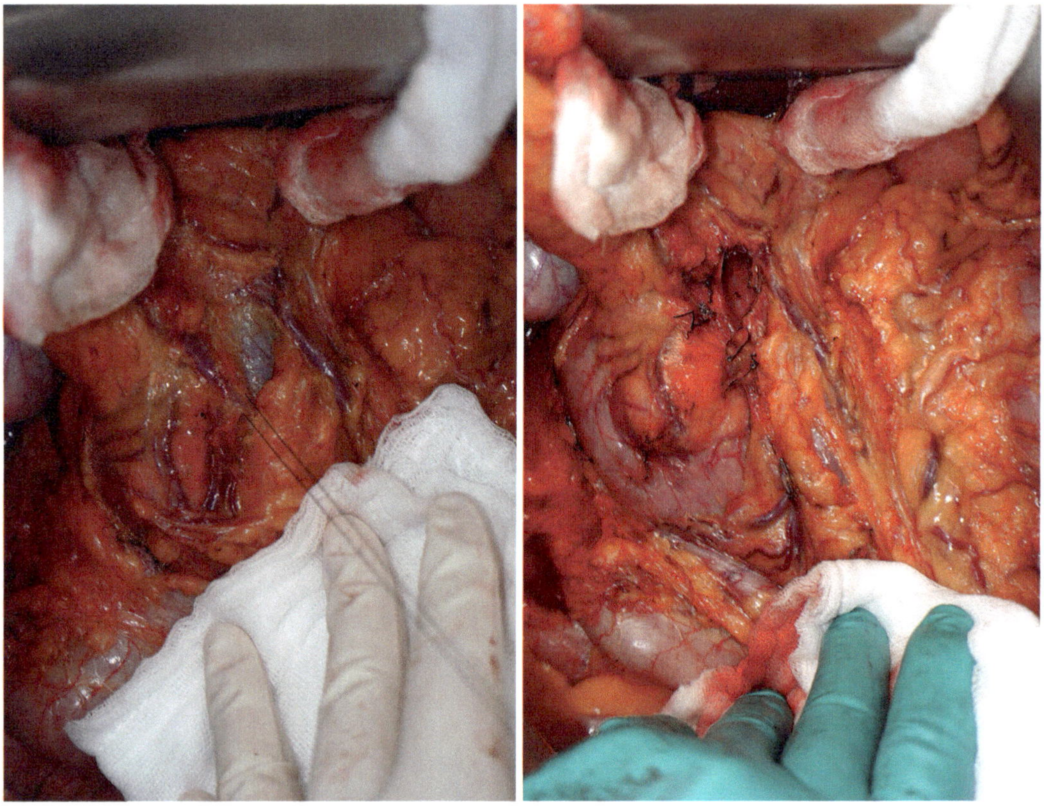

Fig. 39.4 Gatrocolic Trunk Approach

39.1.7 Mobilization of the Ligament of Treitz and SMA Dissection

The ligament of Treiz is mobilized, and the tissues to the right of the IMV are incised. The bowel is then transilluminated approximately 20 cm beyond the ligament of Treitz, and a mesenteric window is fashioned. The bowel is stapled and transected. With anterior and lateral traction on duodenum, the dissection is carried to a point at which the uncinate process is visible. Vein retractors are then applied to the SMV-PV confluence, and the PV is retracted to the patient's left, which allows retraction of the SMV-PV confluence to the left and anteriorly and provides access to the anterior aspect of the SMA. The adventitia of the SMA is incised carefully, exposing the SMA, followed by dissection posteriorly along the right side of the pancreas. It should be noted that the arterial branches originating from the posterolateral aspect of the SMA are very friable, easily avulsed, and may trigger annoying hemorrhage (Fig. 39.11a, b).

39.1.8 Reconstruction and Pancreaticojejunostomy

An opening is made in the mesocolon to the right of the middle colic vessels, through which

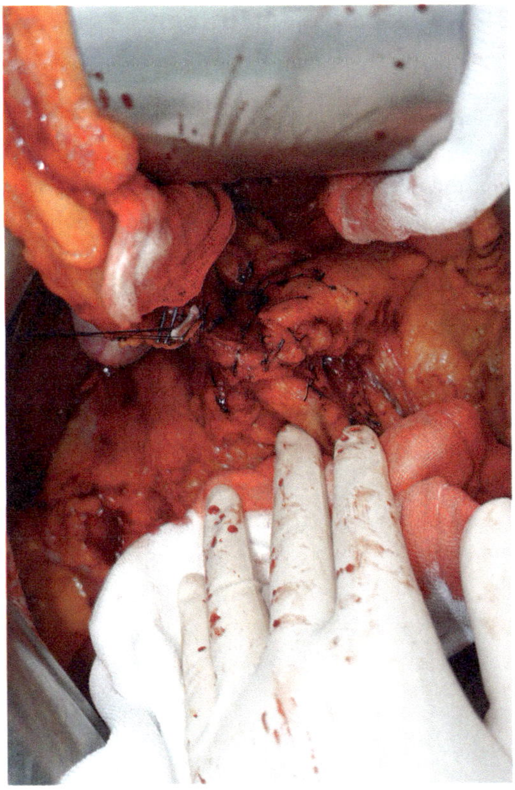

Fig. 39.5 Rt. gastroepiploic artery/Vein ligation

the jejunum passes. Preparations are made for the end-to-side pancreaticojejunostomy. The anastomosis is facilitated by mobilizing the pancreatic stump to elevate the stump anteriorly. With interrupted 4-0 vicryl sutures, the pancreatic parenchyma is sutured transversely to the seromuscular layer of the jejunum. A small opening is made with an insulated point cautery in a full-thickness stitch in the jejunum adjacent to the pancreatic duct. A silastic catheter with a diameter somewhat smaller than the pancreatic duct is inserted into the jejunal opening. The duct-to-mucosa anastomosis is created with interrupted 5-0 non-absorbable sutures with the posterior row completed tied. The silastic catheter is then advanced into the pancreatic duct to facilitate the anterior row of sutures and to prevent inadvertent suturing of anterior and posterior walls of the anastomosis. The sutures are placed inside-out on the jejunum and outside-in on the pancreatic duct, and tied. The anterior row of the anastomosis is completed with interrupted 4-0 vicryl sutures (Fig. 39.12a, b, c, d).

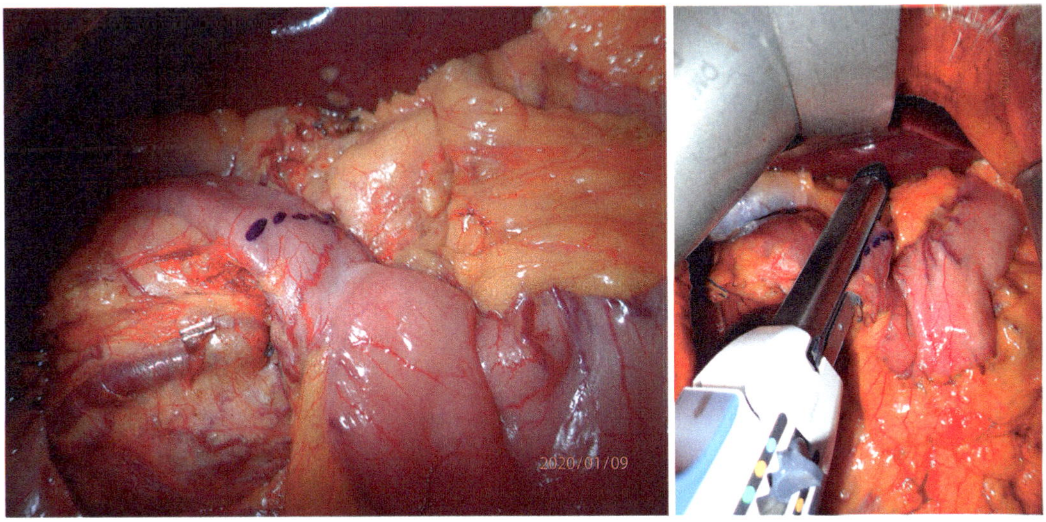

Fig. 39.6 Duodenal divided with GIA

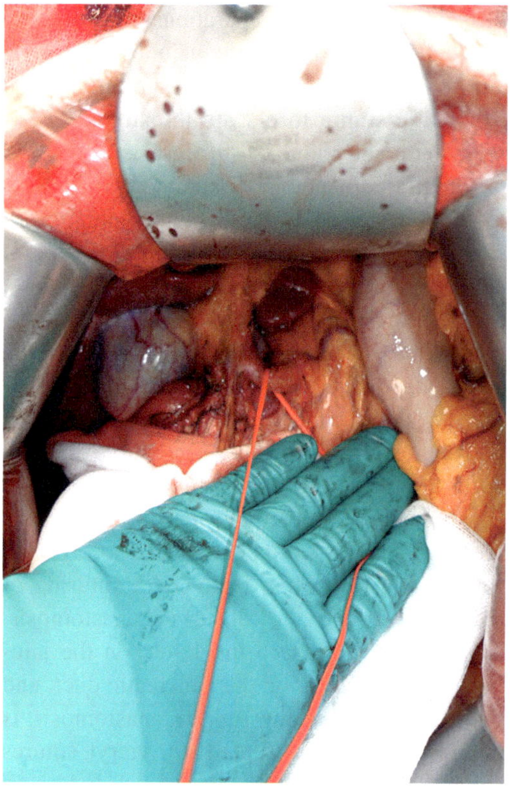

Fig. 39.7 Dissection of Lesser SAC

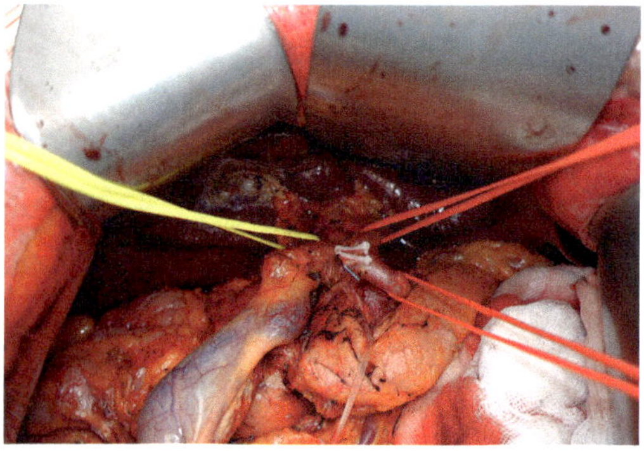

Fig. 39.8 Identify of CBD

39.1.9 Hepaticojejunostomy and Duodenostomy

Approximately 8–10 cm distal to the pancreaticojejunostomy, an end-to-side biliary enteric anastomosis is performed. A single layer of non-absorbable interrupted suture is used through all layers (Fig. 39.13). Approximately 25–30 cm distally, an end-to-side duodenojejunal anastomosis is created in two layers: an inner layer with a running suture of vicryl and an outer layer with permanent interrupted sutures (Fig. 39.14). Two JP drains are placed posterior to the biliary and pancreatic anastomoses.

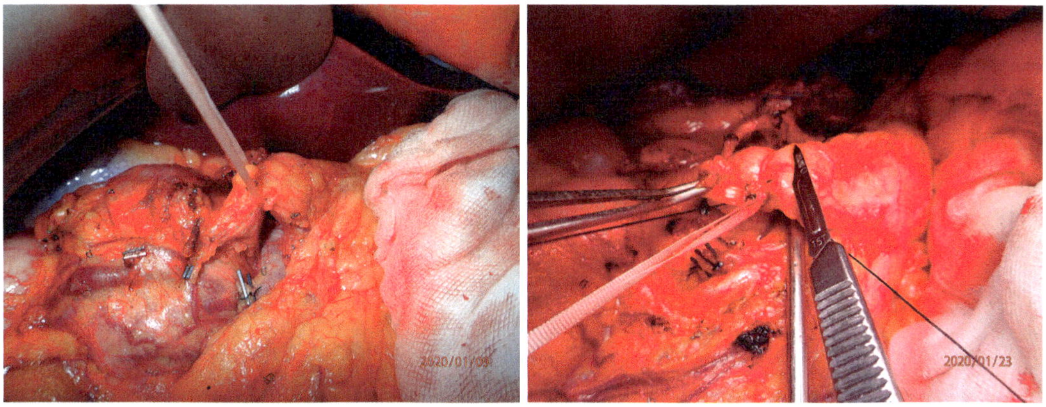

Fig. 39.9 Division of Pancreas

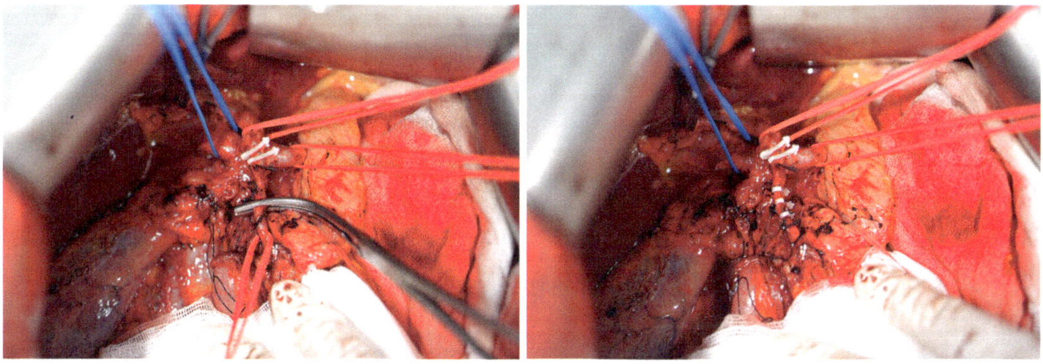

Fig. 39.10 GDA ligation

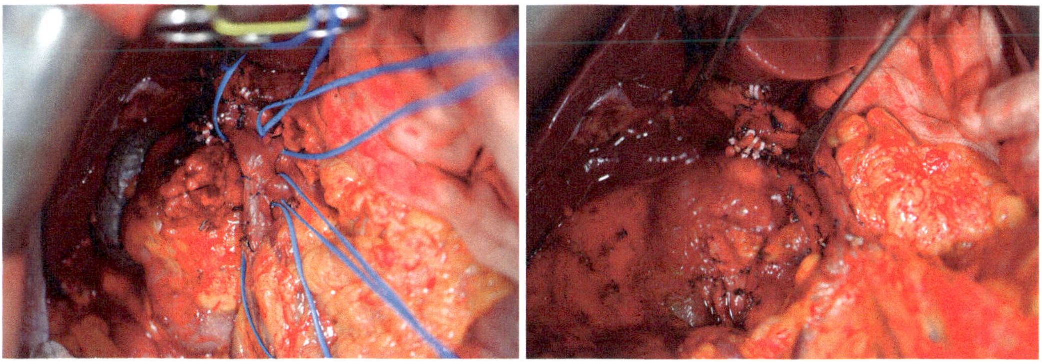

Fig. 39.11 SMV and SMA dissection

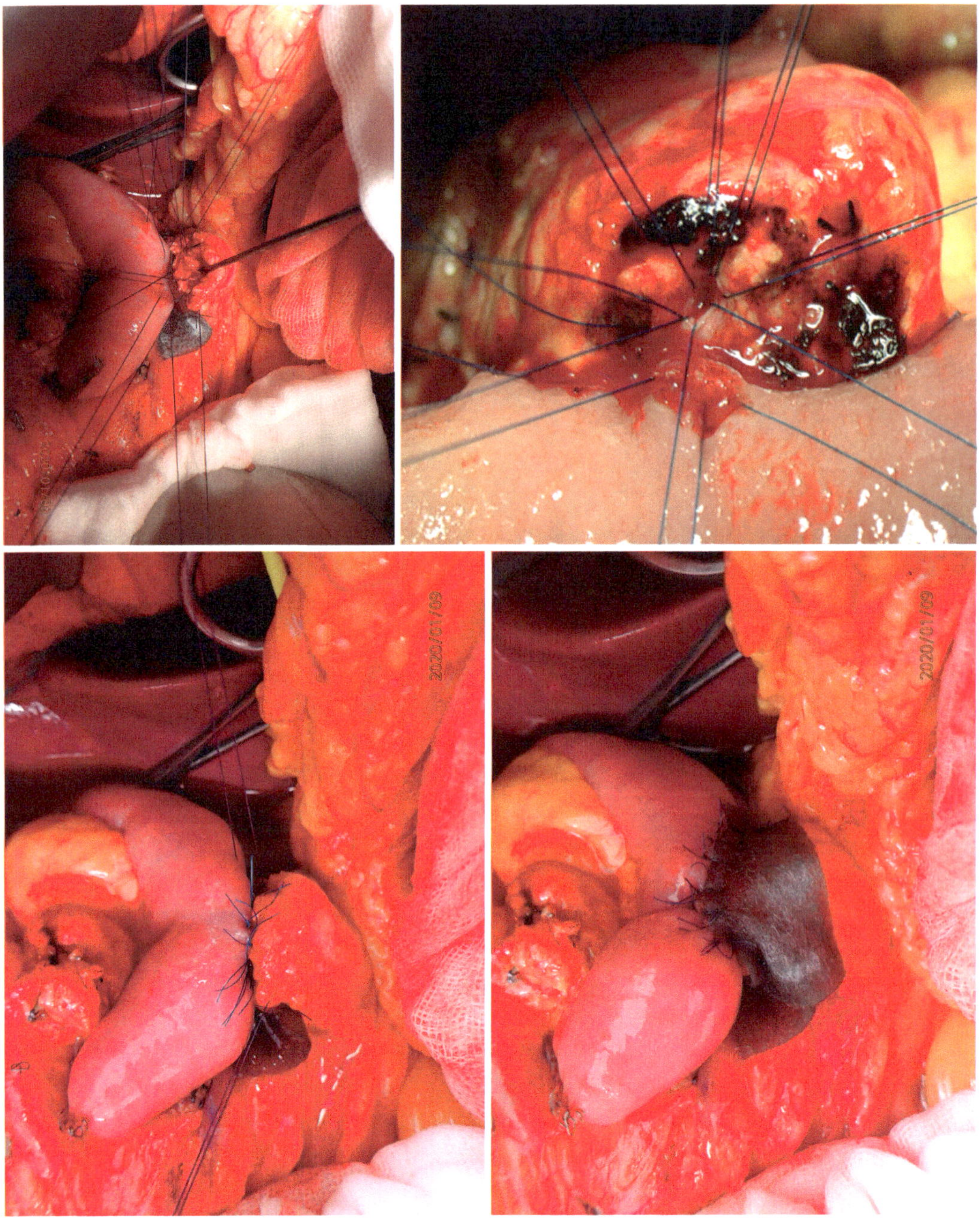

Fig. 39.12 Pancreatojejunostomy

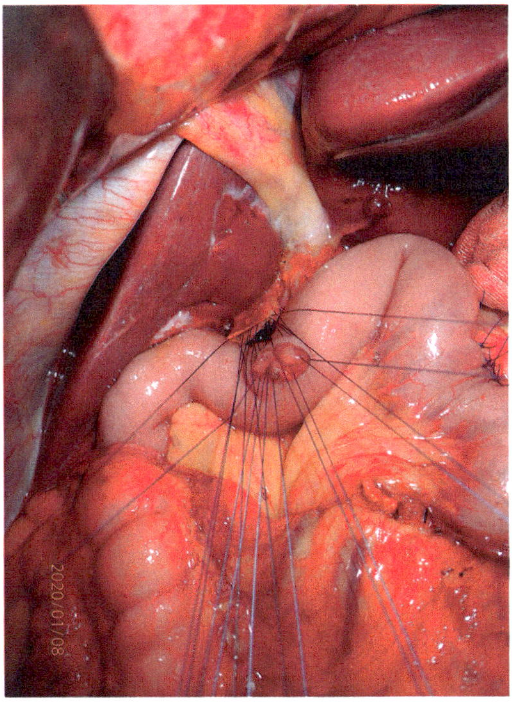

Fig. 39.13 Hepaticojejunostomy

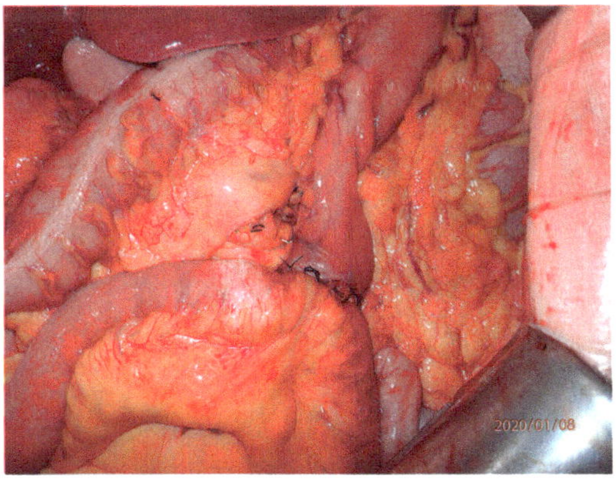

Fig. 39.14 Duodenojejunostomy

References

1. Traverso LW, Longmire WP Jr. Preservation of the protrusion pancreatoduodenectomy. Surg Gynecol Obstet. 1978;146:959–62.
2. Yeo CJ, Cameron JL, Sohn TA, et al. Six hundred fifty consecutive pancreatoduodenectomies in the 1990s: pathology, complications, and outcomes. Ann Surg. 1997;226:248–60.

40 Radical Antegrade Modular Pancreatosplenectomy (RAMPS)

Sung Su Yun and Dong-Shik Lee

Abstract

Conventional distal pancreatectomy for pancreatic cancer in the body or tail proceeds in a left-to-right retrograde fashion, which results in mobilization of the spleen and pancreas before dissection for the lymph node removal and vessel ligation. This approach has been associated with high positive margin rates and low lymph node (celiac and superior mesentery artery node) retrieval rate due to limitation of visualization for posterior plane of pancreas dissection. To overcome these problems, Strasberg et al., in 2003, introduced a novel method of operation for pancreatic cancer in the body and tail—radical antegrade modular pancreatosplenectomy (RAMPS). (Steven et al. Surgery. 133:521–7, 2003; Strasberg and Fields, Cancer J. 18:562-70, 2012; Hyo Jun Park et al. World J Surgery, 38: 86–193, 2014) RAMPS proceeds in a right-to-left antegrade fashion, with early parenchymal transection of pancreas, ligation of splenic vessels, dissection of celiac, and SMA lymph node. This procedure ensures the full visualization of the retroperitoneal plane of dissection and enables high negative resection margin and a large number of lymph node retrieval.

Keywords

RAMPS · Pancreas body · Tail cancer

40.1 The Procedure

40.1.1 Skin Incision

'L'-shaped incision or midline incision usually is performed.

40.1.2 Expose of Pancreas

The omentum between the colon and the stomach is separated with vessel sealing device which provides advantages such as shorter operating times and less bleeding during the entire operation process. When the omental dissection is completed, the gastrosplenic ligament is completely excised so that the stomach can be driven to the right from spleen. The short gastric vessels contained in gastrosplenic ligament are common causes of postoperative bleeding, so they must be safely ligated using hemolock clip or metal clip

Supplementary Information The online version contains supplementary material available at https://doi.org/10.1007/978-981-16-1996-0_40.

S. S. Yun (✉) · D.-S. Lee
Department of Surgery, Yeungnam University, College of Medicine, Daegu, South Korea
e-mail: ssyun@med.yu.ac.kr; dslee9@ynu.ac.kr

H. C. Yu (ed.), *Hepato-Biliary-Pancreatic Surgery and Liver Transplantation*,
https://doi.org/10.1007/978-981-16-1996-0_40

along the stomach side. The colon is separated from the spleen by dividing the splenocolic ligament. When we can see the whole pancreas, the location and boundary of the tumor are confirmed through palpation and ultrasound.

40.1.3 Kocherization

A Kocher maneuver is performed until we can expose the anterior surface of the left renal vein and the left of the aorta. Strasberg et al. recommended to put the gauze in the plane between left renal vein and pancreas. This procedure will provide easier to find dissection plane of dorsal border of RAMP in later.

40.1.4 Dividing Neck of the Pancreas

Retroperitoneal dissection of the lower border of the pancreas is performed near the neck of the pancreas to find the superior mesenteric vein. And then dissect as much as possible between the posterior surface of the pancreas and the superior mesenteric vein to expose the splenic vein and portal vein. After the lesser omentum is opened to find the proper and common hepatic artery, the right gastric artery is divided to facilitate lymph node dissection and expose ~~of~~ surrounding vascular structures. After dissection toward the common hepatic artery and proper hepatic artery, the lymph node around the common hepatic artery and the left margin of the portal vein are removed and then mobilize the common hepatic artery from the upper border of the pancreas. After this process, we can get a non-vascular tunnel between the pancreas and SMV. How to divide neck of the pancreas depends on the surgeon's preference. In these days, most surgeons like to use a stapler which depends on the hardness and thickness of the pancreas.

40.1.5 Ligation of Splenic Vessels and Dissection of Lymph Node

In the extension line of lymph node dissection around the common hepatic artery, celiac node dissection can be done around the origins of the left gastric, hepatic, and splenic arteries, but ligation of the left gastric artery should be judged depending on the progression of disease. In this way, the origin of the splenic artery is identified and divided. And then, the splenic vein is isolated at its junction with the superior mesenteric vein and divided. The further dissection is carried, dividing fat, and fibrous tissue until we can see the left side of the superior mesenteric artery. The left sides of the superior mesenteric and celiac arteries should now be visible down to the point that they come off the aorta. The lymph nodes anterior to the aorta between the celiac artery and superior mesenteric artery and those anterior and to the left of the superior mesenteric artery are taken with this step.

40.1.6 Determination of Posterior Plane of Dissection

When a rim of normal pancreas remains posterior to the tumor, the anterior RAMPS is chosen (Fig. 40.1). When the posterior margin of the tumor contacts or seems to break through the posterior capsule of the pancreas, the posterior RAMPS is selected (Fig. 40.2).

1. Anterior RAMPS

   The left renal vein is the point for the inferior line of the RAMPS technique. The left renal vein should be found during dissection of the lymph nodes and fibrous tissues around the left margin of the superior mesenteric artery and aorta. The adrenal veins are

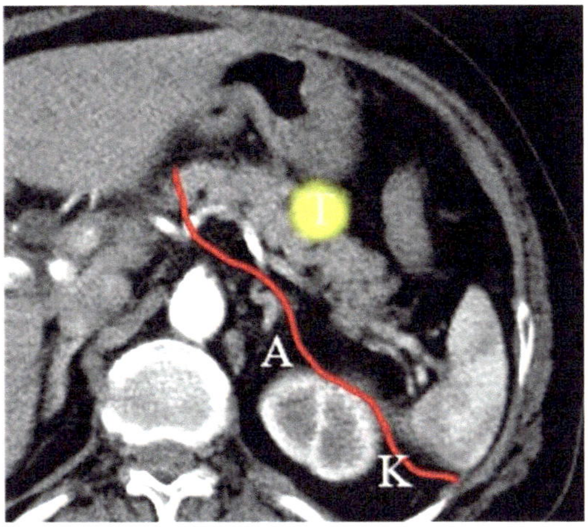

Fig. 40.1 Red line shows planned plane of posterior dissection as shown in preoperative CT scan in anterior RAMPS in which the tumor has not penetrated the posterior capsule of the pancreas. A left adrenal gland; K kidney; T tumor

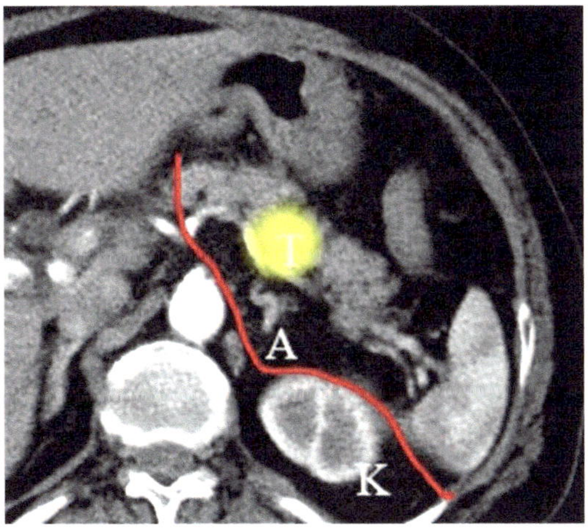

Fig. 40.2 Red line shows planned plane of posterior dissection as shown in preoperative CT scan in posterior RAMPS in which the tumor has penetrated the posterior capsule of the pancreas. A left adrenal gland; K kidney; T tumor

preserved and dissection begins in the anterior plane of the adrenal gland, continued laterally, usually taking Gerota's fascia. The superior and inferior attachments of the pancreas are divided as the dissection proceeds to the left. The inferior mesenteric vein is transected. Division of the several splenic ligaments is the last step in the procedure

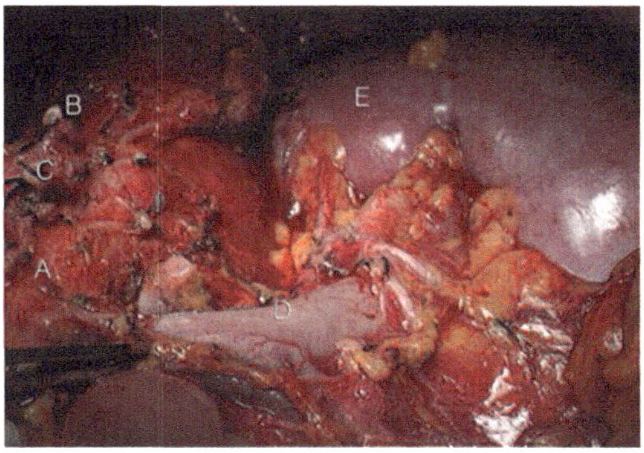

Fig. 40.3 Real picture taken after posterior RAMPS. A aorta; B left gastric artery; C splenic artery; D renal vein; E kidney

2. Posterior RAMPS

   In the posterior RAMPS, the adrenal vein is divided at its termination into the left renal vein, and the dissection is carried to the left and posteriorly behind the adrenal gland and onto the surface of the kidney. The view at the end of the dissection is shown in Fig. 40.3 [1]

40.1.7 Combined Resection of Other Organs

If there is local invasion to the surrounding organs, such as the stomach, large intestine, and mesentery of the colon, combined resection should be considered.

Reference

1. Yun SS, Lee DS, Kim HJ. Hepatobiliary & pancreatic surgery. Seoul: koonja; 2015. p. 237–40.

Further Reading

Strasberg SM, Drebin JA, Linehan D. Radical antegrade modular pancreatosplenectomy. Surgery. 2003;133:521–7.

Strasberg SM, Fields R. Left-sided pancreatic cancer: distal pancreatectomy and its variants: radical antegrade modular pancreatosplenectomy and distal pancreatectomy with celiac axis resection. Cancer J. 2012;18(6):562–70.

Park HJ, Do You D, Choi DW, Heo JS, Choi SH. Role of radical antegrade modular pancreatosplenectomy for adenocarcinoma of the body and tail of the pancreas. World J Surgery. 2014;38:86–193.

Spleen-Preserving Distal Pancreatectomy

41

Yong Hoon Kim

Abstract

Exposure to blood-borne antigens elicits immune response of spleen primarily. Spleen plays an important role in the patient's immune system. Spleen preservation is beneficial to the patient in the absence of oncological contraindication for distal pancreatic resection. However, because the splenic vessels are weak and the pancreatic parenchyma carries several short branches, it is easily damaged during surgery.

Keywords

Distal pancreatectomy · Spleen-preserving · Splenic vessel

41.1 Introduction

41.1.1 Terminology

The two types of spleen-preserving distal pancreatectomy include conservation of the splenic artery and vein, and the sacrifice of splenic vessels. The blood supply to spleen is maintained by the remaining short gastric artery [1]. In the latter case, partial necrosis of the splenic parenchyma may occur after surgery, but splenic infarction was reported in 1.9% of cases in a recent long-term follow-up series and gastric varices were detected in 25% of patients [2]. However, no cases of gastrointestinal bleeding or splenic hypertrophy were reported. Rather, the operation duration is short; the bleeding is minor and associated with few complications, which reduces the length of hospital stay [3]. We will only discuss distal pancreatic resection that preserves the spleen and splenic vessel (artery and vein).

41.1.2 Definition

During distal pancreatic resection, the pancreatic transection line may vary depending on the tumor location but usually refers to resection in the superior left portion of the pancreas at the junction of portal and superior mesenteric veins.

41.1.3 Indications

Pancreatic resection is indicated for benign tumors requiring surgery, pancreatic cystic neoplasm, and borderline malignant tumors in the body and tail of the pancreas without adjacent organ infiltration (Fig. 41.1).

Y. H. Kim (✉)
Department of Surgery, Keimyung University School of Medicine, Dongsan Medical Center, Daegu City, South Korea

H. C. Yu (ed.), *Hepato-Biliary-Pancreatic Surgery and Liver Transplantation*,
https://doi.org/10.1007/978-981-16-1996-0_41

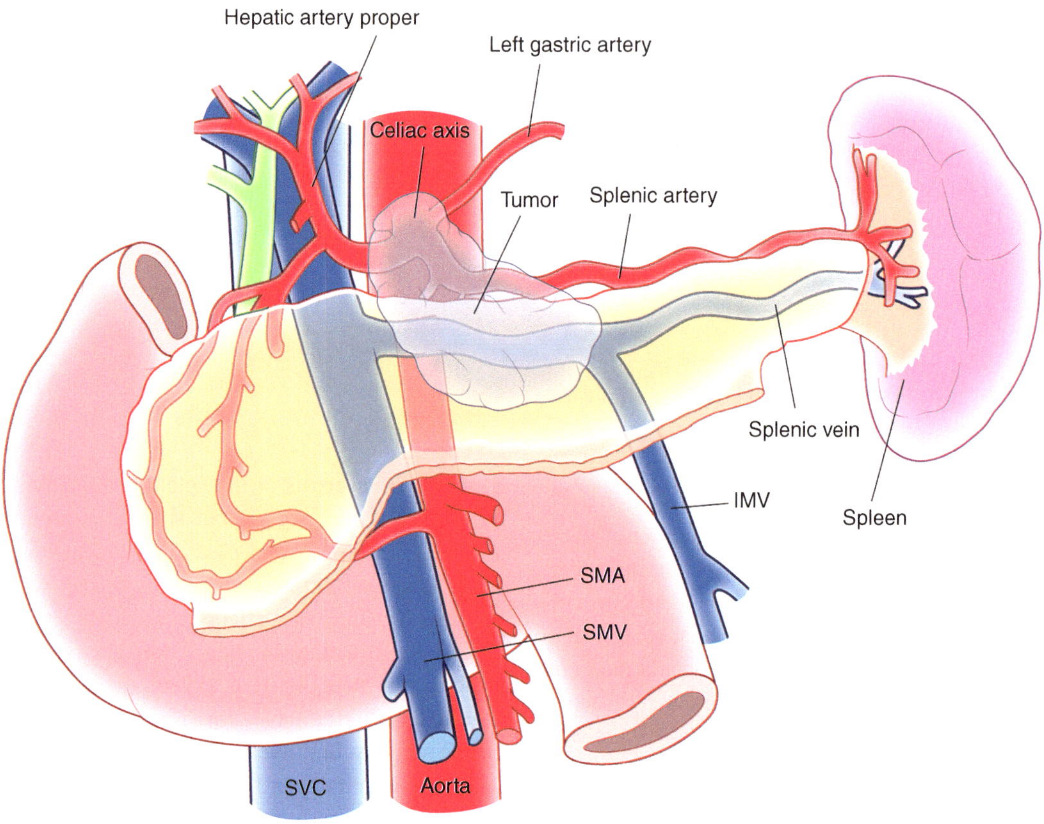

Fig. 41.1 Anatomical structure and blood vessels around the pancreas

41.2 Surgical Technique

41.2.1 Incision

Laparotomy may be performed with an upper midline incision or a left subcostal incision, and a lower midline incision or a right-side subcostal incision may be additionally performed depending on the patient's condition, the tumor location, and the anatomical structure.

41.2.2 Exposure of Pancreas and Confirmation of Pancreatic Tumor Location

After exploration of the entire abdominal cavity, the gastrocolic ligament is separated and opened to ensure sufficient visibility to the posterior gastric wall and anterior pancreas to identify the pancreatic head, body, and tail, and spleen. At this time, dissection is performed carefully to prevent damage to the short gastric vessel and the gastroepiploic arcade (Fig. 41.2a, b).

The proximal part is resected, followed by dissection toward the splenic hilum. Another method entails detaching the pancreatic tail from the splenic hilum and dissecting it toward the proximal part (from left to right) of the pancreas. There is a high possibility of damage to the small vascular branch of the spleen when the initial pancreatic parenchyma is separated from the spleen (left-to-right dissection). Therefore, it is safe to dissect it from the right to the left side.

The normal pancreatic region to be excised is selected proximally, and the peritoneum surrounding the pancreas is separated from the upper and lower pancreatic borders. Stay sutures are applied to both the upper and lower borders of the pancreas. The pancreas is blunt dissected

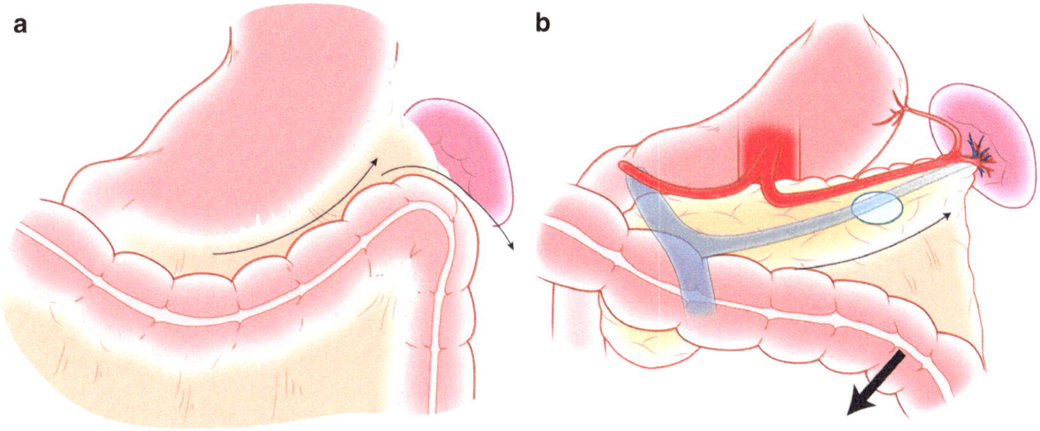

Fig. 41.2 (**a**) Gastrocolic ligament is sufficiently separated to expose the anterior part of the pancreas (**b**) The transverse colon from the spleen is separated and dropped down to secure the field of view

dorsally by lifting the supporting sutured pancreas upwards until the splenic vein is confirmed. The splenic vein runs parallel along the distal region deep inside the upper portion of the pancreatic parenchyma from the back of the pancreas. If it is difficult to identify the splenic vein, it is easier to examine the portal vein-splenic vein junction, underneath the pancreatic neck, and detached to the splenic hilum. The splenic artery is usually located along the upper border of the pancreas. After the spleen artery and vein are separately taped with a vascular loop, the pancreas can be excised and dissected to the distal portion.

1. The gastrocolic ligament is separated, and the transverse colon is dropped downwards to expose the anterior pancreatic surface.
2. Caution is needed to avoid damage to the gastroepiploic arcade.
3. Blunt dissection and taped back of the pancreas are followed by upper and lower stay suture.
4. After the pancreas is transected, the dissection proceeds while lifting from the right side to the splenic hilum. When lifting the pancreas upward, caution is necessary to prevent tears in the branch of the short splenic vein by applying excessive force.

41.2.3 Pancreatic Dissection

The umbilical tape is hung after deciding the expected pancreatic cutting area and tunneling the back of the pancreas. A support stay suture is applied to the upper and lower portions of the pancreas, and the pancreas is incised while pulling upward. The transection is usually initiated with electrocautery, and the last incision is made using a knife around the main pancreatic duct for accurate identification (Fig. 41.3). In addition, the pancreas may be cut using ultrasonic shears instead of electrocautery or it may be excised at once with a linear stapling device.

41.2.4 Management of the Pancreatic Remnant

The most common complication after distal pancreatic resection is pancreatic fistula. Several methods have been reported to treat the remaining pancreatic stump after resection and to prevent the leakage of pancreatic duct from the divided pancreas, but there is no way to consistently reduce the pancreatic fistula. In a meta-analysis comparing hand-sewn ligation suture and automatic suture (staple) for treatment of pancreatic remnants after pancreatic resection,

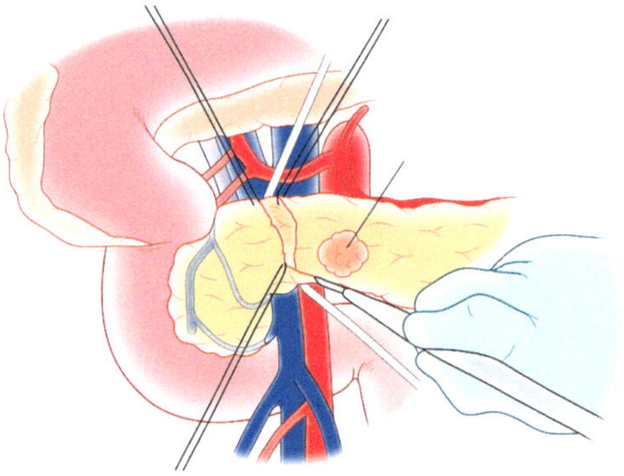

Fig. 41.3 The expected portion of the pancreatic cut is placed on the U-tape and a support suture is applied on the cutting surface

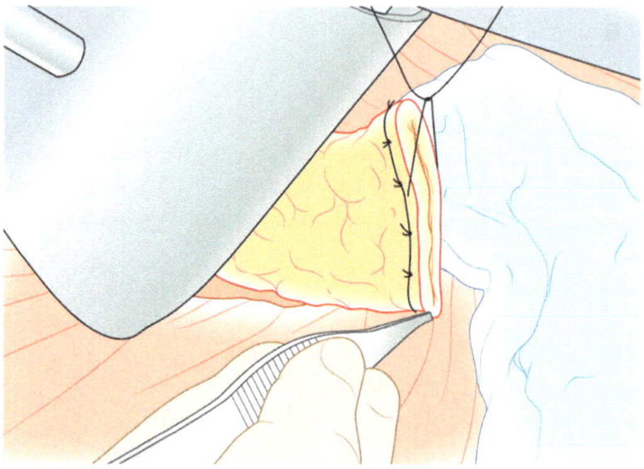

Fig. 41.4 The remaining cut surface of the pancreas is closed with a non-absorbable suture in the form of a fish mouth to prevent pancreatic fistula

no statistically significant difference was found in the incidence of pancreatic fistula between the two methods. When the two methods were compared in a multicenter prospective comparative study conducted in a European group, no significant difference was found in the occurrence of pancreatic fistula between the two groups. Our institute prefers application of a fibrin sealant after cutting with an automatic suture (staple) or suture ligating the cut surface of the pancreatic duct.

1. Direct ligation or suture of the main pancreatic duct: When the pancreas is cut with a surgical knife, the remaining cut surface is interrupted with a mattress suture and sealed in a fish-mouth form. At this time, it is important to examine the main pancreatic duct and ligate it separately (Fig. 41.4).
2. Using a linear stapling device: If the pancreas is relatively soft and not so thick, it is better to cut with an automatic suture device (staple), because the stapling line tightly holds the cutting surface in a tight row. It can prevent the leakage of microscopic pancreatic ducts. The self-sealing cartridge of appropriate height can be used according to the thickness of the pancreas, and the appropriate one can be selected based on the color of manufacture [4].
3. Other methods include anastomosis of the main pancreatic duct with jejunum, and covering the pancreatic stump with the greater omentum, the small bowel, or the falciform ligament of the liver.
4. Sealing with a fibrin sealant: After treating the cut surface with method A or B, the fibrin sealant may be used additionally to prevent pancreatic fistula [5].

41.2.5 Pancreatic Detachment from the Splenic Vein

After the pancreas is transected, the dissection is performed by lifting the pancreas to the upper left side. Small branches, usually from the splenic vein, are weak and often enter the pancreatic parenchyma briefly, which can lead to severe bleeding during the dissection. It is common to ligate and separate both sides of a small vein branch. However, if the branch is short and the space is narrow for clamping, the remaining side is ligated with a suture or a hemostatic clip ensuring safe hemostasis of the pancreatic side excised with ultrasonic shears.

Vascular sutures may be performed using non-absorbable monofilament 5-0 suture material if there is bleeding from the venous branch during dissection of the splenic vein. Dissection can be performed from the proximal to the distal part (spleen) until the pancreatic tail is separated from the splenic hilum (Fig. 41.5). At this time, the surgery is in the final stage. The surgeon should be careful not to pull the pancreas excessively

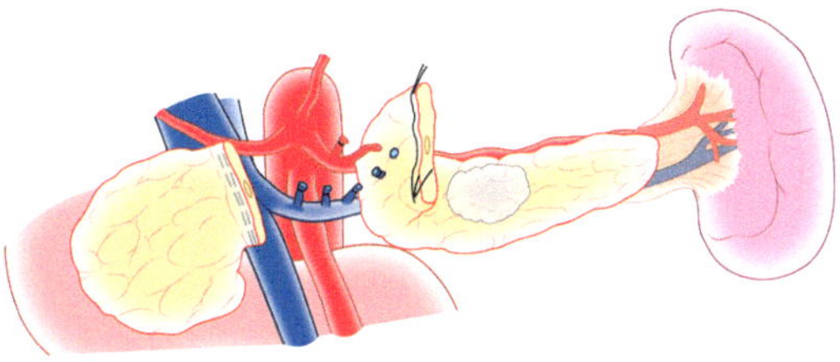

Fig. 41.5 The pancreas is transected and raised from the right to the left during the dissection, avoiding excessive traction to prevent damage to the splenic vein branch

upward to prevent tearing of short gastric or left gastroepiploic vessels and bleeding. It is a good practice to avoid mobilizing the spleen and lifting it to the right, which can increase the risk of iatrogenic splenic injury.

41.3 The Surgical Field of View Is Evaluated before Completing the Surgery and Post-Operative Patient Care

Following the pancreatic resection, a re-evaluation of bleeding in the surgical field is necessary, and if unclear, hemostasis should be carefully performed via ligation and electrocautery. It is important to ensure that no bleeding occurs in the small branch of the preserved splenic vein. After sufficiently washing the abdominal cavity with physiological saline and confirming the absence of gauze on the back of the spleen or the back of the stomach, the closed suction drain is placed around the remaining pancreatic stump. The stomach and omentum are covered with the front of the pancreas to close the open abdominal wall.

Immediately after surgery, the patient's hemodynamic status is monitored to ensure that there is no rapid bleeding. The nature (color, viscosity, amount of drainage) of the drainage catheter is evaluated daily and the amylase level measured to determine the occurrence of pancreatic fistula.

References

1. Warshaw AL. Conservation of the spleen with distal pancreatectomy. Arch Surg. 1988;123(5):550–3. https://doi.org/10.1001/archsurg.1988.01400290032004. PMID: 3358679
2. Ferrone CR, Konstantinidis IT, Sahani DV, Wargo JA, Fernandez-del Castillo C, Warshaw AL. Twenty-three years of the Warshaw operation for distal pancreatectomy with preservation of the spleen. Ann Surg. 2011;253(6):1136–9. https://doi.org/10.1097/SLA.0b013e318212c1e2. PMID: 21394008
3. Jain G, Chakravartty S, Patel AG. Spleen-preserving distal pancreatectomy with and without splenic vessel ligation: a systematic review. HPB (Oxford). 2013;15(6):403–10. https://doi.org/10.1111/hpb.12003. Epub 2012 Dec 2. PMID: 23458666; PMCID: PMC3664043
4. Tieftrunk E, Demir IE, Schorn S, Sargut M, Scheufele F, Calavrezos L, Schirren R, Friess H, Ceyhan GO. Pancreatic stump closure techniques and pancreatic fistula formation after distal pancreatectomy: meta-analysis and single-center experience. PLoS One. 2018;13(6):e0197553. https://doi.org/10.1371/journal.pone.0197553. PMID: 29897920; PMCID: PMC5999073
5. Wilson C, Robinson S, French J, White S. Strategies to reduce pancreatic stump complications after open or laparoscopic distal pancreatectomy. Surg Laparosc Endosc Percutan Tech. 2014;24(2):109–17. https://doi.org/10.1097/SLE.0b013e3182a2f07a. PMID: 24686344

Laparoscopic Pancreaticoduodenectomy

42

Song Cheol Kim and Ki Byung Song

Abstract

During the past 25 years, the feasibility and safety of minimally invasive pancreatic surgery have been established progressively. Although laparoscopic pancreaticoduodenectomy (LPD) is one of the most technically challenging procedures, it is safe, feasible, and oncologically acceptable when performed in a high-volume center. Studies have demonstrated the several advantages of minimally invasive approaches compared with the open approach for pancreatic resection, namely, less blood loss, shorter hospital stay, and early recovery. LPD requires long and steep learning curve.

Keywords

Laparoscopic pancreaticoduodenectomy · Pancreatic head tumor

Supplementary Information The online version contains supplementary material available at https://doi.org/10.1007/978-981-16-1996-0_42.

S. C. Kim (✉) · K. B. Song
Division of Hepatobiliary and Pancreatic Surgery, Department of Surgery, Asan Medical Center, University of Ulsan College of Medicine, Seoul, South Korea
e-mail: drksc@amc.seoul.kr

42.1 Historical Background

- Pancreaticoduodenectomy has been considered one of the most challenging abdominal surgeries. Because of the complexity of the techniques used, surgeons require more training time than in other abdominal surgeries, in order to gain adequate experience.
- Gagner and Pomp were the first to describe laparoscopic pancreaticoduodenectomy (LPD) in 1994 [1]. During the first 10 years, the progress of LPD was slow due to widespread controversy and opposition.
- Over the past 2 decades, advances in LPD have resulted in major improvements in perioperative and oncologic outcomes in high-volume centers [2, 3]. LPD represents a potential alternative to open approach following the learning curve.

42.2 Surgical Management

- Positioning and trocar placement

  The patient is placed in the supine position. An anti-Trendelenburg (10–30°) is used to expose the operation field. Two monitors are placed at the sides of the operator and first assistant. The primary surgeon and the second assistant, who holds the laparoscope, stand to the right of the patient. The first assistant and the scrub nurse are positioned to the left of the

H. C. Yu (ed.), *Hepato-Biliary-Pancreatic Surgery and Liver Transplantation*,
https://doi.org/10.1007/978-981-16-1996-0_42

patient. Alternatively, a split-leg positioning can be used for LPD. In this position, the operator stands between the legs of the patient and the assistants stand on either side of the patient. Open technique is used to establish the pneumoperitoneum using a 12-mm trocar on the umbilicus. A 30° angled vision scope is used to visualize the deep portion. The trocar locations are shown in Fig. 42.1. Three-dimensional visualization improves image quality and accuracy in spatial distance and hand–eye coordination, which enhances performance and surgical manipulation. Additional four trocars are placed under direct vision. Two to three 5-mm trocars (one on the right flank for the left hand of the surgeon and one to two on the left flank for surgical assistance, if necessary) and two 12-mm trocars (one for the laparoscope and one on the umbilicus for the right hand of the surgeon) are employed. Abdominal pressure is maintained at 12 mmHg using carbon dioxide (CO_2) gas insufflation. It is impor-

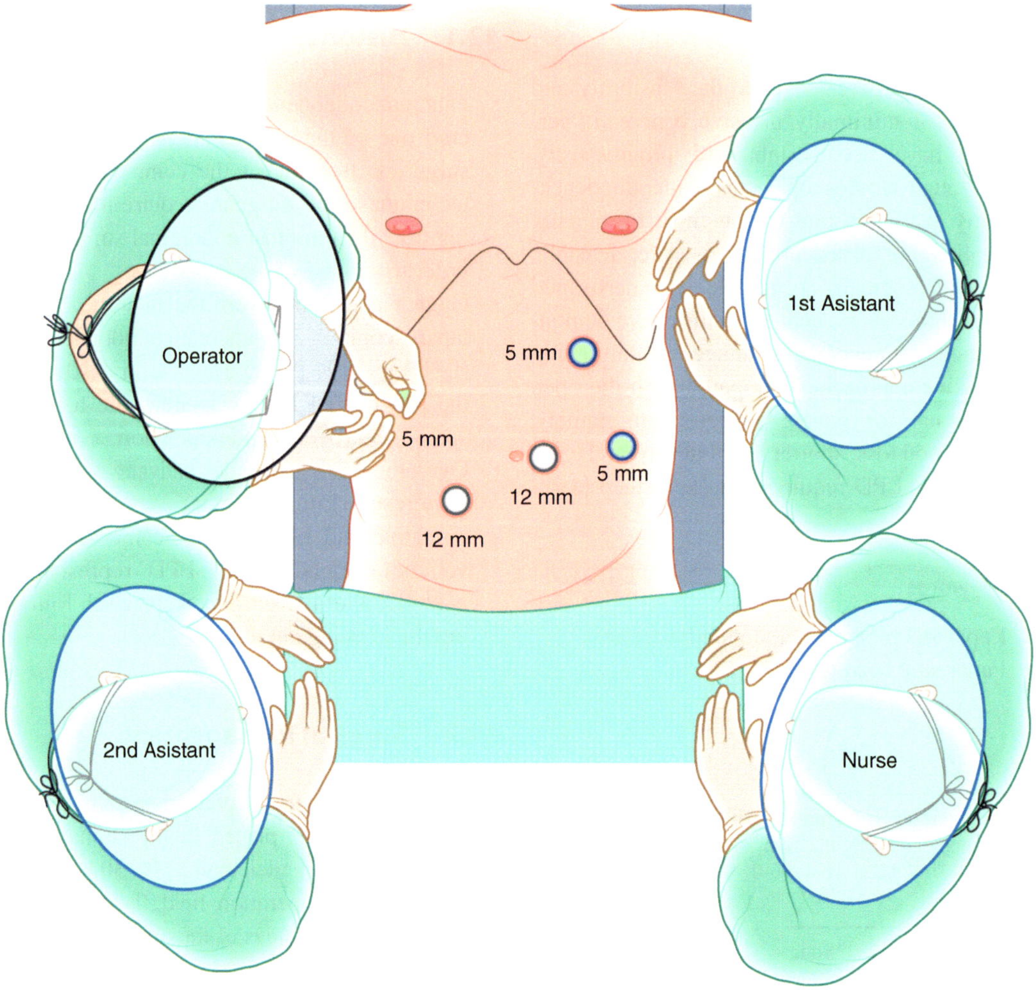

Fig. 42.1 Location of trocar for laparoscopic PD. Three 5-mm trocars (one on the right flank for the left hand of the surgeon and two on the left flank for surgical assistance) and two 12-mm trocars (one for the laparoscope and one on the umbilicus for the right hand of the surgeon) are employed. (PD, pancreaticoduodenectomy)

tant to minimize accumulation of CO_2 gas by maintaining the abdominal inflation pressure low, not more than 12 mmHg.

- Identification of the portal vein and division of the duodenum or stomach

Any abnormalities or metastasis in the entire abdomen is examined. The entire hepatic and peritoneal surfaces should be inspected. The gastrocolic omentum is dissected to allow entry into the lesser sac. Intraoperative ultrasound may be used for further examination to identify the location of the lesion. The portal vein (PV) is identified at the inferior border of the pancreas by distally following the gastroepiploic vein (GEV) along its insertion into the SMV. The GEV is clipped and divided at its entry into the SMV. The anterior aspect of the retropancreatic segment of the PV/SMV is dissected, and a tunnel is created (Fig. 42.2). The gastrohepatic omentum is opened to expose the hepatic artery coursing cephalad to the pancreas. The right gastric artery is ligated using a metal clip and divided using a Harmonic scalpel. After dividing the branches of the right gastroepiploic vessels along the duodenum, the duodenum is divided 2 cm distal to the pylorus using an endoscopic linear stapler. Alternatively, resection of the gastric antrum can be performed according to surgical preference or when an adequate margin cannot be acquired. The stomach is placed in the left upper abdomen, providing better surgical view around the pancreatic head. The upper border of the pancreas is dissected to establish a triangular zone formed by the common hepatic artery, upper border of the pancreatic neck, and the gastroduodenal artery (GDA) (Fig. 42.3). The GDA is ligated at its origin and then divided with a vascular staple load. The author recommends marking this vessel as well using a clip. The PV tunnel is completed and gentle upward traction of the isolated pancreas is applied using an umbilical tape in preparation for pancreatic division.

- Mobilization of the right colon and duodenum, and identification of the superior mesenteric vein

The peritoneum of the hepatic flexure of the right colon is incised. The right colon is mobilized downward and to the left side of the patient to fully expose the second and third portions of the duodenum. The dissection between the mesocolon and the duodenum/pancreatic head is continued along the avascular surgical plane and is facilitated by the first assistant pulling the mesentery of the

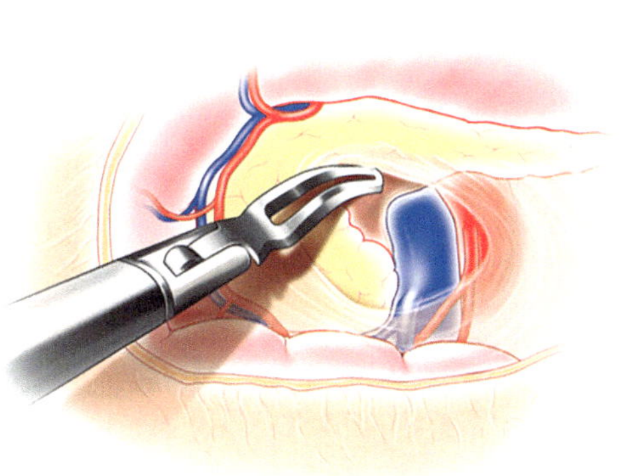

Fig. 42.2 Identification of PV and SMV. The SMV is identified at the inferior border of the pancreas and dissected up to the retropancreatic PV. (PV, portal vein; SMV, superior mesenteric vein)

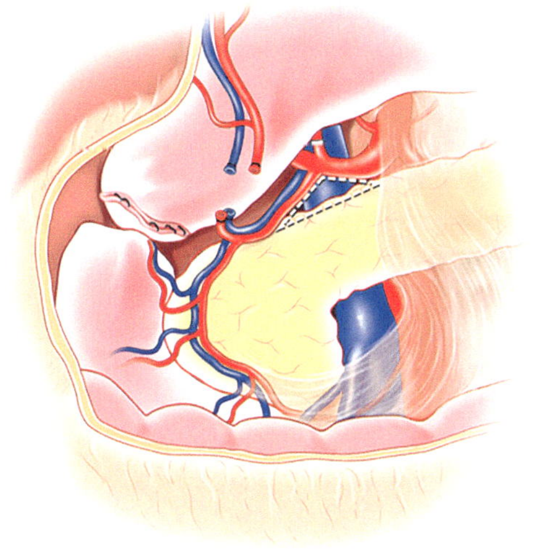

Fig. 42.3 Triangular zone. The common hepatic artery, upper border of the pancreatic neck, and GDA form a triangle for the tunnel behind the pancreatic neck. The triangular space is dissected to isolate the pancreas from the PV (tunneling) and a gentle upward traction of the isolated pancreas is applied using a cotton tape in preparation for pancreatic division (GDA, gastroduodenal artery)

right colon toward the patient's right lower quadrant. The third and fourth portions of the duodenum are mobilized (Kocher maneuver), including the division of the ligament of Treitz (Fig. 42.4). Dissection is continued to the left of the aorta and up to the origin of the superior mesenteric artery (SMA). The third and fourth portions of the duodenum must be fully exposed prior to the division of the mesentery to the duodenum.

- Dissection of the porta hepatis

  Cholecystectomy is performed. The lymphatic dissection occurs distally from the divided origin of the GDA until the bifurcation of the proper hepatic artery. Careful dissection of the bile duct should be performed to avoid injury to the accessory or replaced hepatic artery from the SMA traveling posterior to the common bile duct or the low-lying right hepatic artery traversing anterior to the bile duct. Preoperative review of the CT scan and careful inspection before division of the bile duct is crucial to avoid unexpected injury to the hepatic artery because palpation of the porta hepatis is impossible in laparoscopic surgery. The common bile duct is divided. The proximal duct is controlled with a bulldog clamp. The distal duct is ligated to prevent contamination and facilitate hemostasis. The PV is now fully exposed by dissecting the soft tissues and lymphatics using ultrasonic shears or monopolar electrocautery.

- Division of the pancreatic neck

  Suture ligation of the longitudinal arteries coursing within the parenchyma along the superior and inferior border of the pancreatic neck can be used to control bleeding from the cut surface during pancreatic transection. We prefer to use ultrasonic shears to divide the pancreatic parenchyma to minimize bleeding. The pancreatic duct is resected using laparoscopic scissors (METZENBAUM ENDO) and identified (Fig. 42.5). A frozen tissue section can be obtained from the margin of the pancreas. The remaining pancreatic stump is further dissected to provide a mobility of 1–2 cm necessary to invaginate the pancreas into the jejunum for the pancreaticojejunostomy (Fig. 42.6).

- Transection of the proximal jejunum

  The jejunal mesentery, 10–15 cm distal to the ligament of Treitz, is divided between vascular arcades and the mesenteric vessels are ligated. The jejunum is transected with an endoscopic linear gastrointestinal stapler. This procedure is performed in its original position (division of the jejunum and mesentery prior to pulling the jejunum into the right side).

- Division between the superior mesenteric artery (SMA) and the uncinate process.

  This step is the most technically difficult part of the procedure and also the most criti-

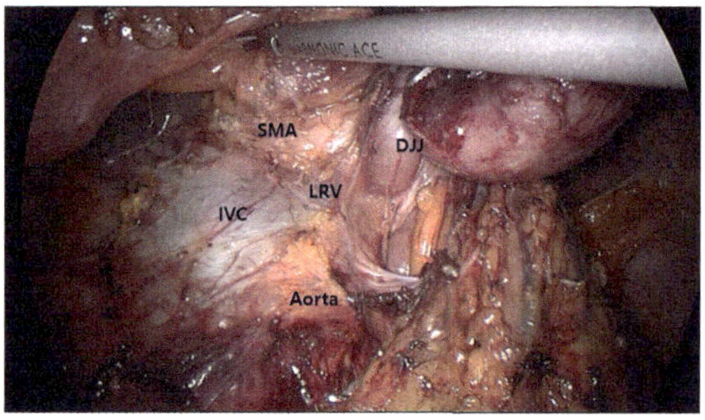

Fig. 42.4 Mobilization of the retroperitoneal duodenum. Kocher maneuver involves the left renal vein and aorta. Careful traction of the duodenum is essential to prevent duodenal perforation. A full mobilization of the retroperitoneal duodenum facilitates the separation of duodenum from the root of the mesentery. (IVC, inferior vena cava; SMA, superior mesenteric artery; LRV, left renal vein; DJJ, duodenojejunal junction)

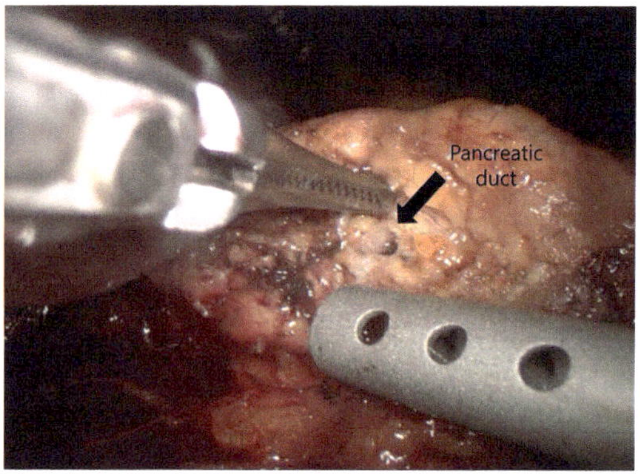

Fig. 42.5 Identification of pancreatic duct

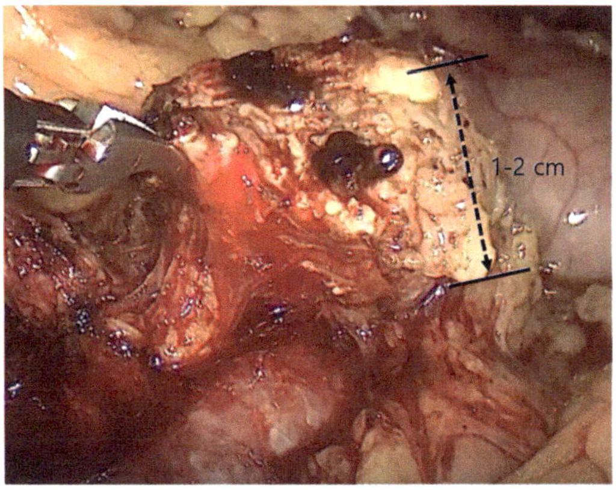

Fig. 42.6 Mobilizing the pancreatic remnant. The remaining pancreatic stump is mobilized by 1–2 cm to facilitate invagination of the pancreas into the jejunum for the pancreaticojejunostomy

cal in terms of obtaining tumor-free margins. Elevation of the specimen reveals detailed features of the remaining attachments, including tributaries of the PV or SMV. The first jejunal vein and pancreaticoduodenal veins drain into the portomesenteric vein (Fig. 42.7). To facilitate the dissection and control any unexpected bleeding from the PV or SMV, vessel loops are applied to the PV and SMV, respectively, immediately above the splenic vein and the first jejunal vein. Traction with vessel loops enables clear visualization of the neurolymphatic soft tissues around the SMA. We prefer an upward dissection to expose the venous branches more effectively than the downward approach. Upward traction of the SMV using vessel loops and caudal traction of the specimen can facilitate the identification of posterior venous tributaries draining from the uncinate process into the first jejunal vein (two or three veins), which can be divided with clips and a Harmonic scalpel. The soft tissue near the SMA should then be dissected to identify one to two inferior pancreaticoduodenal arteries. The remaining dissection of the soft tissue between the SMA and the uncinate should be dictated by the oncologic status. The dissection can be performed near the uncinate process without risk of injury to the SMA in diseases other than pancreatic ductal adenocarcinoma. However, in case of pancreatic ductal adenocarcinoma, a clear dissection of the neurolymphatic soft tissues of the right side of the SMA is needed to obtain a margin-negative specimen (Fig. 42.8). The specimen is placed in a specimen bag and retrieved at the end of procedure, either through the 2–3 cm extension of the umbilical port or a separate incision.

- Reconstruction

  Pancreatojejunostomy (PJ) was performed using a double-layered, end-to-side, duct-to-mucosa method using laparoscopic sutures. PJ involving the first layer of the anastomosis was performed between the posterior wall of the pancreas and the seromuscular layer of the jejunum with a running suture (non-absorbable 4-0). The second layer was sutured

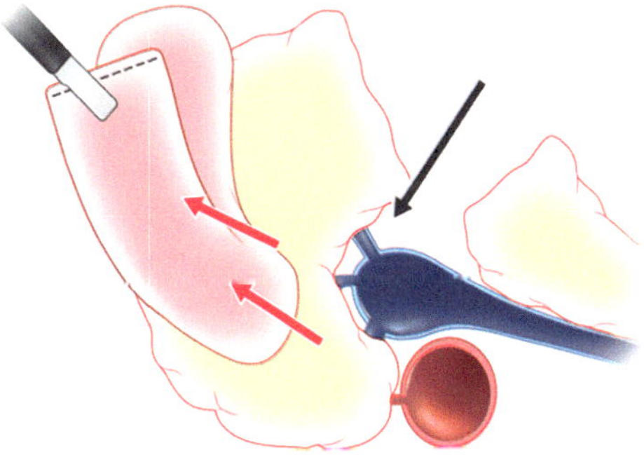

Fig. 42.7 Lateral and anterior retraction of the specimen is useful to identify the first jejunal vein and pancreaticoduodenal veins (PDV) draining into the portomesenteric vein

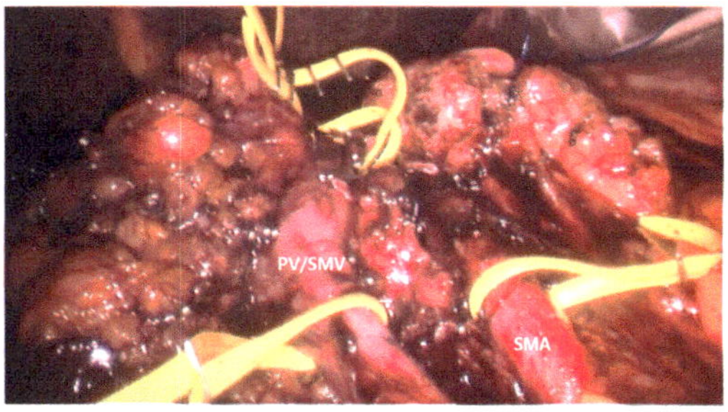

Fig. 42.8 A clear dissection of the neurolymphatic soft tissues of the right side of the SMA is needed to obtain a margin-negative pancreatic cancer specimen (SMA, superior mesenteric artery)

between the posterior wall of the main pancreatic duct and the full layer of the jejunum with interrupted suture (non-absorbable 4-0). A hole was created in the jejunum using the electronic coagulator and a polyethylene internal stent was temporarily inserted into the main pancreatic duct. Duct-to-mucosa PJ entailed more than four stitches of sutures (absorbable 5-0). The third layer of the anastomosis was sutured between the anterior wall of the main pancreatic duct and the anterior wall of the jejunum with a running suture (non-absorbable 4-0). The fourth layer was sutured between the anterior wall of the pancreatic stump and the seromuscular layer of the jejunum with interrupted sutures (non-absorbable 4-0).

End-to-side hepaticojejunostomy was performed via laparoscopic continuous suturing (non-absorbable 5-0) at the posterior wall and interrupted or continuous suturing at the anterior wall. Duodenojejunostomy or gastrojejunostomy with Braun anastomosis was carried out intracorporeally or extracorporeally via the specimen extraction site. Two to three closed suction drains were placed at the superior and inferior borders of the pancreatojejunostomy site.

References

1. Gagner M, Pomp A. Laparoscopic pylorus-preserving pancreatoduodenectomy. Surg Endosc. 1994;8(5):408–10.
2. Conrad C, Basso V, Passot G, Zorzi D, Li L, Chen HC, Fuks D, Gayet B. Comparable long-term oncologic outcomes of laparoscopic versus open pancreaticoduodenectomy for adenocarcinoma: a propensity score weighting analysis. Surg Endosc. 2017;31(10):3970–8.
3. Song KB, Kim SC, Hwang DW, Lee JH, Lee DJ, Lee JW, Park KM, Lee YJ. Matched case-control analysis comparing laparoscopic and open pylorus-preserving Pancreaticoduodenectomy in patients with Periampullary tumors. Ann Surg. 2015;262(1):146–55.

Laparoscopic Distal Pancreatectomy

43

Chang Moo Kang

Abstract

Laparoscopic distal pancreatectomy (LPD) is one of the potential options for benign and low-grade malignant tumors in the left-sided pancreas. Many experiences and a recent prospective randomized control study (RCT) have confirmed that LPD is safe, effective, and provide the benefit of minimally invasive surgery. Recently, with advancements in the laparoscopic technique, LPD is being actively applied even to resectable left-sided pancreatic cancer, and it has shown comparable perioperative and long-term oncologic outcomes to open surgery. In addition, the robotic surgical system was introduced and is currently available. Surgeons could take advantage of this system in well-selected cases. In this chapter, detailed surgical techniques for LPD are discussed with special clinical issues, such as spleen-preserving technique, clinical application to left-sided pancreatic cancer, and an innovative robotic approach for minimally invasive distal pancreatectomy.

Keywords

Laparoscopic · Robotic · Distal pancreatectomy · Spleen · Pancreatic cancer

43.1 Introduction

Adaptation of laparoscopic surgery for pancreatic resection was late compared with other types of general surgery [1]. Considering the limitations of laparoscopic surgery, the pancreas is not easy to access laparoscopically, because of its location in the retroperitoneal space. In particular, the pancreas is supplied with abundant blood from major blood vessels. Therefore, even a small disruption of tributary vessels around the pancreas results in severe bleeding, obscuring the surgical field. In addition, postoperative pancreatic fistula (POPF) [2] is associated with fatal complications for the patient. However, accumulating laparoscopic surgical experience, development of new surgical techniques, energy devices, and advances in perioperative patient care have contributed to the safety and effectiveness of laparoscopic pancreatic resection.

Laparoscopic distal pancreatectomy (LDP) was first introduced in 1994 by Soper et al. [3], who reported successful LDP in pig pancreas. In

Supplementary Information The online version contains supplementary material available at https://doi.org/10.1007/978-981-16-1996-0_43.

C. M. Kang (✉)
Division of Hepatobiliary and Pancreatic Surgery, Department of Surgery, Yonsei University College of Medicine, Seoul, South Korea
e-mail: cmkang@yuhs.ac

H. C. Yu (ed.), *Hepato-Biliary-Pancreatic Surgery and Liver Transplantation*,
https://doi.org/10.1007/978-981-16-1996-0_43

1996, Cuschieri [4] and Gagner [5] reported 5 and 12 patients with LDP, respectively, suggesting the technical feasibility and safety of LDP. In Korea, Yoon, et al. [6] first performed LDP in 2001. Min et al. [7] reported the first two cases of LDP by conserving both splenic artery and vein in 2003, opening the door to function-preserving minimally invasive pancreatic surgery.

Many recent clinical investigations showed that LDP is effective and appropriate in treating benign and low-grade malignant tumors of the pancreas, compared with open DP [8]. Moreover, short-term and long-term oncologic outcomes of LDP were not inferior to those of open DP even in left-sided pancreatic cancer [9]. Especially, rapid recovery after LDP potentially increases the possibility of non-delayed postoperative adjuvant chemotherapy. Recently, a multicenter, prospective randomized control study was performed to compare LDP with open DP. In cases involving well-selected pancreatic tumors limited to the pancreas, Rooij, et al. [10] reported that minimally invasive DP significantly reduced the time leading to functional recovery, reducing delayed gastric emptying without increasing costs, and maintaining high quality of life. Therefore, LDP is currently established as a standard technique. In this chapter, technical aspects of LDP with special clinical considerations will be discussed.

43.2 Indications

LDP is indicated not only for benign and low-grade malignant tumors of left-sided pancreas that can be treated via standard surgical approaches, but also well-selected left-sided pancreatic cancer (see below). However, large tumors in contact with major blood vessels or associated with multiple organs may lead to intraoperative complications such as bleeding of major blood vessels and peripheral organ damage or inevitable intraoperative conversion to open surgery. Therefore, the indication for LDP should be carefully and safely evaluated according to the operator's experience and technique.

In particular, rather than performing LDP for all patients who have resectable pancreatic cancer, it is more reasonable to perform selective, minimally invasive DP in patients with left-sided pancreatic cancer to improve quality of life and long-term oncologic safety. Accordingly, clinically significant *Yonsei criteria* were proposed [11]. *Yonsei criteria* are based on the concept of appropriate tumor conditions to achieve bloodless and margin-negative resection using a laparoscopic approach in light of past surgical experience of resected distal pancreatic cancer. The criteria include the following: (1) tumors confined to pancreas; (2) intact fascia layer of posterior pancreas; and (3) 1–2 cm apart from the origin of celiac and splenic arteries. In fact, the *Yonsei criteria* were cited to include tumor conditions for pancreatic cancer in the previous multicenter prospective randomized clinical trials [10]. Accordingly, the indications for LDP in pancreatic cancer may be gradually expanded following advances in surgeons' experience and techniques,

43.3 Preoperative Factors

Similar to other surgeries, the following three factors should be considered before performing LDP.

43.3.1 Patient Assessment

It is critical to evaluate patients preoperatively and understand their physical and functional capacity. Especially, it is not uncommon that LDP entails prolonged operation and bleeding. Long-term pneumoperitoneum can result in adverse cardiopulmonary effects. In addition, in preparation for lower extremity venous thrombosis and pulmonary embolism due to stagnant venous blood in the lower extremity during surgery, a low-molecular heparin is considered during surgery and within 48 h after surgery. When concomitant splenectomy is highly expected, vaccination to prevent OPSI should be considered at least 7–10 days before surgery. In particular, as the number of elderly patients is increasing, it is necessary to determine the appropriate surgical extent and operation time, considering the tumor biology and the physiological capacity of the elderly patients.

43.3.2 Tumor Assessment

Before surgery, patients usually undergo a number of radiological examinations for accurate preoperative diagnosis, and decision-making regarding the extent of surgical resection. It is thought that preoperative abdominal computed tomography (CT) facilitates determination of the tumor location relative to blood vessels and other organs. Based on the CT images, the surgeon can preoperatively estimate whether the pancreatic mass is malignant, the location of the pancreatic mass, running course of the major blood vessels (splenic artery and vein), the anatomic relationship between the tumor and the splenic vessels, or surrounding organs, such as stomach, colon, or left kidney/adrenal gland, and even between the pancreatic tail and spleen hilum, which are essential factors in surgical design.

43.3.3 Planning Operation

Surgeons need to develop their own strategies for LDP based on preoperative imaging studies, and prepare several alternative options in the event of unexpected operative findings. A personal checklist when preparing for elective LDP in clinical practice is presented in Table 43.1. The appropriate surgical approach should be based on patients' safety and surgical merit depending on the tumor location, biological characteristics, and anatomical relationship between tumor and surrounding vascular structure.

Table 43.1 Preoperative factors determining LDP

Tumor location
• Potential division line of the pancreas (neck/body/tail).
Feasibility of spleen preservation
• Appropriate for splenic vessel conserving.
• Appropriate for splenic vessel sacrificing (Warshaw's procedure)?
Combined splenectomy
• Preoperative vaccination and schedule of elective surgery
• Feasibility of robotic single-site plus ONE-port approach
Malignancy
• Resectable within Yonsei criteria/ out of Yonsei criteria
• Open vs. laparoscopic approach
• Combined resection of left-adrenal gland, colon, and stomach
• Perigastric collateral vessels

43.4 Operative Technique

43.4.1 Patient Posture

Surgeons may prefer the right lateral decubitus position when performing LDP. However, the author recommends a supine position for the following reasons.

The preparation for supine position is simple. Supine position does not waste unnecessary time and energy before surgery. Right lateral decubitus is a useful method for securing the surgical field for left-sided pancreas using gravity, but this condition differs from the open surgery. Therefore, even in the case of laparoscopic surgery, based on the supine posture, the surgeon can operate in the same surgical field and under conditions similar to open surgery. Therefore, even a beginner may be quick to adapt to laparoscopic surgery. Surgeons cannot access the whole pancreas, especially pancreatic neck and head area in a patient with right lateral decubitus, because omentum and small intestine fall into dependent position due to gravity, resulting in hidden duodenum and proximal pancreatic head area. Therefore, the supine position can resolve all these issues, ensuring adequate operation field and ensuring dissection of SMV-SV-PV confluence and pancreatic neck, even in the pancreaticoduodenal unit. A supine position can expand the surgical indication of LDP, even in well-selected cases of distal pancreatic cancer, and laparoscopic pancreaticoduodenectomy (LPD). It is easy to switch rapidly to open conversion during laparoscopic surgery. In addition, in the right lateral decubitus position, spleen preservation may be difficult because the spleen is pressed against the pancreatic tail due to the weight of the spleen and the spleen is directed toward the abdominal cavity along with the pancreatic tail. However, supine position facilitates spleen-preserving procedures because spleen is located in the dependent position.

When the patient is supine, the patient operating table may be adjusted (for example, head-side up or left-side up) to create appropriate surgical field for LDP. Although some surgeons may stand between the legs of the patient, the author performs the operation on the right side of the patient. A typical operating room layout for LDP is shown in Fig. 43.1.

43.4.2 Trocar Placement

In general, two 5-mm trocars and three 12-mm trocars are used. However, the location and the number of trocars can be adjusted according to the tumor location and size. For example, in case of pancreatic tail lesions, a minimum of one left-sided 5-mm and another one 12-mm trocar are used for LDP with concomitant splenectomy (Fig. 43.2a). However, when the tumor is in the neck or near the proximal body of the pancreas, an additional right-sided 5-mm and another 12-mm trocar need to be inserted for effective surgical manipulation (Fig. 43.2b). Therefore, the trocar position of LPD can be adjusted according to the patient's condition, operator's experience, and tumor location.

In the past, small trocars (5 mm) and a minimum number of trocars (3 trocars including umbilical site trocar for laparoscope) were preferred. However, larger trocars (12 mm) have been actively used recently. If it is properly applied, (1) the access angle of laparoscopic working instruments can be adjusted as needed by changing the position of laparoscopic camera, and (2) active laparoscopy is feasible while inserting the gauze into abdominal cavity (via 12-mm trocars) under direct laparoscopic vision. In addition, (3) advanced laparoscopic instruments are appropriate for larger trocars.

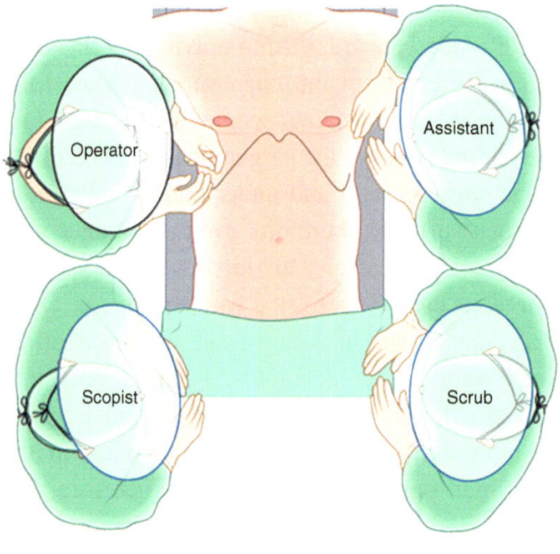

Fig. 43.1 Patient posture and OR setup for LDP

43.4.3 Access to Pancreas

Access to pancreas is similar in open and laparoscopic surgery. With the stomach lifted, the division of gastrocolic ligament with an energy device (ultrasonic shears or vessel sealer) can create surgical access to the whole pancreas from the pancreas body to the tail (Fig. 43.3). When planning for concomitant splenectomy, gastrosplenic ligament should be divided in this stage. When planning for spleen-preserving DP, gastrosplenic ligament need to be conserved briefly because splenic vessel-sacrificing spleen-preserving DP (so-called, Warshaw's procedure) can be selected when splenic vessel-conserving DP procedure is difficult and impossible due to chronic inflammation and frequent bleeding.

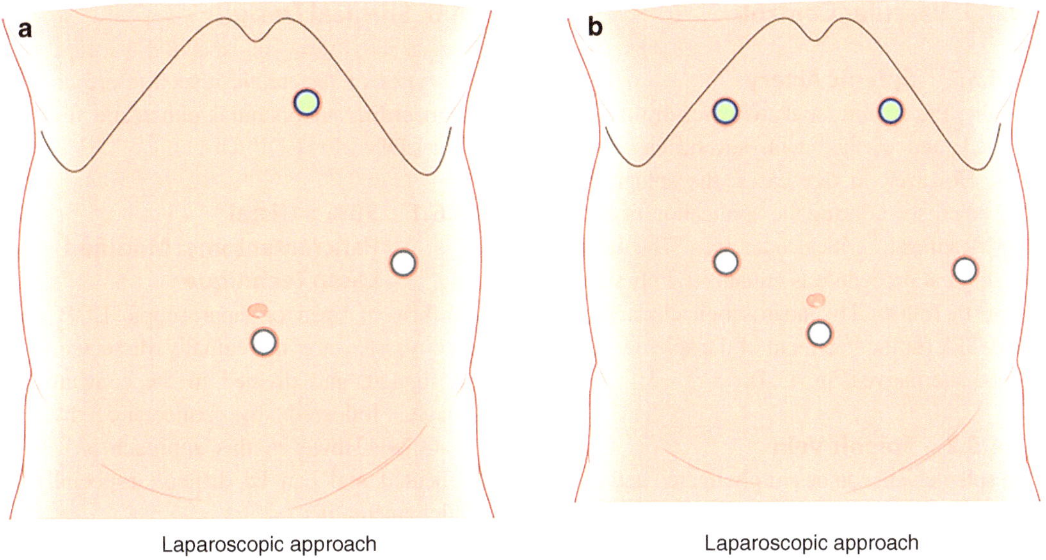

Fig. 43.2 Trocar placement in LDP. (**a**) In case of pancreatic tail lesion with concomitant splenectomy (**b**) In case of division of pancreatic neck or proximal body of the pancreas. Please note the right flank-sided trocar. These configurations of trocar placement are universal for all standard pancreatic resections. Trocar placement can be adjusted according to the patient's condition (body shape, operator's experience, and tumor location)

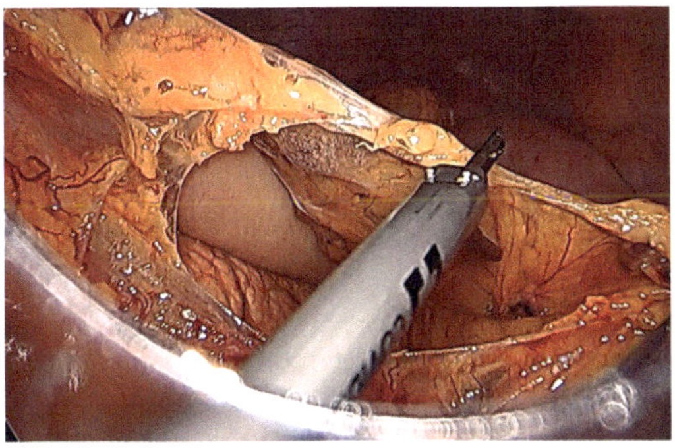

Fig. 43.3 Division of gastrocolic ligament to access to pancreas

43.4.4 Pancreatic Division

43.4.4.1 Endo-GIA Stapler

Studies reported no statistical difference in postoperative outcomes between manual resection of the pancreas and surgical stapling in DP [12]. As a result, laparoscopic endo-GIA is widely used for LDP.

According to recent clinical studies, pancreatic thickness [13] and firing time [14] of endo-GIA are a challenge in reducing postoperative pancreatic fistula. Crushing of the pancreas during endo-GIA may result in POPF. Therefore, it is recommended that surgeons should slow down the firing time in endo-GIA.

In addition, vascular endo-GIA reduced POPF [15]. However, this author divides the pancreas via endo-GIA with staple size ranging from 3 to 3.5–4 mm, which is appropriate for medium or thick tissue.

43.4.4.2 Ultrasonic Sheers

In some cases, the pancreas can be divided using an ultrasonic sheer [16], especially, when there is insufficient space between pancreas and splenic vessels to use an endo-GIA, or endo-GIA cannot be closed because the pancreas is hard and thick. When pancreas is divided by ultrasonic sheers, the author closes the cut pancreatic surface with sutures as much as possible before the operation is complete. In addition, a few studies demonstrated the feasibility and safety of pancreatic resection using other energy devices [17], but the effectiveness of this surgical technique should be carefully evaluated in the future based on scientific evidence.

43.4.5 Vascular Control

43.4.5.1 Splenic Artery

Usually, the splenic artery is carefully dissected, isolated, and divided with several laparoscopic clips. However, in rare cases, the splenic artery may be crushed during the application of surgical clips, leading to critical outcomes. The safety of the surgical procedure is enhanced with a laparoscopic tie followed by laparoscopic clips. Vascular endo-GIA for the treatment of the splenic artery is a good alternative (Fig. 43.4).

43.4.5.2 Splenic Vein

The splenic vein can be simply ligated and treated with several clips, or vascular endo-GIA. However, this author usually applies surgical clips following a laparoscopic tie (Fig. 43.5).

43.4.5.3 Small Tributary Vessels

Careful dissection of the small blood vessels running into the pancreas around the splenic artery and the splenic veins is followed by control with small clips and scissors, or energy devices with small clips on the capillaries of the splenic artery or splenic vein (Fig. 43.6). These capillaries can also be simply treated with a vessel-sealing energy device [18]. The treatment approach can be individualized.

43.4.6 Surgical Design

Three types of pancreatic resection are considered according to potential pancreatic division line for LDP.

43.4.6.1 50% > Distal Pancreatectomy: Modified Lasso Technique

Regardless of open or laparoscopic LDP, both splenic vessels are individually dissected, isolated, ligated, and divided in the conventional approach, followed by pancreatic division (Fig. 43.7a). However, this approach is a little complicated and can be difficult especially in chronic pancreatitis.

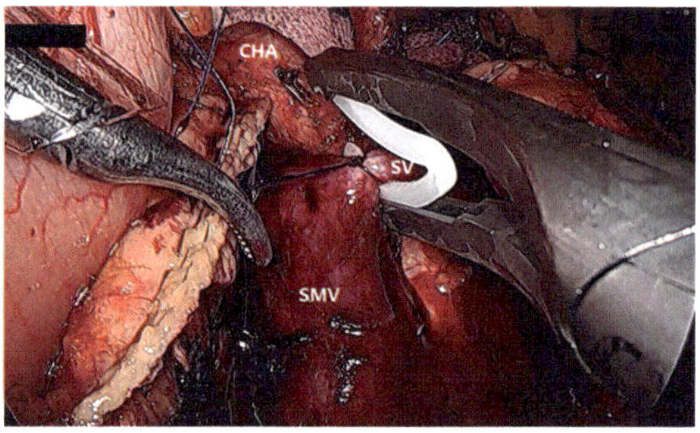

Fig. 43.5 Splenic vein control

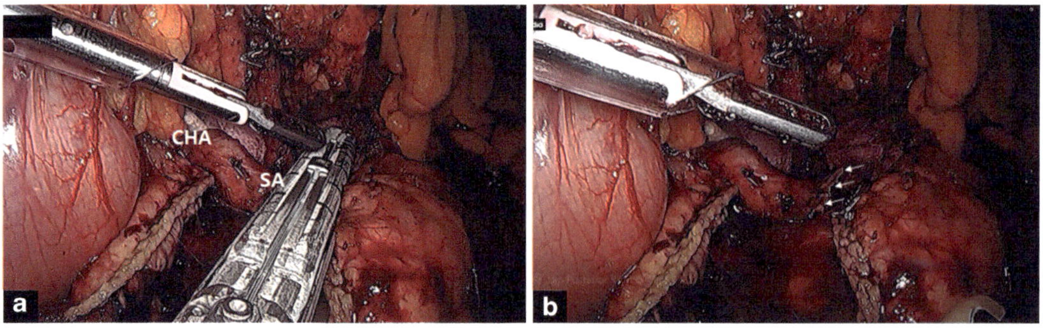

Fig. 43.4 Splenic artery control using vascular stapler. Vascular stapler is applied (**a**), Note stapled line (white arrow) after division of SA (**b**) *CAH* common hepatic artery, *SA* splenic artery

Therefore, to facilitate LDP, Velanovich [19] introduced the "lasso" technique. In brief, when LDP is performed, the distal pancreas with both splenic vessels (splenic artery and vein) is lifted altogether from the retroperitoneum using a Penrose drain. The pancreas and both the splenic vessels are divided once via endo-GIA (Fig. 43.7b). It was argued that it was technically easy and available for LDP, so that the potential indications for LDP will be expanded. However, no further follow-up studies have been published since then.

In fact, the author once used "simply" endo-GIA to control pancreaticosplenic ligament in laparoscopic splenectomy [20]. As expected, surgical procedure is very simple, but one patient experienced severe postoperative bleeding immediately after surgery and managed via interventional radiologic coil embolization. Since then, splenic artery ligation either by clips or by laparoscopic tie is conducted first before applying endo-GIA to pancreaticosplenic ligament in laparoscopic splenectomy in an effort to enhance procedural safety.

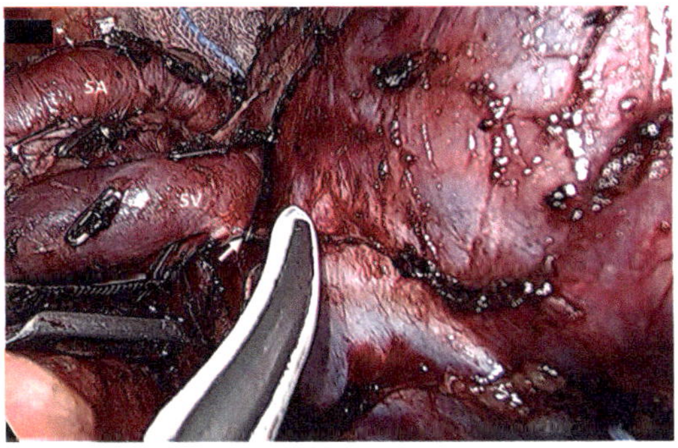

Fig. 43.6 Control of small tributaries from splenic vessels

It is true that the "lasso" technique in LPD is very simple and quite easy; however, the original "lasso" technique may also carry a potential risk of bleeding-related complications due to the stapled splenic artery, based on the author's personal experience involving laparoscopic splenectomy. Therefore, splenic artery control using either a tie or clips is always completed before the original lasso technique is performed (modified lasso technique, Fig. 43.7c). Recently, Kawasaki and Kang, et al. [21] reported that this modified lasso technique had favorable effects on the operation time, intraoperative bleeding, postoperative morbidity rate, and the length of the postoperative hospital stay, suggesting that the modified lasso technique is simple, safe, and effective in LDP.

43.4.6.2 70% Distal Pancreatectomy: "Subtotal (Extended)" Distal Pancreatosplenectomy

When pancreatic lesion is located on the pancreatic neck or in the proximal pancreatic body, the pancreatic neck above the SMV-SV-PV confluence is divided and the distal portion of the pancreas (subtotal/ extended distal pancreatectomy) is considered. The division of pancreatic neck laparoscopically has clinical implications. First, it is possible to extend the indications of

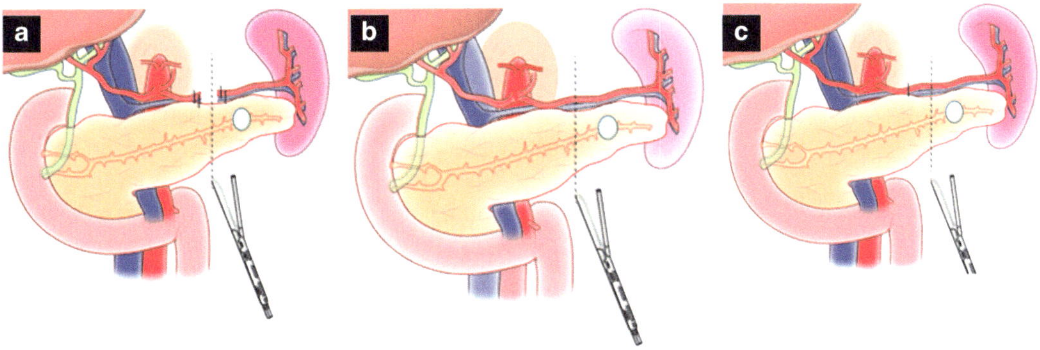

Fig. 43.7 Surgical concept of modified lasso technique in laparoscopic DPS (**a**) Usual technique for distal pancreatectomy. (**b**) Lasso technique. (**c**) Modified lasso technique

LDP. Second, it is a basic technique for performing LPD or central pancreatectomy.

The space between the pancreatic neck and the SMV-SV-PV confluence is generally known as avascular plane, but very rarely, small blood vessels enter directly from the pancreas into venous confluence, suggesting the need for caution. Although the preferences of every surgeon for dissection of pancreatic neck may differ, the following technique will guide surgeons to isolate the pancreatic neck safely and effectively.

- Dissection of upper part of the pancreatic neck first can be helpful. Soft tissue between the common hepatic artery and upper part of the pancreatic neck portion can be carefully dissected to identify the portal vein (PV) at the bottom of this space (Fig. 43.8).
- Carefully dissection following the right gastroepiploic vein is essential to locate the part of superior mesenteric vein (SMV).
- In some cases, the SMV can be found directly at the lower pancreatic neck by estimating the running course of SMV based on the location of PV, which was previously located at the upper part of pancreatic neck.

Once SMV is found, the area between the pancreatic neck and the SMV-SV-PV confluence represents an avascular plane (as mentioned above). Blunt dissection can be used to create a window between pancreatic neck and SMV-SV-PV confluence (Fig. 43.9) and hang the pancreatic neck covered with nylon tape. The division of the pan-

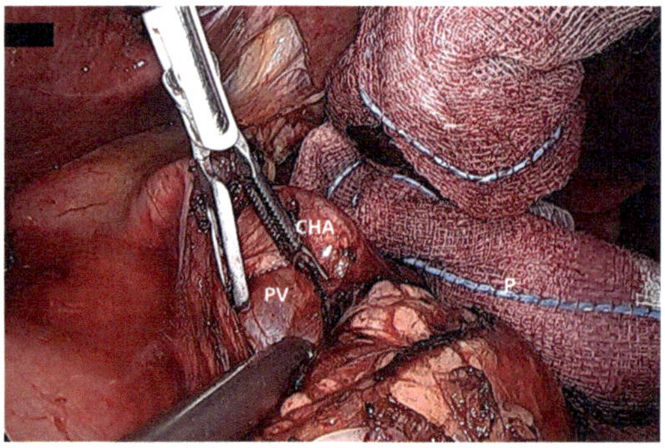

Fig. 43.8 Laparoscopic dissection around upper part of the pancreatic neck

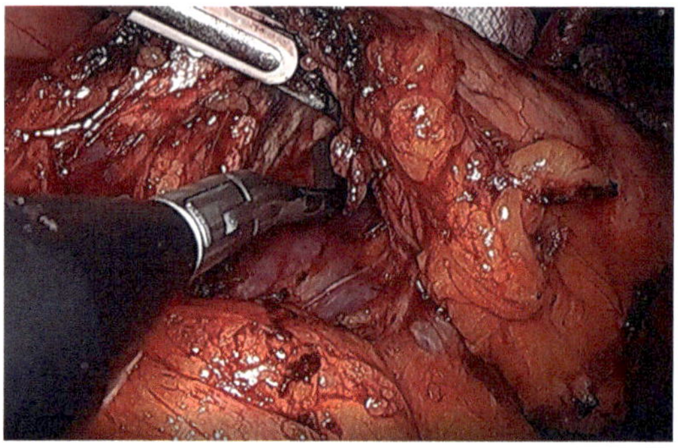

Fig. 43.9 A window between pancreatic neck and SMV-SV-PV confluence

creatic neck portion is ready. At this moment, if not careful, the common hepatic artery may be encircled with pancreatic neck together and divided with pancreatic neck. Therefore, dissection of the upper part of the pancreatic neck portion to identify the PV before creating the window between pancreatic neck and venous confluence will facilitate pancreatic neck encircling.

In addition, when dissecting pancreatic neck, small tributary vessels connecting pancreas with SV, SMV, or SMA should be controlled using clips in the large blood vessels, but not on the pancreatic side. Most of the blood vessels in the pancreatic side can be controlled with an energy device without clips. Endo-GIA may be difficult for division of the pancreas due to the use of some clips on the pancreatic side to control small tributary vessels. These small clips may not be allowed to securely close the endo-GIA during the division of the pancreas.

The splenic artery and vein are safely ligated using a laparoscopic tie first, followed by clips when controlling the splenic vessels in 70% LDP. Vascular endo-GIA application to control splenic vessels is also an alternative option, especially in splenic artery (Figs. 43.4 and 43.5). When the pancreas is detached from the peritoneum, it does not matter if the inferior mesenteric vein (IMV) enters the SMV, but if it enters the SV, the IMV must be ligated and divided during pancreatic resection.

In most benign or low-grade malignant tumors located in the neck or proximal body of the pancreas, function-preserving pancreatectomy (spleen-preserving procedures or limited pancreatectomy, such as central pancreatectomy) is desirable. The application of laparoscopic radical DPS in pancreatic cancer will be discussed briefly later.

43.4.6.3 50% Distal Pancreatectomy

This surgical extent is thought to be one of the most difficult surgical designs. During 50% distal pancreatectomy, the origin of splenic artery needs to be dissected first, but is not that easy because of several reasons. First, the origin of splenic artery is usually behind the pancreas or embedded in the pancreas. Second, neural tissue covers the origin of the splenic artery. These two factors interfere with the dissection of splenic artery in the modified lasso technique. In addition, the potential line of division of the pancreas is wide and thick in the pancreas, resulting in frequent POPF. Therefore, technically, for 50% distal pancreatectomy, the general approach might be similar to subtotal distal pancreatectomy.

43.4.7 Spleen-Preserving Procedure

The role of spleen is still controversial in adult patients. Spleen is the largest immunologic organ in our body. In the past, splenectomy was performed during distal pancreatectomy for technical convenience due to anatomical intimacy between the pancreatic tail and the spleen. As the role of the spleen is established [22], the frequency of spleen-preserving distal pancreatectomy (SpDP) has increased recently. The two methods to preserve the spleen to date are as follows.

1. Splenic vessel conserving

   Since the splenic vessels (splenic artery and vein) anatomically supply blood to the spleen and pancreas simultaneously, splenic vessel conservation (SVC) may facilitate spleen-preserving distal pancreatectomy (SpDP). However, it is not easy to control individual small blood vessels from the splenic vessels using a laparoscopic approach. This technique usually requires a lot of time, effort, and advanced surgical techniques. Particularly, during pancreatitis or large tumors in wide contact with the splenic vessels, it is often necessary to combine splenectomy due to frequent and severe bleeding during the spleen-preserving procedure. Recently, minimally invasive SVC-SpDP can be performed effectively before using a special energy device or robotic surgical system.
2. Splenic vessel sacrificing

   In 1988, Warshaw introduced alternative spleen-preservation technique, the so-called Warshaw procedure, in which splenic vessel sacrificing (SVS, segmental excision of splenic vessels with resected distal pancreas) SpDP was performed to increase the technical feasibility of SpDP. As mentioned briefly above. However, the SVC procedure is technically challenging or even impossible in the presence of chronic pancreatitis. In this scenario, segmental resection of both splenic artery and vein with distal pancreas are alternative options for spleen preservation. As a result, the spleen blood supply is facilitated via short gastric vessels and left gastroepiploic artery instead of excised main splenic artery and vein. Subsequently, this procedure may involve two issues to be addressed.

   - The substantial risk of spleen infarction after surgery: In the original article published by Warshaw [23], 4% (1 out of 25) required additional splenectomy due to spleen abscess following spleen infarction, limiting the application of this procedure in the case of a large spleen.
   - There may be a risk of gastrointestinal bleeding from the perigastric collateral vessels due to impaired venous circulation via excision of splenic vein. However, based on 23 years of experience of the Warshaw group [24], only 3 (1.9%) of the 158 patients in the Warshaw study underwent additional splenectomy due to splenic infarction. In addition, among 65 patients, only 16 patients (25%) carried perigastric collateral veins, but no clinical gastrointestinal bleeding or

splenic hypertension was noted, suggesting that the operation was a safe procedure.

43.5 Methods to Prevent POPF after Distal Pancreatectomy

Several studies demonstrating reduced POPF following DP are summarized (Table 43.2). Based on the studies, in the era of LDP, the application of PGA and glue [25], perioperative IV hydrocortisone [26], and pasireotide [27] is recommended to reduce POPF following distal pancreatectomy.

43.6 Intraoperative Peritoneal Drainage

Surgical drains are frequently used in LDP to evacuate blood, pancreatic juice, lymphatic fluid, and small necrotic debris after surgery. However, it should be balanced with the potential risk of ascending infection. Several studies [40, 41] found no significant differences in the incidence of POPF compared with DP with and without a surgical drain. A prospective, randomized multicenter trial of distal pancreatectomy with and without routine intraperitoneal drainage was per-

Table 43.2 Recent RCTs to investigate surgical approach to reduce POPF following DP

Authors, Year	Intervention	N	POPF (%)	*p*-value
Kondo, 2018 [28]	Reinforced stapler	61	16.3	
	Bare stapler	61	27.1	0.15
Cuncha, 2015 [29]	TachoSil®	135	41(30.6)	
	Control	135	33(24.3)	0.279
Park, 2016 [30]	TachoSil®	48	11(22.9)	
	Control	53	15(28.3)	0.536
Jang,2017 [25]	PGA (Neoveil®)	44	5(11.4)	
	Control	53	15(28.3)	0.04
Shubert, 2016 [31]	SIMGUARD®	32	4(12.5)	
	TISSELINK®	35	8(22.9)	0.35
Kawai, 2016 [32]	PJ	62	24 (38.7)	
	Stapler closure	61	23 (37.7)	0.332
Hassenpfulg, 2016 [33]	Tres ligament patch	76	17(22.4)	
	Control	76	25(32.9)	0.1468
Montorsi, 2012 [34]	TachoSil®	145	12(9)	
	Control	130	18(14)	0.139
Carter, 2013 [35]	Falciform ligament patch + glue	50	9(18)	
	Control*	51	9(18)	1
Frozanpor, 2012 [36]	Preoperative transpapillary pancreatic stent	29	11(42.3)	
	Control	29	6(22.2)	0.122
Diener, 2011 [37]	Stapler	221	24(43)	
	Hand-sewn closure	229	16(33)	0.27
Suc, 2003 [38]	Fibrin glue occlusion	24	4	
	Control	20	3	>0.05
Uemura, 2017 [39]	PG	36	7(19.4)	
	Control (hand-sewn)	37	7(18.9)	1
Antila, 2019 [26]	Hydrocortisone, iv	17	1(6)	
	Control	14	6(43)	0.028
Allen, 2014 [27]	Pasireotide, iv	41	(7)	
	Control	39	(23)	0.006

formed [42]. It was noted that about 44% of the patients underwent LDP (229 out of 528 enrolled patients). No statistical differences were found in terms of POPF and mortality, suggesting that clinical outcomes are comparable in DP with or without routine intraperitoneal drainage. However, early drain removal strategy is a practical and reasonable approach after pancreatectomy. Further studies are needed.

43.7 Special Consideration

43.7.1 The Role of Spleen in Adult Patients

In the past, Shoup et al. [22] reported the potential role of spleen in distal pancreatectomy. Splenic preservation was strongly recommended because it decreased perioperative infectious complications, reduced the rate of severe complications, and decreased the length of hospital stay. However, this conclusion was based on historical data (October 1, 1983, to July 1, 2000). Recent studies reported contrary findings, suggesting that both LDPS and LSPDP were associated with similar perioperative complications and could be performed safely [43]. OPSI in patients with DPS [44] is thought to be necessary, but POSI, in fact, is very rare in patients with elective PDS for nonhematologic pathologic conditions, and preoperative vaccination is thought to be adequate for preventing critical long-term complications. The potential role of spleen in adult patients requires further investigation.

43.7.2 Application in Left-Sided Pancreatic Cancer

The theoretical advantages of LDP over open DP for left-sided pancreatic cancer include the following:

- Reduced inflammatory response during the recovery phase following surgical intervention to prevent the progression of potential residual cancer cells because the cytokines associated with inflammation act as cancer progressing factor [45].
- Possible association with increased use of postoperative adjuvant chemotherapy due to early fast recovery [46].

It is still controversial, but laparoscopic radical distal pancreatectomy in well-selected pancreatic cancer is technically feasible and ontologically safe. Lee, and Kang et al. [47] recently reported long-term oncologic outcomes of LDP in left-sided pancreatic cancer comparable to those of open DP. In addition, a recent systematic review and meta-analysis investigated 21 studies with 11,246 patients who underwent DP for pancreatic ductal adenocarcinoma (PDAC). They concluded that in patients with PDAC, MIDP is associated with comparable survival (hazard ratio 0.86; 95% confidence interval (CI) 0.73–1.01; p = 0.06), R0 resection (odds ratio (OR) 1.24; 95% CI 0.97–1.58; p = 0.09), and use of adjuvant chemotherapy (OR 1.07; 95% CI 0.89–1.30; p = 0.46) [9]. However, these studies are based on retrospective observational studies. Selection bias and subsequent oncologic effectiveness still remain to be resolved. Prospective, randomized controlled studies are necessary. However, well-selected patients and experienced surgeons should be involved to ensure patients' safety [10]. Large-scale, multicenter studies investigating the long-term survival and oncologic efficacy of pancreatic resection in pancreatic cancer have been reported [48–50].

43.7.3 Role of Robotic Surgical System in Laparoscopic Distal Pancreatectomy

Theoretically, the robotic surgical system was introduced for effective and safe minimally invasive surgery by addressing the limitations of the conventional laparoscopic surgery, such as two-dimensional surgical field of view, attenuated touch sensation, limitation of intra-abdominal movement, increased hand tremor, and fulcrum effect.

Accordingly, SpDP is considered to be the best indication for robotic surgery. In particular, laparoscopic SVC-SpDP requires highly sophisticated manipulation to effectively and safely control the capillaries distributed between spleen vessels and the pancreas, which is mostly compensated by the robotic surgical system. In addition, during SVS-SpDP, the robot may facilitate the safe excision of splenic vessels via effective dissection of the pancreas near the spleen hilum.

Indeed, the authors reported that, in spite of longer operation time compared to laparoscopic surgery, the success rate of spleen preservation in patients using robots was statistically significant and very high (95% vs. 64%, $p = 0.027$) when the SpDP was initially planned and attempted [51]. However, accumulating evidence of laparoscopic techniques suggests that the efficacy of spleen preservation was similar in robotic and laparoscopic DP without statistical difference [52], which is also noted in recently published meta-analysis [53, 54].

Therefore, robotic DP is a safe and effective surgical option. Depending on surgeons' experience, the pancreatic pathology and the economic conditions of the patient, a safe minimally invasive DP can be performed using either a laparoscopic or robot approach. However, as the cost of robotic surgery is high, a cost-benefit analysis is needed [53, 55].

43.7.4 Robotic Single-Site *plus* ONE-Port Distal Pancreatectomy

The robotic approach may be technically feasible in reducing the port DP. Advances in laparoscopic techniques have continued to reduce the number of access routes for LDP. In fact, several studies suggesting technical feasibility and safety of laparoscopic single-, or, reduced port distal pancreatectomy have been published [56–58]. However, it is technically difficult and a limited number of expert surgeons can perform this surgery. In theory, robot has been introduced to overcome the limitation of laparoscopic surgery.

Kim and Kang [59, 60] introduced a cutting-edge surgical technique involving robotic-single site plus ONE-port distal pancreatectomy. A recent Korean multicenter study [61] supported the technical feasibility and safety of this new technique. Especially, Han and Kang [62] compared laparoscopic and robotic approaches reduced port distal pancreatectomy. It was found that both techniques are technically feasible and safe. However, the robotic approach is superior to laparoscopic approach in terms of operation time, blood loss, severe complications, and hospital stay, suggesting the need for further investigation.

References

1. Sussman LA, Christie R, Whittle DE. Laparoscopic excision of distal pancreas including insulinoma. Aust N Z J Surg. 1996;66(6):414–6. https://doi.org/10.1111/j.1445-2197.1996.tb01222.x.
2. Young S, Sung ML, Lee JA, DiFronzo LA, O'Connor VV. Pasireotide is not effective in reducing the development of postoperative pancreatic fistula. HPB (Oxford). 2018;20(9):834–40. https://doi.org/10.1016/j.hpb.2018.03.007.
3. Soper NJ, Brunt LM, Dunnegan DL, Meininger TA. Laparoscopic distal pancreatectomy in the porcine model. Surg Endosc. 1994;8(1):57–60.; discussion 60–51. https://doi.org/10.1007/bf02909495.
4. Cuschieri A, Jakimowicz JJ, van Spreeuwel J. Laparoscopic distal 70% pancreatectomy and splenectomy for chronic pancreatitis. Ann Surg. 1996;223(3):280–5.
5. Gagner M, Pomp A, Herrera MF. Early experience with laparoscopic resections of islet cell tumors. Surgery. 1996;120(6):1051–4. https://doi.org/10.1016/s0039-6060(96)80054-7.
6. Yoon DKHH, Kim YW, Choi YM. A case report of laparoscopic distal pancreatectomy. J Korean Endosc Laparosc Soc. 2000;3:4.
7. Min SKHH, Choi YM. Laparoscopic spleen preserving distal pancreatectomy with the conservation of the splenic artery and the vein. J Korean Surg Soc. 2003;64(6):5.
8. Yi X, Chen S, Wang W, Zou L, Diao D, Zheng Y, et al. A systematic review and meta-analysis of laparoscopic and open distal pancreatectomy of nonductal Adenocarcinomatous pancreatic tumor (NDACPT) in the pancreatic body and tail. Surg Laparosc Endosc Percutan Tech. 2017;27(4):206–19. https://doi.org/10.1097/sle.0000000000000416.
9. van Hilst J, Korrel M, de Rooij T, Lof S, Busch OR, Groot Koerkamp B, et al. Oncologic outcomes of minimally invasive versus open distal pancreatectomy for pancreatic ductal adenocarcinoma: a systematic review and meta-analysis. Eur J Surg Oncol. 2019;45(5):719–27. https://doi.org/10.1016/j.ejso.2018.12.003.

10. de Rooij T, van Hilst J, van Santvoort H, Boerma D, van den Boezem P, Daams F, et al. Minimally invasive versus open distal pancreatectomy (LEOPARD): a multicenter patient-blinded randomized controlled trial. Ann Surg. 2019;269(1):2–9. https://doi.org/10.1097/sla.0000000000002979.
11. Kang CM, Lee SH, Lee WJ. Minimally invasive radical pancreatectomy for left-sided pancreatic cancer: current status and future perspectives. World J Gastroenterol. 2014;20(9):2343–51. https://doi.org/10.3748/wjg.v20.i9.2343.
12. Zhang H, Zhu F, Shen M, Tian R, Shi CJ, Wang X, et al. Systematic review and meta-analysis comparing three techniques for pancreatic remnant closure following distal pancreatectomy. Br J Surg. 2015;102(1):4–15. https://doi.org/10.1002/bjs.9653.
13. Chang YR, Kang JS, Jang JY, Jung WH, Kang MJ, Lee KB, et al. Prediction of pancreatic fistula after distal pancreatectomy based on cross-sectional images. World J Surg. 2017;41(6):1610–7. https://doi.org/10.1007/s00268-017-3872-3.
14. Ariyarathenam AV, Bunting D, Aroori S. Laparoscopic distal pancreatectomy using the modified prolonged Prefiring compression technique reduces pancreatic fistula. J Laparoendosc Adv Surg Tech A. 2015;25(10):821–5. https://doi.org/10.1089/lap.2015.0200.
15. Sahay SJ, Lykoudis PM, Al Midani A, Haswell A, Rahman SH. Vascular stapler for transection of pancreatic parenchyma in laparoscopic distal pancreatectomy. Am Surg. 2019;85(6):e275–6.
16. Hanly EJ, Mendoza-Sagaon M, Hardacre JM, Murata K, Bunton TE, Herreman-Suquet K, et al. New tools for laparoscopic division of the pancreas: a comparative animal study. Surg Laparosc Endosc Percutan Tech. 2004;14(2):53–60. https://doi.org/10.1097/00129689-200404000-00002.
17. Okano K, Suto H, Oshima M, Ando Y, Asano E, Kishino T, et al. Pure laparoscopic pancreas parenchymal dissection using CUSA for distal pancreatectomy. Minim Invasive Ther Allied Technol. 2019;28(3):194–7. https://doi.org/10.1080/13645706.2018.1479272.
18. Kim S, Yoon YS, Han HS, Cho JY, Choi Y, Hyun IG, et al. A blunt dissection technique using the LigaSure vessel-sealing device imprtcomes and postoperative splenic-vessel patency after laparoscopic spleen- and splenic-vessel-preserving distal pancreatectomy. Surg Endosc. 2018;32(5):2550–8. https://doi.org/10.1007/s00464-018-6140-1.
19. Velanovich V. The lasso technique for laparoscopic distal pancreatectomy. Surg Endosc. 2006;20(11):1766–71. https://doi.org/10.1007/s00464-004-8704-5.
20. Choi SH, Kang CM, Hwang HK, Lee WJ. Reappraisal of anterior approach to laparoscopic splenectomy: technical feasibility and its clinical application. Surg Laparosc Endosc Percutan Tech. 2011;21(5):353–7. https://doi.org/10.1097/SLE.0b013e31822d6c8c.
21. Kawasaki Y, Hwang HK, Kang CM, Natsugoe S, Lee WJ. Improved perioperative outcomes of laparoscopic distal pancreatosplenectomy: modified lasso technique. ANZ J Surg. 2018;88(9):886–90. https://doi.org/10.1111/ans.14351.
22. Shoup M, Brennan MF, McWhite K, Leung DH, Klimstra D, Conlon KC. The value of splenic preservation with distal pancreatectomy. Arch Surg. 2002;137(2):164–8.
23. Warshaw AL. Conservation of the spleen with distal pancreatectomy. Arch Surg. 1988;123(5):550–3. https://doi.org/10.1001/archsurg.1988.01400290032004.
24. Ferrone CR, Konstantinidis IT, Sahani DV, Wargo JA, Fernandez-del Castillo C, Warshaw AL. Twenty-three years of the Warshaw operation for distal pancreatectomy with preservation of the spleen. Ann Surg. 2011;253(6):1136–9. https://doi.org/10.1097/SLA.0b013e318212c1e2.
25. Jang JY, Shin YC, Han Y, Park JS, Han HS, Hwang HK, et al. Effect of Polyglycolic acid mesh for prevention of pancreatic fistula following distal pancreatectomy: a randomized clinical trial. JAMA Surg. 2017;152(2):150–5. https://doi.org/10.1001/jamasurg.2016.3644.
26. Antila A, Siiki A, Sand J, Laukkarinen J. Perioperative hydrocortisone treatment reduces postoperative pancreatic fistula rate after open distal pancreatectomy. A randomized placebo-controlled trial. Pancreatology. 2019;19(5):786–92. https://doi.org/10.1016/j.pan.2019.05.457.
27. Allen PJ, Gönen M, Brennan MF, Bucknor AA, Robinson LM, Pappas MM, et al. Pasireotide for postoperative pancreatic fistula. N Engl J Med. 2014;370(21):2014–22. https://doi.org/10.1056/NEJMoa1313688.
28. Kondo N, Uemura K, Nakagawa N, Okada K, Kuroda S, Sudo T, et al. A multicenter, randomized, controlled trial comparing reinforced staplers with bare staplers during distal pancreatectomy (HiSCO-07 trial). Ann Surg Oncol. 2019;26(5):1519–27. https://doi.org/10.1245/s10434-019-07222-0.
29. Sa Cunha A, Carrere N, Meunier B, Fabre JM, Sauvanet A, Pessaux P, et al. Stump closure reinforcement with absorbable fibrin collagen sealant sponge (TachoSil) does not prevent pancreatic fistula after distal pancreatectomy: the FIABLE multicenter controlled randomized study. Am J Surg. 2015;210(4):739–48. https://doi.org/10.1016/j.amjsurg.2015.04.015.
30. Park JS, Lee DH, Jang JY, Han Y, Yoon DS, Kim JK, et al. Use of TachoSil(®) patches to prevent pancreatic leaks after distal pancreatectomy: a prospective, multicenter, randomized controlled study. J Hepatobiliary Pancreat Sci. 2016;23(2):110–7. https://doi.org/10.1002/jhbp.310.
31. Shubert CR, Ferrone CR, Fernandez-Del Castillo C, Kendrick ML, Farnell MB, Smoot RL, et al. A multicenter randomized controlled trial comparing pancreatic leaks after TissueLink versus SEAMGUARD after distal pancreatectomy (PLATS) NCT01051856. J Surg Res. 2016;206(1):32–40. https://doi.org/10.1016/j.jss.2016.06.034.

32. Kawai M, Hirono S, Okada K, Sho M, Nakajima Y, Eguchi H, et al. Randomized controlled trial of Pancreaticojejunostomy versus stapler closure of the pancreatic stump during distal pancreatectomy to reduce pancreatic fistula. Ann Surg. 2016;264(1):180–7. https://doi.org/10.1097/sla.0000000000001395.
33. Hassenpflug M, Hinz U, Strobel O, Volpert J, Knebel P, Diener MK, et al. Teres ligament patch reduces relevant morbidity after distal pancreatectomy (the DISCOVER randomized controlled trial). Ann Surg. 2016;264(5):723–30. https://doi.org/10.1097/sla.0000000000001913.
34. Montorsi M, Zerbi A, Bassi C, Capussotti L, Coppola R, Sacchi M. Efficacy of an absorbable fibrin sealant patch (TachoSil) after distal pancreatectomy: a multicenter, randomized, controlled trial. Ann Surg. 2012;256(5):853–9.; discussion 859–860. https://doi.org/10.1097/SLA.0b013e318272dec0.
35. Carter TI, Fong ZV, Hyslop T, Lavu H, Tan WP, Hardacre J, et al. A dual-institution randomized controlled trial of remnant closure after distal pancreatectomy: does the addition of a falciform patch and fibrin glue improve outcomes? J Gastrointest Surg. 2013;17(1):102–9. https://doi.org/10.1007/s11605-012-1963-x.
36. Frozanpor F, Lundell L, Segersvärd R, Arnelo U. The effect of prophylactic transpapillary pancreatic stent insertion on clinically significant leak rate following distal pancreatectomy: results of a prospective controlled clinical trial. Ann Surg. 2012;255(6):1032–6. https://doi.org/10.1097/SLA.0b013e318251610f.
37. Diener MK, Seiler CM, Rossion I, Kleeff J, Glanemann M, Butturini G, et al. Efficacy of stapler versus hand-sewn closure after distal pancreatectomy (DISPACT): a randomised, controlled multicentre trial. Lancet. 2011;377(9776):1514–22. https://doi.org/10.1016/s0140-6736(11)60237-7.
38. Suc B, Msika S, Fingerhut A, Fourtanier G, Hay JM, Holmières F, et al. Temporary fibrin glue occlusion of the main pancreatic duct in the prevention of intra-abdominal complications after pancreatic resection: prospective randomized trial. Ann Surg. 2003;237(1):57–65. https://doi.org/10.1097/00000658-200301000-00009.
39. Uemura K, Satoi S, Motoi F, Kwon M, Unno M, Murakami Y. Randomized clinical trial of duct-to-mucosa pancreaticogastrostomy versus handsewn closure after distal pancreatectomy. Br J Surg. 2017;104(5):536–43. https://doi.org/10.1002/bjs.10458.
40. Behrman SW, Zarzaur BL, Parmar A, Riall TS, Hall BL, Pitt HA. Routine drainage of the operative bed following elective distal pancreatectomy does not reduce the occurrence of complications. J Gastrointest Surg. 2015;19(1):72–9. https://doi.org/10.1007/s11605-014-2608-z.
41. Paulus EM, Zarzaur BL, Behrman SW. Routine peritoneal drainage of the surgical bed after elective distal pancreatectomy: is it necessary? Am J Surg. 2012;204(4):422–7. https://doi.org/10.1016/j.amjsurg.2012.02.005.
42. Van Buren GI, Bloomston M, Schmidt CR, Behrman SW, Zyromski NJ, Ball CG, et al. A prospective randomized multicenter trial of distal pancreatectomy with and without routine intraperitoneal drainage. Ann Surg. 2017;266(3):421–31. https://doi.org/10.1097/sla.0000000000002375.
43. Kwon W, Jang JY, Kim JH, Chang YR, Jung W, Kang MJ, et al. An analysis of complications, quality of life, and nutritional index after laparoscopic distal pancreatectomy with regard to spleen preservation. J Laparoendosc Adv Surg Tech A. 2016;26(5):335–42. https://doi.org/10.1089/lap.2015.0171.
44. Cullingford GL, Watkins DN, Watts ADJ, Mallon DF. Severe late postsplenectomy infection. BJS. 1991;78(6):716–21. https://doi.org/10.1002/bjs.1800780626.
45. Coussens LM, Werb Z. Inflammation and cancer. Nature. 2002;420(6917):860–7. https://doi.org/10.1038/nature01322.
46. Anderson KL Jr, Adam MA, Thomas S, Roman SA, Sosa JA. Impact of minimally invasive vs. open distal pancreatectomy on use of adjuvant chemoradiation for pancreatic adenocarcinoma. Am J Surg. 2017;213(4):601–5. https://doi.org/10.1016/j.amjsurg.2017.01.005.
47. Lee SH, Kang CM, Hwang HK, Choi SH, Lee WJ, Chi HS. Minimally invasive RAMPS in well-selected left-sided pancreatic cancer within Yonsei criteria: long-term (>median 3 years) oncologic outcomes. Surg Endosc. 2014;28(10):2848–55. https://doi.org/10.1007/s00464-014-3537-3.
48. Magge D, Gooding W, Choudry H, Steve J, Steel J, Zureikat A, et al. Comparative effectiveness of minimally invasive and open distal pancreatectomy for ductal adenocarcinoma. JAMA Surg. 2013;148(6):525–31. https://doi.org/10.1001/jamasurg.2013.1673.
49. van Hilst J, de Rooij T, Klompmaker S, Rawashdeh M, Aleotti F, Al-Sarireh B, et al. Minimally invasive versus open distal pancreatectomy for ductal adenocarcinoma (DIPLOMA): a pan-European propensity score matched study. Ann Surg. 2019;269(1):10–7. https://doi.org/10.1097/sla.0000000000002561.
50. Sulpice L, Farges O, Goutte N, Bendersky N, Dokmak S, Sauvanet A, et al. Laparoscopic distal pancreatectomy for pancreatic ductal adenocarcinoma: time for a randomized controlled trial? Results of an all-inclusive National Observational Study. Ann Surg. 2015;262(5):868–73.; discussion 873–864. https://doi.org/10.1097/sla.0000000000001479.
51. Kang CM, Kim DH, Lee WJ, Chi HS. Conventional laparoscopic and robot-assisted spleen-preserving pancreatectomy: does da Vinci have clinical advantages? Surg Endosc. 2011;25(6):2004–9. https://doi.org/10.1007/s00464-010-1504-1.
52. Yang SJ, Hwang HK, Kang CM, Lee WJ. Revisiting the potential advantage of robotic surgical system in spleen-preserving distal pancreatectomy over conventional laparoscopic approach. Ann Transl Med. 2020;8(5):188. https://doi.org/10.21037/atm.2020.01.80.

53. Xu SB, Jia CK, Wang JR, Zhang RC, Mou YP. Do patients benefit more from robot assisted approach than conventional laparoscopic distal pancreatectomy? A meta-analysis of perioperative and economic outcomes. J Formos Med Assoc. 2019;118(1 Pt 2):268–78. https://doi.org/10.1016/j.jfma.2018.05.003.
54. Zhao W, Liu C, Li S, Geng D, Feng Y, Sun M. Safety and efficacy for robot-assisted versus open pancreaticoduodenectomy and distal pancreatectomy: a systematic review and meta-analysis. Surg Oncol. 2018;27(3):468–78. https://doi.org/10.1016/j.suronc.2018.06.001.
55. Souche R, Herrero A, Bourel G, Chauvat J, Pirlet I, Guillon F, et al. Robotic versus laparoscopic distal pancreatectomy: a French prospective single-center experience and cost-effectiveness analysis. Surg Endosc. 2018;32(8):3562–9. https://doi.org/10.1007/s00464-018-6080-9.
56. Kim EY, You YK, Kim DG, Lee SH, Han JH, Park SK, et al. Dual-incision laparoscopic spleen-preserving distal pancreatectomy. Ann Surg Treat Res. 2015;88(3):174–7. https://doi.org/10.4174/astr.2015.88.3.174.
57. Park P, Han HJ, Song TJ, Choi SB, Kim WB, Yoo YD, et al. Single-port versus conventional laparoscopic distal pancreatectomy: a propensity score matched analysis and a learning curve of single-port approach. J Hepatobiliary Pancreat Sci. 2019;26(9):401–9. https://doi.org/10.1002/jhbp.646.
58. Machado MA, Surjan RC, Makdissi FF. Laparoscopic distal pancreatectomy using single-port platform: technique, safety, and feasibility in a clinical case series. J Laparoendosc Adv Surg Tech A. 2015;25(7):581–5. https://doi.org/10.1089/lap.2015.0032.
59. Kim SH, Kang CM, Lee WJ. Robotic single-site plus ONE port distal pancreatectomy. Surg Endosc. 2017;31(10):4258–9. https://doi.org/10.1007/s00464-017-5476-2.
60. Chong JU, Kang CM. Robotic single-site plus one port: pancreas enucleation. J Gastrointest Surg. 2019;23(7):1527–8. https://doi.org/10.1007/s11605-019-04183-3.
61. Park G, Choi SH, Lee JH, Lim JH, Lee H, Lee JH, et al. Safety and feasibility of robotic reduced-port distal pancreatectomy: a multicenter experience of a novel technique. J Gastrointest Surg. 2020;24(9):2015–20. https://doi.org/10.1007/s11605-019-04330-w.
62. Han HJ, Kang CM. Reduced port minimally invasive distal pancreatectomy: single-port laparoscopic versus robotic single-site plus one-port distal pancreatectomy. Surg Endosc. 2019;33(4):1091–9. https://doi.org/10.1007/s00464-018-6361-3.

Video Articles

Choi SH, Kang CM, Lee WJ, Chi HS. Robot-assisted spleen-preserving laparoscopic distal pancreatectomy. Ann Surg Oncol. 2011;18(13):3623. https://doi.org/10.1245/s10434-011-1816-y.

Choi SH, Kang CM, Lee WJ, Chi HS. Laparoscopic modified anterior RAMPS in well-selected left-sided pancreatic cancer: technical feasibility and interim results. Surg Endosc. 2011;25(7):2360–1. https://doi.org/10.1007/s00464-010-1556-2. Epub 2011 Feb 7

Choi SH, Hwang HK, Kang CM, Yoon CI, Lee WJ. Pylorus- and spleen-preserving total pancreatoduodenectomy with resection of both whole splenic vessels: feasibility and laparoscopic application to intraductal papillary mucin-producing tumors of the pancreas. Surg Endosc. 2012;26(7):2072–7. https://doi.org/10.1007/s00464-011-2113-3.

Choi SH, Kang CM, Hwang HK, Lee WJ, Chi HS. Robotic anterior RAMPS in well-selected left-sided pancreatic cancer. J Gastrointest Surg. 2012;16(4):868–9. https://doi.org/10.1007/s11605-012-1825-6. Epub 2012 Jan 19

Choi SH, Kang CM, Kim JY, Hwang HK, Lee WJ. Laparoscopic extended (subtotal) distal pancreatectomy with resection of both splenic artery and vein. Surg Endosc. 2013;27(4):1412–3. https://doi.org/10.1007/s00464-012-2605-9.

Chong JU, Kang CM. Robotic Single-Site Plus One Port Pancreas Enucleation. J Gastrointest Surg. 2019;23(7):1527–8.

Kawasaki Y, Hwang HK, Kang CM, Natsugoe S, Lee WJ. Improved perioperative outcomes of laparoscopic distal pancreatosplenectomy: modified lasso technique. ANZ J Surg. 2018;88(9):886–90.

Kim SH, Kang CM, Lee WJ. Robotic single-site plus ONE port distal pancreatectomy. Surg Endosc. 2017;31(10):4258–9.

Ntourakis D, Marzano E, De Blasi V, Oussoultzoglou E, Jaeck D, Pessaux P. Robotic left pancreatectomy for pancreatic solid pseudopapillary tumor. Ann Surg Oncol. 2011;18(3):642–3. https://doi.org/10.1245/s10434-010-1376-6. Epub 2010 Nov 19

44 Laparoscopic Central Pancreatectomy

Yoo-Seok Yoon

Abstract

Central pancreatectomy was introduced as a surgical procedure to replace distal pancreatectomy or pancreaticoduodenectomy in patients with lesions around the pancreatic neck. This procedure was first performed by Dagradi and Serio in 1984 and widely implemented since Warshaw published a case series involving 12 patients. The procedure is superior to other pancreatic resections in that it can preserve pancreatic exocrine and endocrine functions by conserving pancreatic parenchyma. It can also preserve the upper gastrointestinal tract, bile ducts, and spleen. The main indications for this procedure are benign or low-malignant tumors located in the neck or proximal body of the pancreas. The resection extends from the left of the gastroduodenal artery to approximately 6 cm or more of the distal pancreas after resection.

Supplementary Information The online version contains supplementary material available at https://doi.org/10.1007/978-981-16-1996-0_44.

Y.-S. Yoon (✉)
Departments of Surgery, Seoul National University Bundang Hospital, Seoul National University College of Medicine, Seongnam, South Korea
e-mail: yoonys@snubh.org

Keywords

Central pancreatectomy · Laparoscopy

44.1 Operative Procedure

44.1.1 Patient Position and Trocar Placement

Under general anesthesia, the patient is placed in the lithotomy position and in the reverse Trendelenburg position. The surgeon stands on the right side of the patient, whereas the assistant stands left of the patient, and the scopist is positioned between the patient's legs. After creation of CO_2 pneumoperitoneum via a 12-mm infraumbilical port, four additional trocars (two 12 mm each and two 5 mm each) are placed on both sides of the upper abdomen in a curvilinear shape around the umbilicus trocar (Fig. 44.1). Two trocars in the right upper abdomen are used as the operator's working ports and two trocars in the upper left abdomen as ports for the assistant. A scope with a 30° angle or a flexible scope can be used to clearly visualize the superior area of the pancreas.

H. C. Yu (ed.), *Hepato-Biliary-Pancreatic Surgery and Liver Transplantation*,
https://doi.org/10.1007/978-981-16-1996-0_44

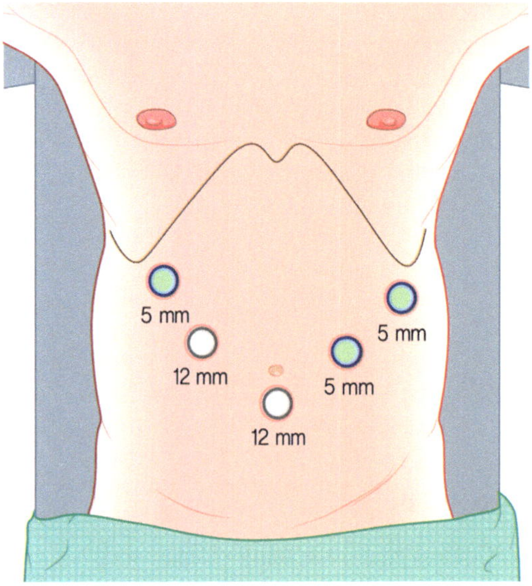

Fig. 44.1 Location of trocars

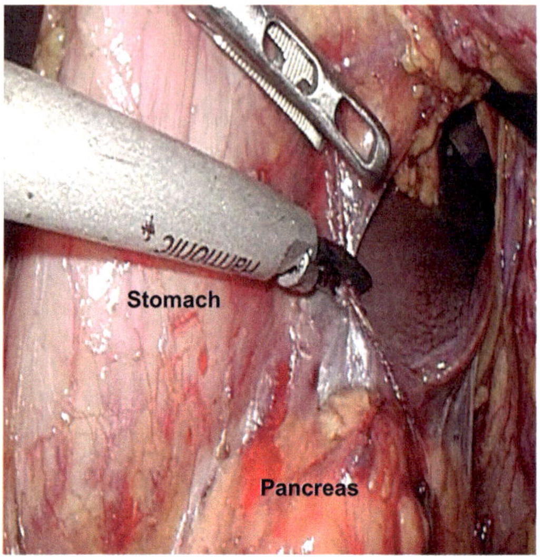

Fig. 44.2 Full gastric mobilization from the anterior side of the pancreas

44.1.2 Approach to the Pancreas

The gastrocolic ligament is first divided at the midline area and widely dissected toward the duodenum and spleen to expose the pancreas. The gastrocolic ligament is divided close to the gastroepiploic vessels so that the bulky omentum on the side of the stomach does not block the surgical field. After the posterior side of the stomach is fully mobilized from the anterior side of the pancreas (Fig. 44.2), the gastric antrum is sutured to the abdominal wall. This procedure can obviate the need for a trocar to maintain the surgical field. If necessary, a laparoscopic ultrasound is performed to determine the location and extent of the tumor.

44.1.3 Dissection of the Pancreas and Exposure of the Superior Mesenteric Vein (SMV) and the Portal Vein (PV)

The inferior pancreatic border is dissected until the SMV is exposed after elevating the pancreatic neck using the grasper. In this procedure, grasping the soft tissues around the pancreas rather than the pancreas itself reduces bleeding due to damaged pancreatic parenchyma. Small branches of the SMV encountered during dissection are controlled with energy devices. Once the SMV is exposed, the posterior surface of the pancreas is dissected from the SMV toward the PV (Fig. 44.3). As there are no branches on the anterior side of the SMV-PV, a retropancreatic tunnel is easily created via blunt dissection using a suction tip.

Thereafter, the superior border of the pancreas is dissected to expose the common hepatic artery (CHA) with downward traction of the pancreas aided by the assistant. The pancreas is further dissected from the CHA to expose the PV (Fig. 44.4). Care is taken to avoid injury to the coronary vein draining into the PV or splenic vein. When the PV is fully dissected from the superior border of the pancreas, a tape is passed around the pancreatic neck through a window between the pancreas and SMV-PV.

44.1.4 Proximal and Distal Pancreatic Division

With traction of the tape, the proximal pancreas is divided using an endoscopic linear stapler (Fig. 44.5). The type of cartridge is selected

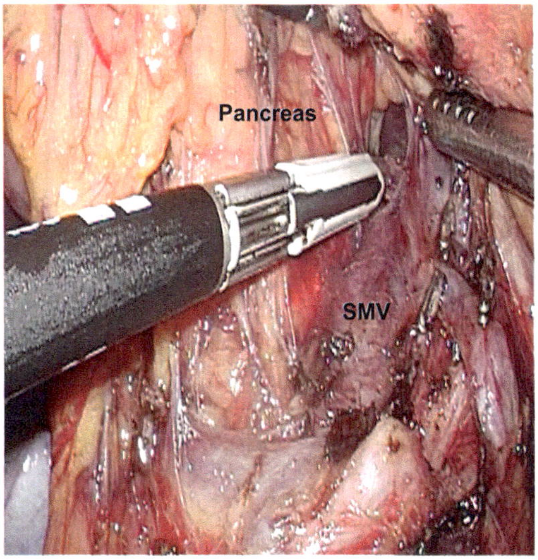

Fig. 44.3 Dissection of the pancreatic surface from the SMV toward the PV

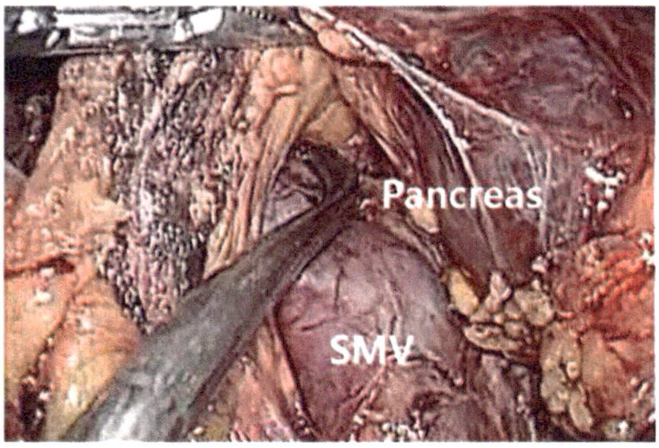

Fig. 44.4 Dissection of the superior border of the pancreas to expose the PV. *CHA* common hepatic artery, *LGA* left gastric artery, *PV*, portal vein

depending on the pancreatic thickness and texture. Thereafter, the pancreas is dissected from the splenic vessels toward the spleen. Small branches of the splenic vessels encountered during dissection are divided using endoclips or energy devices (Fig. 44.6). The distal pancreas is divided with an ultrasonic shear after mobilizing the pancreas from the splenic vessels approximately 2 cm away from the expected distal margin (Fig. 44.7). Parenchymal transection is performed with ultrasonic shears at a peripheral site and scissors in the presumed area of the pancreatic duct to obtain a clear duct margin.

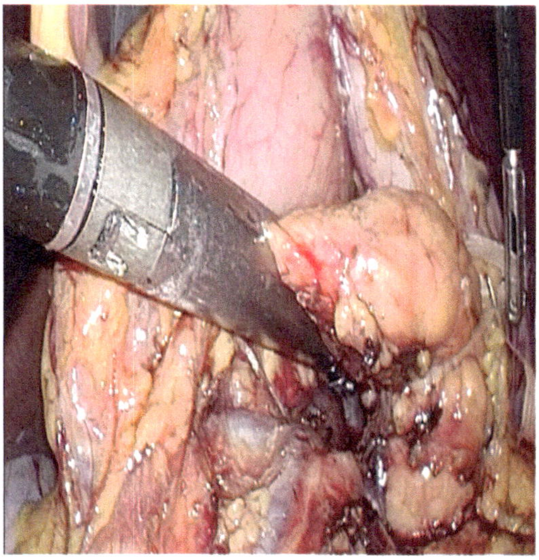

Fig. 44.5 Division of the proximal pancreas using an endoscopic linear stapler

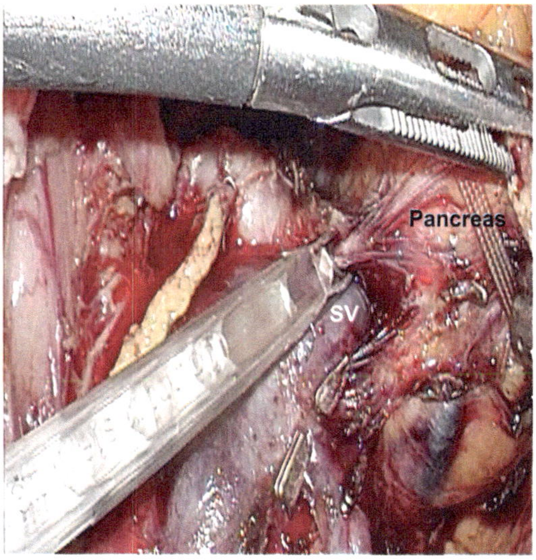

Fig. 44.6 Pancreatic dissection from the splenic vessels toward the spleen: small branches of the splenic vessels are divided using endoclips. *SV* splenic vein

44.1.5 Pancreatic Anastomosis

The proximal jejunum is transected approximately 20 cm distal to the ligament of Treitz with an endoscopic linear stapler. The transected proximal jejunum is brought up to the remnant pancreas via an opening in the mesocolon. Pancreatic reconstruction is performed

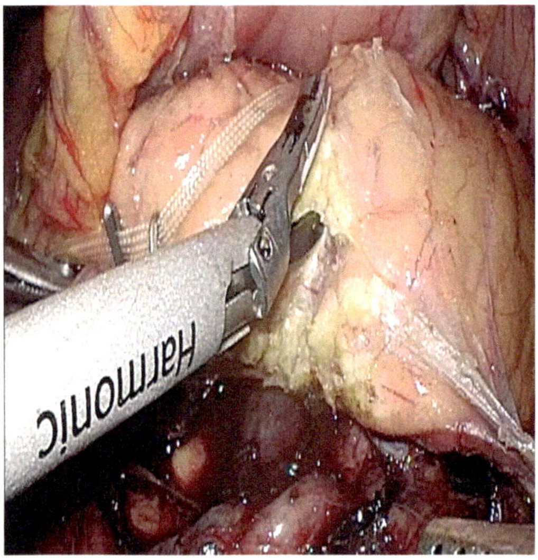

Fig. 44.7 Division of the distal pancreas using an ultrasonic shear

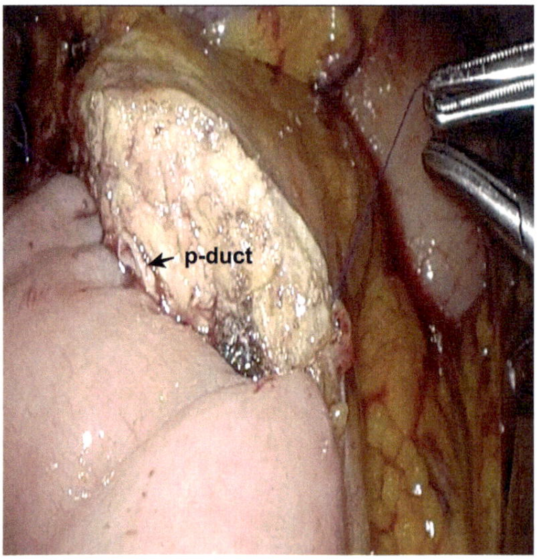

Fig. 44.8 Pancreaticojejunostomy: outer-layer anastomosis between the pancreatic parenchyma and the seromuscular layer of the jejunum using a continuous running suture

by the operator standing between both legs of the patient and the camera inserted through the right lower 12 mm trocar. A two-layer duct-to-mucosa pancreaticojejunostomy is performed in an end-to-side fashion (Figs. 44.8 and 44.9). Continuous running 4–0 Prolene sutures are used for outer-layer anastomosis between the pancreatic parenchyma and the seromuscular layer of the jejunum. Five to eight polydioxanone (PDS) 5–0 sutures are used for duct-to-mucosa anastomosis depending on the size of the pancreatic duct. After completion of the PJ, a polyglycolic acid mesh is placed circumferentially around the anastomosis, and fibrin glue is applied. Thereafter, a side-to-side jejunojejunostomy is performed using an endoscopic linear stapler, approximately 40 cm distal to the pancreaticojejunostomy. The enterotomy is closed using continuous 4–0 V-loc sutures (Fig. 44.10).

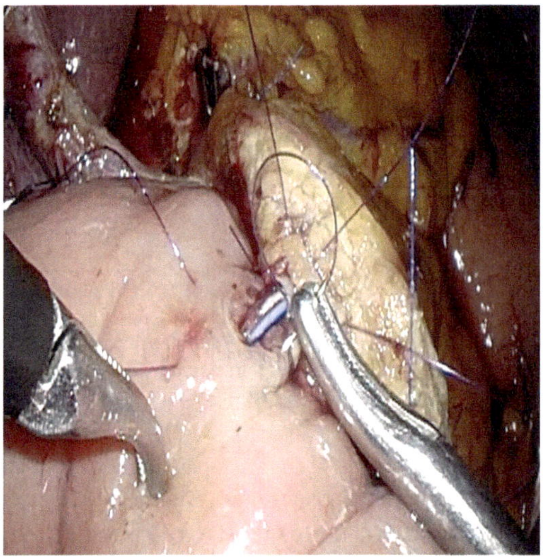

Fig. 44.9 Pancreaticojejunostomy: duct-to-mucosa anastomosis using interrupted sutures

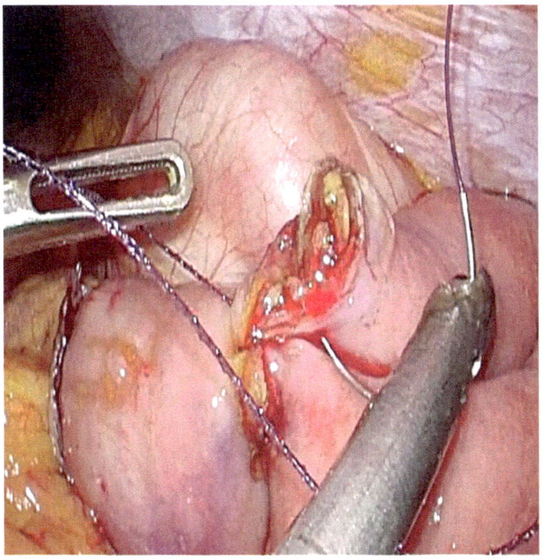

Fig. 44.10 Side-to-side jejunojejunostomy: closure of the enterotomy using a continuous running suture

44.1.6 Drain Placement

Two Jackson-Pratt drains are placed near the pancreatic stump and pancreaticojejunostomy. The surgical specimen is retrieved in a vinyl bag and extracted through a small incision by extending a port-site incision.

Transduodenal Ampullectomy of Ampullary Adenoma

45

Jinseok Heo and Wooil Kwon

Abstract

Transduodenal ampullectomy remains a valid surgical procedure for ampullary adenoma, despite the emergence of endoscopic papillectomy. It is a relatively simple procedure; however, there are critical issues that are associated with serious outcomes, if overlooked. Therefore, hepatobiliary and pancreatic surgeons should be familiar with the procedures. The procedures of transduodenal ampullectomy are briefly discussed here.

Keywords

Transduodenal ampullectomy · Ampulla of Vater · Adenoma · Local excision · Papillectomy

Supplementary Information The online version contains supplementary material available at https://doi.org/10.1007/978-981-16-1996-0_45.

J. Heo (✉)
Department of Surgery, Samsung Medical Center, Sungkyunkwan University School of Medicine, Seoul, Korea

W. Kwon
Department of Surgery, Samsung Medical Center, Sungkyunkwan University School of Medicine, Seoul, Korea

Department of Surgery, Seoul National University Hospital, Seoul, Korea
e-mail: willdoc@snu.ac.kr

45.1 Introduction

Surgical resection is the mainstay of treatment for tumors of ampulla of Vater (AoV). It is needless to say that radical resection such as pancreaticoduodenectomy is required for AoV cancer. Ampullary adenomas, although benign, still require resection as they are known to be associated with concomitant adenocarcinoma in 25–60% of cases with potential risk of malignant transformation [1, 2]. For these benign premalignant lesions, pancreatoduodenectomy appears superfluous given the high rate and severity of complications and its adverse effects on the patient's quality of life. In this regard, transduodenal ampullectomy is more adequate for ampullary adenoma considering the shorter operation duration, shorter hospital stay, and lower morbidity and mortality rate [3].

Endoscopic papillectomy is another alternative. However, it cannot be performed on some lesions with certain morphology and has limited extent of resection [4]. Therefore, transduodenal ampullectomy has a role in the treatment of tumors of AoV.

H. C. Yu (ed.), *Hepato-Biliary-Pancreatic Surgery and Liver Transplantation*,
https://doi.org/10.1007/978-981-16-1996-0_45

45.2 Indications and Contraindications

Transduodenal ampullectomy is indicated for villous adenoma, tubulovillous adenoma, adenoma with high-grade dysplasia, and carcinoma in situ of AoV [5].

By contrast, the feasibility of transduodenal ampullectomy in adenocarcinoma is disputed due to the risk of recurrence and regional lymph node metastasis [6]. Those who advocate transduodenal ampullectomy in adenocarcinoma argue that it may be used for well-differentiated, polypoid, T1 tumors of grade 1–2, without lymphatic spread, and measuring less than 3 cm [7, 8]. However, it is generally not recommended due to the high risk of recurrence [6, 9, 10]. However, transduodenal ampullectomy may be reserved for cancer patients who are contraindicated for radical surgery with either curative or palliative purpose.

45.3 Preoperative Evaluation

Endoscopic retrograde cholangiopancreatography (ERCP) plays an important role in diagnosis and treatment [11]. The lesion can be directly visualized with a side-viewing endoscope. Loss of symmetry, mucosal erosion or ulceration, and hard texture on probing imply adenocarcinoma than adenoma. Notably, histopathological diagnosis can be established through biopsy using ERCP.

Endoscopic ultrasonography facilitates diagnosis and is particularly useful in evaluating the extent of pancreatic or bile duct involvement [12–14].

45.4 Surgical Procedures

45.4.1 Incision

Under general anesthesia, the patient is placed in supine position. Midline incision is preferred over right subcostal incision as it provides adequate field even when the operation is converted to pancreatoduodenectomy. An upper midline from the xyphoid process to supraumbilicus is adequate but may be extended beneath the umbilicus. After laparotomy, intraperitoneal space, including pelvic cavity, peritoneum, mesentery, and liver, should be carefully examined and palpated for unexpected findings such as seeding.

45.4.2 Kocher Maneuver

Kocher maneuver should be performed mostly and preferably to the left of inferior vena cava. Caudally, duodenum should be completely dissected from the mesocolon to fully expose the third portion of duodenum. Generous dissection and mobilization of the duodenum facilitate the incision and closure of duodenum and the approach to AoV.

45.4.3 Incision of the Duodenum

The location of AoV can be confirmed by palpation if the tumor is large or by palpating the endoscopic retrograde biliary drainage tube if it was placed preoperatively. In such case, incision can be made over the palpated location. If the AoV cannot be confirmed, an incision in the lower third of the second portion of duodenum should provide good exposure of the AoV. A longitudinal incision of 3–4 cm is made with electrocautery to expose the duodenal lumen and the AoV. Placing traction sutures along both sides of the incision and at each end of the incision may result in better field (Fig. 45.1).

45.4.4 Excision of the AoV

The line of excision around the AoV is determined to ensure sufficient safety margin. Regarding the cephalic direction of the AoV as 12 o'clock, traction sutures are made inside and outside of the excision line at 3 and 9 o'clock positions. Applying traction on these sutures generates tension on the line of excision. Using an electrosurgical needle

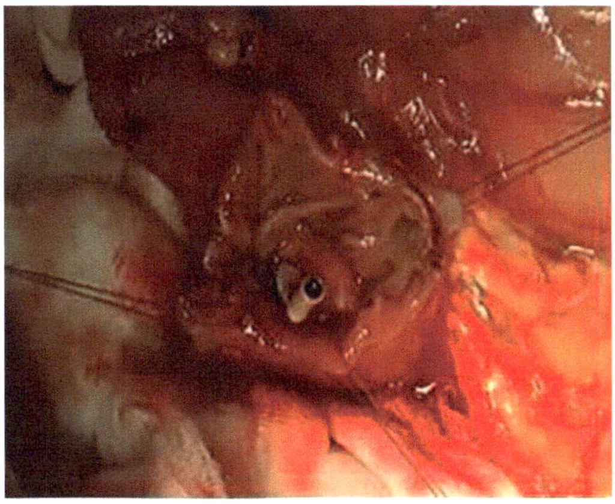

Fig. 45.1 Ampulla of Vater can be easily exposed after incising the lower third of the second portion of duodenum. Four traction sutures are applied to the incision on both sides and each end

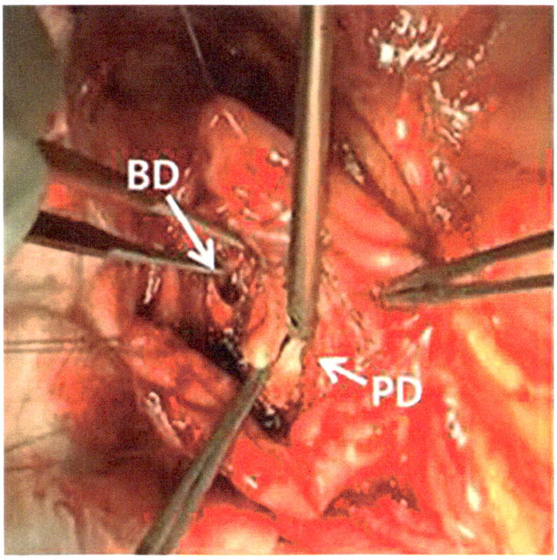

Fig. 45.2 With adequate excision of the ampulla of Vater, the openings of the bile duct (BD) and the pancreatic duct (PD) can be visualized separately

tip, the AoV is excised circumferentially. Using a cutting mode rather than coagulation mode causes less damage and disfiguration of the margin, which will facilitate evaluation of the margin status and reconstruction. However, hemostasis may be less efficient and bleeding points should be focally cauterized using the coagulation mode. In addition to the traction sutures, the operator and the assistant should apply counter-traction with fine forceps to create tension over the excision line along with the resection.

In terms of the depth of excision, the operator should ensure that the AoV is completely excised to include the common channel of bile and pancreatic ducts. If the AoV is excised to adequate depth, the separate openings of the common bile duct and the pancreatic duct should be visible at the deep margin after removing the specimen (Fig. 45.2). The pancreatic duct is caudal to the common bile duct. Frozen section should be sent to evaluate the margin status. Lateral margins should also be checked from the mucosae at 3, 6, 9, 12 o'clock positions or any other parts deemed necessary. The bile duct and pancreatic duct margins should also be sent for frozen section. Additional resection should be performed if margin is not clear. Conversion to pancreatoduodenectomy should not be delayed if the margin cannot be secured or malignancy is confirmed.

45.4.5 Ductoplasty of the Bile and Pancreatic Ducts

Upon complete excision, the bile and pancreatic ducts should be formed into a common duct by suturing the adjacent walls using 5-0 polydioxanone (PDS) sutures (Fig. 45.3). They can be sutured either continuously or interrupted according to the preference of the operator.

45.4.6 Implantation of Common Duct into Duodenum

The common duct should be implanted into the mucosa of the duodenum. The common duct is sutured in interrupted manner to the duodenal mucosa around its circumference at regular intervals using 5-0 PDS (Fig. 45.4). Authors find 8–16 sutures to be sufficient.

Before closing the duodenum, the retroperitoneal side of duodenum should be carefully examined for any wall defects, as duodenal wall may be perforated easily if the AoV is resected too wide or deep. If a wall defect is identified, primary repair should be done.

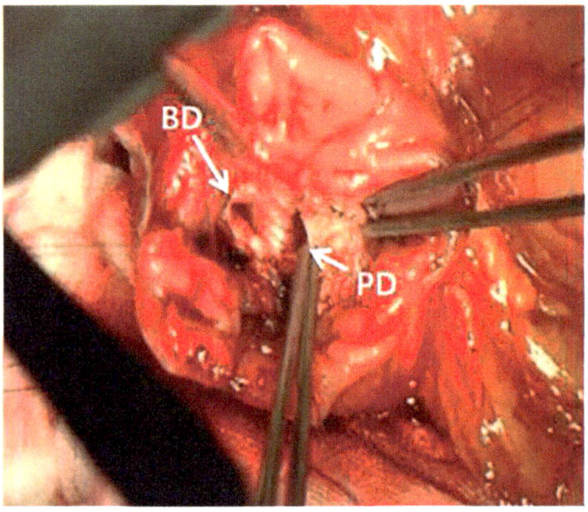

Fig. 45.3 Common channel is formed by suturing the bile duct (BD) and the pancreatic duct (PD) using 5–0 polydioxanone

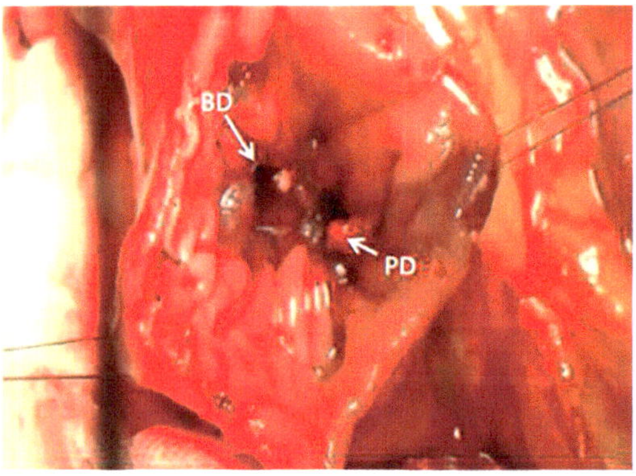

Fig. 45.4 Common channel of the bile duct (BD) and the pancreatic duct (PD) is implanted into the duodenum. The patency of both openings is well preserved

45.4.7 Closure of Duodenostomy

Duodenostomy should be closed in 2 layers after evaluating the patency of the bile and pancreatic ducts with probes (Fig. 45.5). Both longitudinal and transverse closure can be done at the operator's discretion. The incision may be closed transversely when there is a risk of possible stricture. However, strictures are rare even after longitudinal closure.

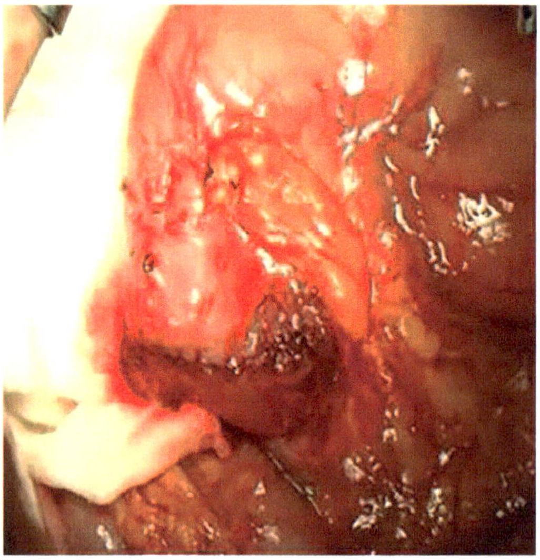

Fig. 45.5 Duodenal opening can be closed either longitudinally or transversely. The transversely closed duodenum is illustrated, but the incidence of stricture is low even after longitudinal closure

45.4.8 Drain Insertion and Abdominal Wall Closure

The duodenum is replaced to its original position and the peritoneal cavity is washed with saline. Authors recommend inserting surgical drain to monitor hemorrhage or duodenal leakage. Closed negative pressure drainage is preferred such as Jackson–Pratt drain. The surgical drain should be placed near the duodenal repair site. However, caution should be taken not to leave the drain in direct contact with the repair site as this may have adverse effect on wound healing.

Abdominal wall is closed in a usual manner.

Tips: Essential Points

1. A generous Kocher maneuver should be performed for better mobilization and exposure of the duodenum and the AoV.
2. The AoV should be excised to adequate depth, and the bile and pancreatic duct openings should be separately identified after resection.
3. The patency of both ducts should be determined after implanting the common duct of bile and pancreatic ducts.
4. Retroperitoneal duodenum should be examined for any wall defects inflicted during the excision.

45.5 Conclusion

Transduodenal ampullectomy is an essential surgical intervention for ampullary adenoma. In addition, it may be offered to AoV cancer patients who are contraindicated for radical operation. Endoscopic papillectomy may have partially replaced transduodenal ampullectomy. However, there are adenomas that are beyond the capability of endoscopic papillectomy. Therefore, transduodenal ampullectomy remains an important component of the treatment for AoV tumors. Hepatobiliary and pancreatic surgeons should have a thorough knowledge of procedures involving transduodenal ampullectomy.

References

1. Posner S, Colletti L, Knol J, Mulholland M, Eckhauser F. Safety and long-term efficacy of transduodenal excision for tumors of the ampulla of Vater. Surgery. 2000;128(4):694–701.
2. Fischer HP, Zhou H. Pathogenesis of carcinoma of the papilla of Vater. J Hepatobiliary Pancreat Surg. 2004;11(5):301–9.
3. de Castro SM, van Heek NT, Kuhlmann KF, Busch OR, Offerhaus GJ, van Gulik TM, et al. Surgical management of neoplasms of the ampulla of Vater: local resection or pancreatoduodenectomy and prognostic factors for survival. Surgery. 2004;136(5):994–1002.
4. van der Wiel SE, Poley JW, Koch AD, Bruno MJ. Endoscopic resection of advanced ampullary adenomas: a single-center 14-year retrospective cohort study. Surg Endosc. 2019;33(4):1180–8.
5. Paramythiotis D, Kleeff J, Wirtz M, Friess H, Buchler MW. Still any role for transduodenal local excision in tumors of the papilla of Vater? J Hepatobiliary Pancreat Surg. 2004;11(4):239–44.
6. Winter JM, Cameron JL, Olino K, Herman JM, de Jong MC, Hruban RH, et al. Clinicopathologic analysis of ampullary neoplasms in 450 patients: implications for surgical strategy and long-term prognosis. J Gastrointest Surg. 2010;14(2):379–87.
7. Beger HG, Treitschke F, Gansauge F, Harada N, Hiki N, Mattfeldt T. Tumor of the ampulla of Vater: experience with local or radical resection in 171 consecutively treated patients. Arch Surg. 1999;134(5):526–32.
8. Klein P, Reingruber B, Kastl S, Dworak O, Hohenberger W. Is local excision of pT1-ampullary carcinomas justified? Eur J Surg Oncol. 1996;22(4):366–71.
9. Sperti C, Pasquali C, Piccoli A, Sernagiotto C, Pedrazzoli S. Radical resection for ampullary carcinoma: long-term results. Br J Surg. 1994;81(5):668–71.
10. Asbun HJ, Rossi RL, Munson JL. Local resection for ampullary tumors. Is there a place for it? Arch Surg. 1993;128(5):515–20.
11. El H II, Cote GA. Endoscopic diagnosis and management of ampullary lesions. Gastrointest Endosc Clin N Am. 2013;23(1):95–109.
12. Rattner DW, Fernandez-del Castillo C, Brugge WR, Warshaw AL. Defining the criteria for local resection of ampullary neoplasms. Arch Surg. 1996;131(4):366–71.
13. Mukai H, Nakajima M, Yasuda K, Mizuno S, Kawai K. Evaluation of endoscopic ultrasonography in the pre-operative staging of carcinoma of the ampulla of Vater and common bile duct. Gastrointest Endosc. 1992;38(6):676–83.
14. Rosch T, Braig C, Gain T, Feuerbach S, Siewert JR, Schusdziarra V, et al. Staging of pancreatic and ampullary carcinoma by endoscopic ultrasonography. Comparison with conventional sonography, computed tomography, and angiography. Gastroenterology. 1992;102(1):188–99.

Essential Tips for Pancreatic and Duodenal Surgery: Vessel Resection

46

Song Cheol Kim and Dae Wook Hwang

Abstract

A combined vascular resection is indicated for a few patients with periampullary cancers and cancers of pancreatic body and tail. In this chapter, we discuss the basic strategy for vessel resection and anastomosis according to the type and location of vascular invasion.

Keywords

Periampullary cancer · Pancreatic cancer · Vascular invasion · Venous resection · Arterial resection · Portal vein · Superior mesenteric vein · Superior mesenteric artery · Celiac axis · Hepatic artery

Supplementary Information The online version contains supplementary material available at https://doi.org/10.1007/978-981-16-1996-0_46.

S. C. Kim (✉) · D. W. Hwang
Division of Hepatobiliary and Pancreatic Surgery, Department of Surgery, Asan Medical Center, University of Ulsan College of Medicine, Seoul, South Korea
e-mail: drksc@amc.seoul.kr

46.1 Combined Venous Resection

46.1.1 End-to-End Anastomosis

En bloc resection is indicated for the tumors in direct contact with the portal vein (PV) or superior mesenteric vein (SMV) in preoperative imaging studies. Preferentially, segmental, cylindrical PV/SMV resection with end-to-end anastomos is can be considered, and even the length of the resected vein can range from 3 to 5 cm [1]. It should be noted that a large enough dissection involving the proximal/distal portion of the resected PV or SMV is required to reduce the tension load on the anastomosis. If resection of the confluence between the PV, SMV, and the splenic vein is needed, anastomosis of the splenic vein is recommended to prevent the potential risk of developing left-sided portal hypertension.

If the cross-section reveals infiltration of less than one-third of the PV or SMV, a primary repair after wedge resection or patch insertion of autogenous/artificial vessels is indicated.

End-to-end anastomosis is not significantly different from general vascular anastomosis, which requires an approximately 5-0 or 6-0-sized nonabsorbable monofilament suture, such as Prolene or Surgipro reflecting growth factors (Fig. 46.1) [2, 3].

H. C. Yu (ed.), *Hepato-Biliary-Pancreatic Surgery and Liver Transplantation*,
https://doi.org/10.1007/978-981-16-1996-0_46

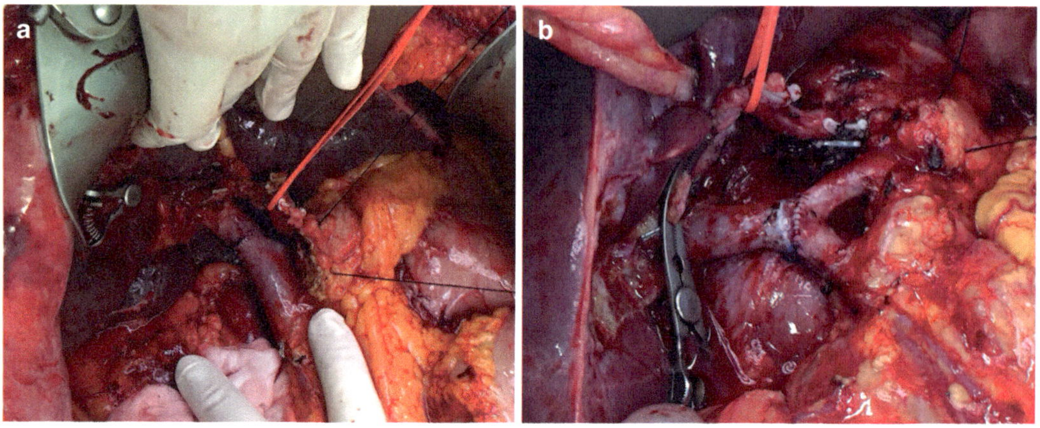

Fig. 46.1 (**a**) End-to-end anastomosis after main portal vein resection. (**b**) End-to-end anastomosis after PV-SMV-SV confluence without SV reconstruction

46.1.2 Interposition Grafting

In case of tumor infiltration longer than 5 cm into the superior mesenteric or the portal vein, interposition grafting can be considered. Although there is no significant difference in the method of anastomosis, it is important to examine the characteristics of each graft for anastomosis. While tension at the anastomotic site should be monitored, the graft should be 60–70% in proportion to the actual length of the resection, in order to avoid kinking or acute angulation around the anastomotic site.

46.1.2.1 Autogenous Vessels

A well-known method utilizes the internal jugular vein, the left renal vein, and the saphenous vein. The actual length is significantly shortened after resection of the veins in many cases, and it should be fully considered before making a decision. This is the best graft due to its biocompatibility and low rates of vascular occlusion associated with thrombosis or anastomotic strictures.

46.1.2.2 Cadaveric Vessels

Cadaveric vessels are similar to autogenous vessels. However, they cannot be used unless they are designed for grafting in liver/kidney/pancreas transplantation.

46.1.2.3 Xenogenic Graft, Bovine Pericardial Patch

Similar to Gore-Tex®, the xenograft (bovine pericardial patch) has excellent biocompatibility without allergic reaction and can be used immediately. Its size and shape can be decided by the operator. In terms of material stiffness, it is closer to autogenous vessels than to Gore-Tex®, thus reducing the risk of subsequent strictures. It is also hemodynamically similar to autogenous vessels. As its stiffness is between that of autogenous vessels and Gore-Tex®, it is difficult to decide the growth factors to use after the suture (the author uses 0.3–0.5). Also, the grafts can cause infection (Fig. 46.2).

46.1.2.4 Artificial Graft: Polytetrafluoroethylene (PTFE, Gore-Tex®) Grafts

Gore-Tex® does not cause allergic reactions and has an excellent biocompatibility and a low rate of thrombogenesis. However, artificial grafts are not histocompatible; they also increase the risk of infection and weak encapsulation. Its size and shape can be decided by the operator and is minimally reduced in length by suture. A constant shape can be maintained. Thus, this method can be used when the autogenous vessels or other grafts are contraindicated [4].

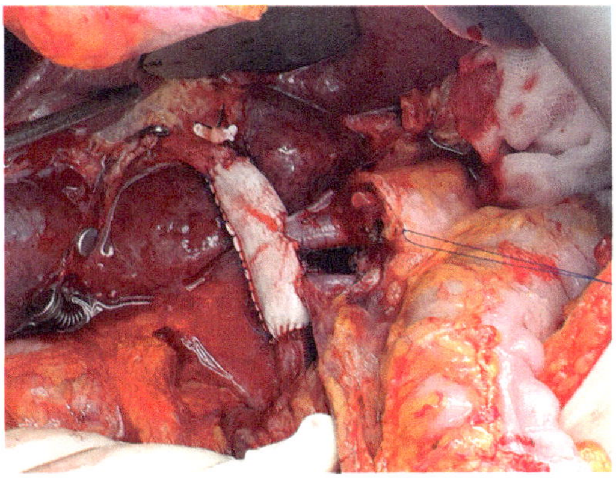

Fig. 46.2 Interposition grafting using bovine pericardial patch, after long segment venous resection

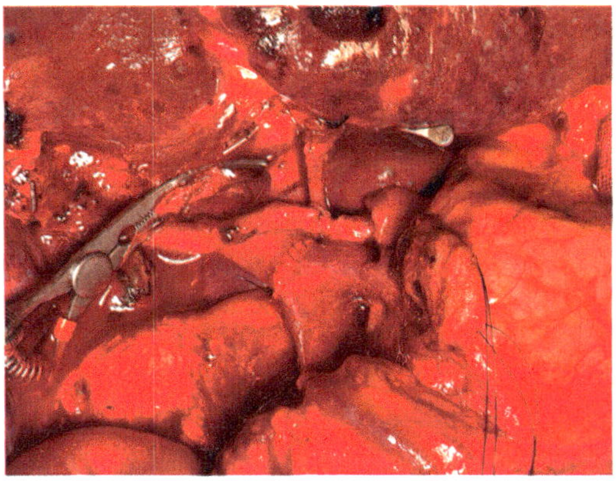

Fig. 46.3 Combined hepatic arterial and portal venous resection with end-to-end anastomosis

46.2 Combined Arterial Resection

46.2.1 Proper Hepatic/Right Hepatic Arterial Resection

Resection of the common hepatic artery or the proper hepatic artery is sometimes required because of tumor infiltration, in which adequate length of the gastroduodenal artery stump should be secured and used to ensure the hepatic arterial flow. If it is not possible to secure the gastroduodenal artery stump, end-to-end anastomosis with or without autogenous vessels/artificial grafts, as described above, can be considered (Fig. 46.3).

The right hepatic artery and common hepatic artery often show variations originating from the superior mesenteric artery. Arterial resection is unavoidable for radical resection during pancreaticoduodenectomy when these arteries course into the pancreatic head. A combined resection can be performed even when tumors infiltrate into the accessory right hepatic artery. The replaced right hepatic artery also rarely causes ischemic challenges in the liver because the hepatic collateral circulation is preserved or collateral circulation occurs later via the hepatic capsular arteries. In case of tumor infiltration into the replaced common hepatic artery, however, an anastomosis is required to secure hepatic arterial flow after the resection, for which end-to-end anastomosis with or without autogenous vessels/artificial grafts can be considered [5].

46.2.2 Distal Pancreatectomy with Celiac Axis Resection (DP-CAR, Appleby Operation)

A combined celiac axis resection can be considered if tumors infiltrate into the celiac axis or the proximal segment of the common hepatic artery, left gastric artery, or splenic artery of the celiac axis. The prerequisites for combined celiac axis resection to ensure negative surgical margins from an oncologic perspective include the following: at least 5-mm-long segment without tumor infiltration at the proximal segment of the celiac axis from the aorta; absence of tumor infiltration into the superior mesenteric artery; and patent gastroduodenal artery. In most cases in which surgery is considered, it is difficult to identify the proximal segment of the celiac axis using the anterior approach. Thus, it is helpful to conduct resection after the identification of the proximal segment of the celiac axis from the aorta via Kocher's maneuver. Further, any infiltration into the proximal portion of the superior mesenteric artery (SMA) should be evaluated using the SMA approach, followed by pancreatic parenchymal resection along the left border of the gastroduodenal artery, and en bloc resection around the celiac axis. If combined resection of the portal vein is required at the same time, the distal/proximal portion of the portal vein should be dissected clearly before resection of pancreatic parenchyma, which facilitates resection of the portal vein and anastomosis.

46.2.3 Resection of Superior Mesenteric Artery

SMA is one of main abdominal arteries and together with hepatic artery and celiac axis, considered in marginal contraindication to resection. However, in some rare cases, the resection of SMA is considered curative. In most of those cases, en bloc resection with primary end-to-end anastomosis can be performed with caution considering the intraoperative and postoperative ischemic changes of small bowel (Fig. 46.4).

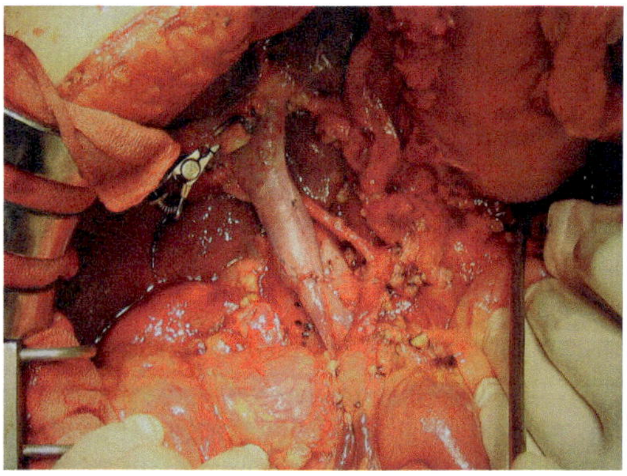

Fig. 46.4 Combined SMA and SMV resection with end-to-end anastomosis

References

1. Kim SC. Surgical management of pancreatic cancer. Korean J Gastroenterol. 2008;51(2):89–100.
2. Yoshitomi H, Kato A, Shimizu H, Ohtsuka M, Furukawa K, Takayashiki T, et al. Tips and tricks of surgical technique for pancreatic cancer: portal vein resection and reconstruction (with videos). J Hepatobiliary Pancreat Sci. 2014;21(9):E69–74.
3. Hwang JW, Kim SC, Song KB, Yoon JH, Nam JS, Lee JH, et al. Significance of radiologic location and extent of portal venous involvement on prognosis after resection for pancreatic adenocarcinoma. Pancreas. 2015;44(4):665–71.
4. Kamenskiy AV, Mactaggart JN, Pipinos GPK II, Dzenis YA. Hemodynamically motivated choice of patch angioplasty for the performance of carotid endarterectomy. Ann Biomed Eng. 2013;41(2):263–78.
5. Michels NA. Newer anatomy of the liver and its variant blood supply and collateral circulation. Am J Surg. 1966;112(3):337–47.

Essential Tips for Reconstruction After Pancreaticoduodenectomy

47

Sung-Sik Han, Dong Eun Park, Koo Jeong Kang, and Young Kyoung You

Abstract

Pancreatico-enteric anastomosis is the most critical procedure in pancreaticoduodenectomy, because post-operative pancreatic fistula (POPF) sometimes causes severe morbidity and even mortality. Since pancreaticoduodenectomy was introduced in 1935, countless techniques were conducted to reduce the POPF. However, until now, no standardized method was established. Any type of anastomosis has advantages as well as disadvantages. Thus, which method to choose may vary depending on the operator's preference and experience. Regarding stent insertion, there are various reports about the choice of internal or external stent. Also, there is controversy regarding the usefulness of stent insertion. Herein, we introduce two most frequently performed techniques of pancreatico-enteric anastomosis and transhepatic external drainage technique of pancreatic juice after anastomosis.

Keywords

Pancreaticoduodenectomy · Pancreatico-jejunostomy · Pancreatico-gastrostomy · Pancreatic stent · External drainage · Modified Blumgart pancreaticojejunostomy · Conventional pancreaticojejunostomy

S.-S. Han (✉)
Center for Liver and Pancreatobiliary Cancer, National Cancer Center, Goyang, South Korea
e-mail: sshan@ncc.re.kr

D. E. Park
Department of Surgery, Wonkwang University college of Medicine, Iksan, South Korea
e-mail: knife@wku.ac.kr

K. J. Kang
Division of Hepatobiliary and Pancreatic Surgery, Department of Surgery, Keimyung University Dongsan Hospital, Daegu, South Korea
e-mail: kjkang@dsmc.or.kr

Y. K. You
Division of Hepatobiliary Pancreas Surgery and Liver Transplantation, Department of Surgery, Seoul St. Mary's Hospital, College of Medicine, The Catholic University of Korea, Seoul, South Korea
e-mail: yky602@catholic.ac.kr

47.1 Pancreaticojejunostomy

Anastomosis of the pancreatic stump with the gastrointestinal tract is considered the most challenging feature of surgery, and is crucial for postoperative healing. Technical failure at this point causes postoperative pancreatic fistula (POPF), a potentially fatal complication. Pancreaticojejunostomy and pancreaticogastrostomy are the most frequently performed procedures for anastomosis between the pancreas and the gastrointestinal tract. Even though more than 80 years have passed since the first pancreaticoduodenectomy was introduced, no safe, effective and universally accepted technique is available to

H. C. Yu (ed.), *Hepato-Biliary-Pancreatic Surgery and Liver Transplantation*,
https://doi.org/10.1007/978-981-16-1996-0_47

minimize pancreatic leakage. The anastomosis appears to depend on the surgeon's preference and the characteristics of the pancreas. Herein, I present the modified Blumgart pancreaticojejunostomy technique and conventional 2-layer pancreaticojejunostomy, which I use most frequently.

47.1.1 Modified Blumgart Duct-to-Mucosa Technique

Blumgart pancreatico-jejunostomy entails the use of transpancreatic and jejunal seromuscular U-sutures (outer layer) to approximate the pancreatic stump and the jejunum combined with duct-to-mucosa (inner layer) anastomosis.

Approximately 20 mm of the pancreatic stump is freed from the splenic vein and surrounding tissues following transection of the pancreatic neck. The jejunal limb is lifted up through the transverse mesocolon next to the right side of the second portion of the duodenum. The ante-mesenteric side of the jejunal limb is placed next to the pancreatic stump. A 3-0 prolene® is used for the transpancreatic and jejunalseromuscular suture. The needle should be straightened before suture in order to easily penetrate the whole thickness of the pancreas. The needle is passed from the anterior to the posterior surface of the pancreas, about 10 mm from its cut edge. It is then passed through the seromuscular layer of the jejunum, parallel to its long axis, and again from the posterior to the anterior surface of the pancreatic parenchyma, about 5 mm away from the initial entry. I place only 3 U-sutures in order to enhance the perfusion of the pancreatic stump and each suture is placed 2–3 mm next to the previous one. These sutures are left untied until the duct-to-mucosa anastomosis is performed (Fig. 47.1). After creating a tiny hole on the jejunum, the PDS® 5-0 is used for the duct-to-mucosa anastomosis with interrupted sutures. The number of PDS® sutures depends on the pancreatic duct size: usually four sutures for non-dilated duct and six sutures for dilated duct (Fig. 47.2). I always insert a plastic stent inside the duct to avoid ductal collapse while doing the U-suture and to ensure the continuity of the anastomosis postoperatively. After the duct-to-mucosa sutures are tied, the straightened needles of these untied U-sutures are passed again through the seromuscular layer of the jejunum, parallel to its long axis, (Fig. 47.3) and tied on the anterior surface of the pancreas.

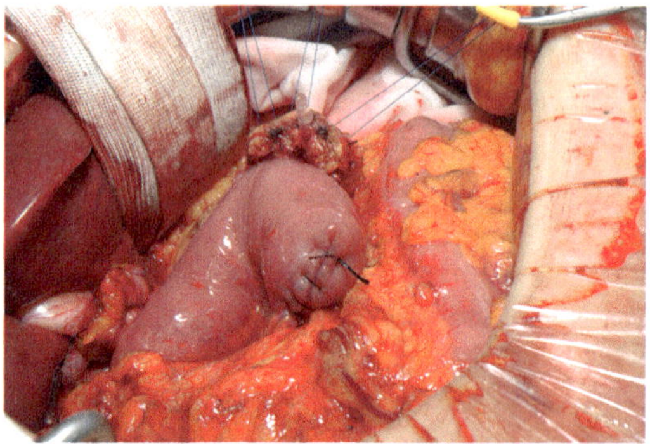

Fig. 47.1 Three U-sutures were applied and hold untied

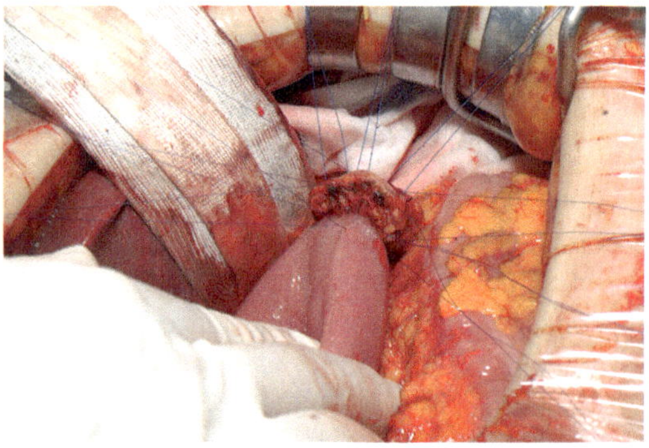

Fig. 47.2 PDS 5-0 interrupted sutures were applied for duct-to-mucosa anastomosis

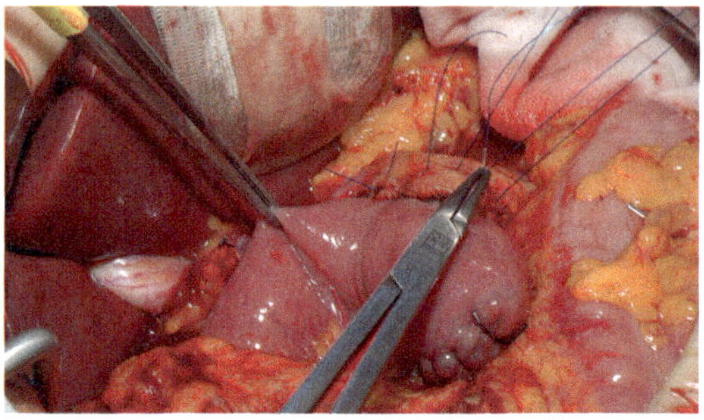

Fig. 47.3 Anterior sero-muscular suture of the jejunum, parallel to its long axis

47.1.2 Conventional 2-Layer Duct-to-Mucosa Technique

The conventional 2-layer duct-to-mucosa anastomosis is still widely performed in many institutions. It entails suturing inner layer of duct-to-mucosa and outer layer of continuous suturing of pancreatic parenchyma with the jejunal seromuscular layer.

A 4-0 prolene® continuous suture is applied from the posterior part of the pancreatic capsule (parallel to the axis of the pancreas, 1 cm from the cut edge) and through the seromuscular layer of the intestine (Fig. 47.4). A smaller intestinal opening than the pancreatic duct is created electrosurgically on the side opposite to the pancreatic duct. The intestinal mucosa is pulled out to perform a precise suture of the mucosa with the duct. The intestinal opening should be smaller than the pancreatic duct opening because the mucosal opening is prone to enlarge during the anastomosis. The 5-0 PDS® interrupted sutures are applied between the pancreatic duct and the whole layer of the intestinal wall. Sutures of the posterior wall of the duct and the intestine are tied and cut. Pancreatic stent is inserted if needed to secure the anastomosis (Fig. 47.5). I usually use a pediatric feeding tube. The anterior wall of the duct and the intestine are sutured and tied after stent insertion. Finally, the anastomosis between the anterior layer of the pancreatic parenchyma and the intestinal wall is performed using the same 4-0 prolene® continuous suture, which was used for the posterior outer layer (Fig. 47.6). Two closed-suction drains are placed anterior and posterior to the anastomotic site.

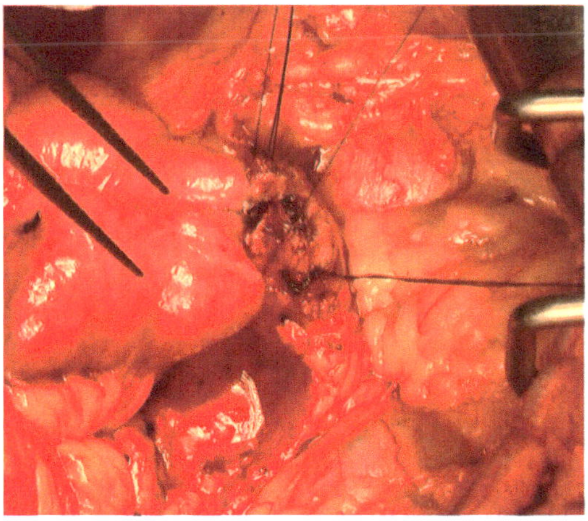

Fig. 47.4 Continuous suture is applied from the posterior part of the pancreatic capsule

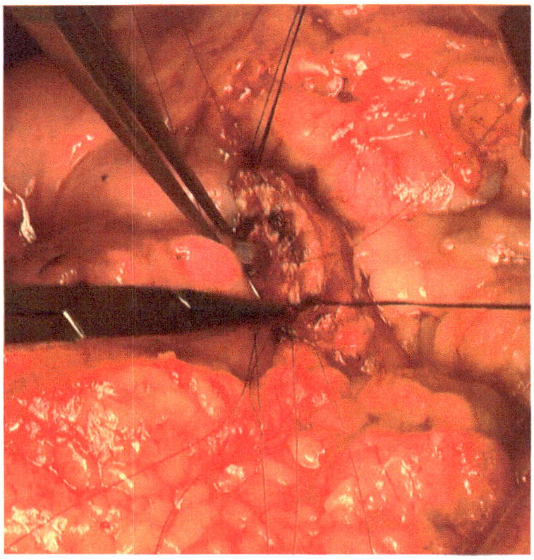

Fig. 47.5 Short pancrератic stent is inserted to secure the anastomosis

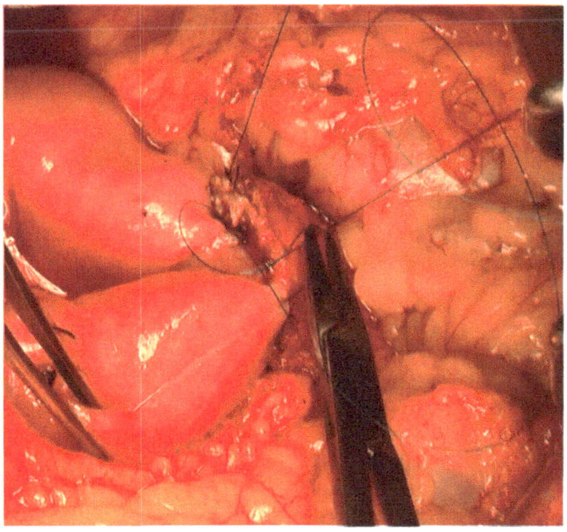

Fig. 47.6 The anterior layer of the pancreatic parenchyma and the intestinal wall are sutured

47.2 External Drainage of Pancreatic Duct

47.2.1 Transjejunal External Drainage of Pancreatic Duct

47.2.1.1 Background

Although there are contrasting opinions about the usefulness of pancreatic stent insertion during pancreatic anastomosis, a recent prospective randomized multicenter study reported that the incidence of the pancreatic fistula was significantly reduced when a stent was used. A short stent is inserted into the pancreatic duct and drained through the jejunal loop. It can be divided into the internal drainage method and the external drainage method, in which it is pulled out of the pancreas for a long time through the jejunum or liver. The internal drainage method is easy to manage, but the stent remains at the site of the duct-to-jejunal anastomosis and can cause atrophy of the residual pancreas. On the other hand, the external drainage can increase the anastomosis stability but the management of the tube is complicated. The choice of the drainage method may depend on the operator's preference. A recent prospective randomized study comparing the internal and external drainage methods reported that the incidence of pancreatic fistula after surgery did not differ according to the drainage method.

47.2.1.2 Surgical Technique

The order of stent insertion differs depending on the methods of pancreatic anastomosis. In the case of the dunking method, a stent is inserted and ligated to the pancreatic duct. In duct-to-mucosa anastomosis, a stent is inserted after the anastomosis of the posterior layer of the pancreatic duct. Here the authors will describe stent insertion mainly in duct-to-mucosa anastomosis. The author mainly uses the so-called novel pancreaticojejunostomy method as proposed by Grobmyer et al. The aim of this procedure is to prevent rupture of the suture site by firmly fixing the pancreas to the jejunum by suturing the entire parenchyma of the remaining pancreas with the jejunum.

1. Interrrupted suture between the entire pancreas and the seromuscular layer of the jejunum

   First, flatten the needle of the absorbable suture (2-0, 3-0 Vicryl®) using forceps. After penetrating the parenchyma of the pancreas from the front to the back at a distance of about 1 cm from the cut surface of the pancreas, suture the seromuscular layer near the mesenteric border of the jejunum. Without ligating the suture, hang it on the forceps with the needle attached. The spacing is approximately 0.75 cm. Four to six interrupted sutures are performed, and it should be noted that the main pancreatic ducts are not sutured together; placing a thin probe in the pancreatic duct is one of the ways to prevent this (Fig. 47.7).

2. The duct-to-mucosa anastomosis and pancreatic stent insertion

   For the duct-to-mucosa anastomosis, a small hole is made in the jejunum, corresponding to the pancreatic duct using an electric cauterizer or scalpel. A stent must be placed prior to the anastomosis. Depending on the inner diameter of the pancreatic duct, a 3–8 Fr silastic tube can be used. The author mainly uses newborns' feeding tubes. Insert a thin explorer through the pre-drilled hole and advance to the lower jejunum to more than 10 cm. After the explorer comes out of the jejunum which is 10 cm lower from the opening, it is tied with a prepared feeding tube. They are pulled out of the opening and the explorer is removed. Next, perform posterior duct-to-mucosa anastomosis with approximately three to four interrupted sutures with absorbable sutures (5-0 PDS). A previously prepared stent is placed in the pancreatic duct. When inserting it, be careful not to exceed 2–3 cm; if it is inserted too deeply, it can cause postoperative pancreatitis. After ligating and fixing the stent using the remaining sutures used for the rear suture, Approximately three or four stiches are needed to perform an anterior duct-to-mucosa anastomosis (Fig. 47.7).

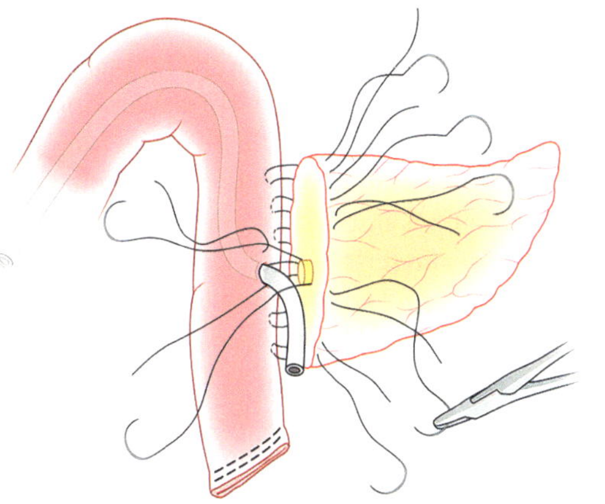

Fig. 47.7 The interrrupted sutures of the whole thickness of pancreas and posterior jejunal seromuscular layer. First, a flattened needle is passed from the front to the back at a distance of 1 cm from the edge of the transected pancreas. Then, after forming a seromuscular suture with the jejunum in a horizontal mattress manner, the needle is again passed from the back to the front of the pancreas. During this process, a probe such as a feeding tube is placed in the duct to prevent occlusion. After posterior duct-to-mucosa anastomosis is performed using PDS 5-0, the stent is fixed by simple suture in the middle thread. Then proceed with anterior duct-to-mucosa anastomosis

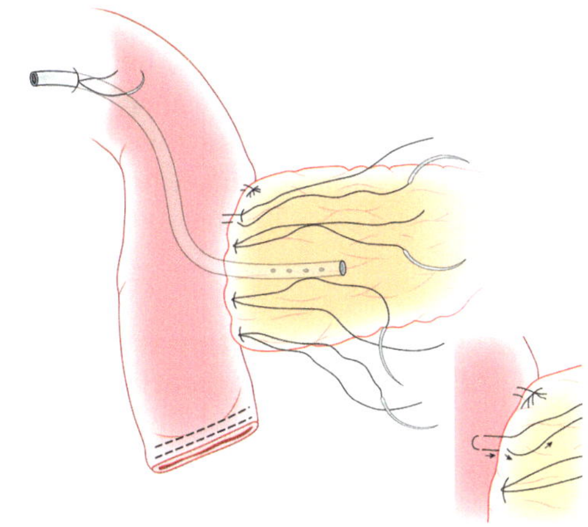

Fig. 47.8 The anterior jejunal seromuscular sutures and stent fixation. After completion of the duct-to-mucosa anastomosis, vicryl sutures are tied down and not to be cut. Using the vicryl sutures, the anterior jejunal seromuscular sutures are completed. The horizontal mattress sutures can allow the jejunum to fold over the anterior surface of the pancreas. The jejunum site where the stent came out is fixed with a purse-string suture, and several seromuscular stitches are made approximately 3–5 cm in length over it

3. The final anterior row of the anastomosis and fixing a external stent.

   After the duct-to-mucosa anastomosis is completed, the remaining posterior sutrues (3-0 Vicryl®) are ligated without pulling too hard and cutting needles. After ligating all the posterior sutures, perform an anterior seromuscular suture of the jejunum using the remaining needle. After the horizontal mattress like the posterior layer is sutured, the needle tip is withdrawn toward the origin of the pancreas, ligated and cut (Fig. 47.8).

   Next, a procedure to fix the external drainage tube is done. Approximately 10 cm below the pancreatic anastomosis site, the drain tube exiting from the jejunum is fixed with a purse-string suture, and the drain tube is covered with a seromuscular suture of approximately 3–5 cm like in gastrostomy. The drainage tube exit from the body through a skin incision in an appropriate area on the right side of the flank. Then, the serosal membrane of the jejunum and the parietal peritoneum from which the drainage tube came out is sewn up using absorbent sutures.

47.2.1.3 Post-Surgery Management

The drainage is drained naturally using a bile bag, etc. The amount of drainage per day varies from patient to patient, but in the case of the authors, approximately 100–200 mL of clear water-like pancreatic juice was drained per day. There are cases where the color of the drainage changes to that of the bile. These cases happen when, first, the stent in the pancreatic duct is naturally removed and is placed in the jejunum, and second, when the pancreatic jejunal anastomosis is leaked. In this case, confirmation through an abdominal CT scan is recommended, and in some cases, 10 cc or less of a contrast medium (gastrographin) is spread using the drain tube. A fistulogram may also be helpful.

Major complications, and the removal time of the external drainage tube differ from operator to operator, but in the case of the author, the removal was performed approximately 2 weeks after the operation, considering the time when the tension of the absorbable suture is reduced by half.

47.2.2 Transhepatic External Drainage of Pancreatic Duct

The rate of postoperative pancreatic fistula (POPF) in case of soft pancreas with a pancreatic duct measuring less than 3 mm in diameter is higher in distal bile duct cancer compared with pancreatic cancer involving a firm pancreatic parenchyma with a pancreatic duct size larger than 3 mm. The external diversion of the pancreatic juice is very safe even in case of POPF because of limited intraperitoneal leakage of the pancreatic juice (1). External drainage occurs via transjejunal and transhepatic routes. Transjejunal drainage may result in leakage of the intestinal juice from the jejunal opening, whereas transhepatic drainage is technically challenging and requires a device (Fig. 47.9a), but it is safer than the transjejunal route. A stylet with a hole at the end of the tip is inserted into the cut bile duct cut and the hepatic surface, and mainly the left lateral section (B2or B3) of the liver is selected. A percutaneous preput polyethylene catheter is pulled after connecting it to the tip of the stylet. The cut end of the common hepatic duct is pulled out and inserted into the pancreatic duct through the jejunum. The tube is fixed tightly with the pancreatic duct using a PDS 5-0 purse-string suture. The schematic diagram after completion of this procedure is shown in Fig. 47.7b. The tube is removed after confirming the absence of postoperative leakage for 2–3 weeks.

The author's algorithm for the transhepatic external drainage or anastomosis without any drainage (internal of external) is depicted in Fig. 47.10.

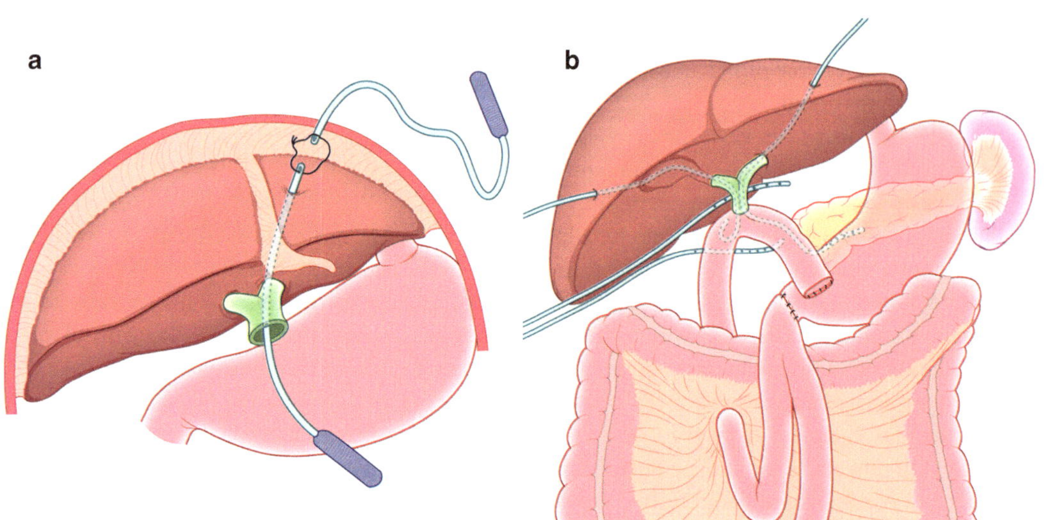

Fig. 47.9 A schematic diagram of pancreaticojejunostomy and transhepatic external drainage of pancreatic juice. (**a**) A stainless steel stylet with a hole at the end and a polyethylene tube is inserted into the bile duct. (**b**) Completion of pancreaticojejunostomy and insertion of transhepatic pancreatic tube and two J-P catheters

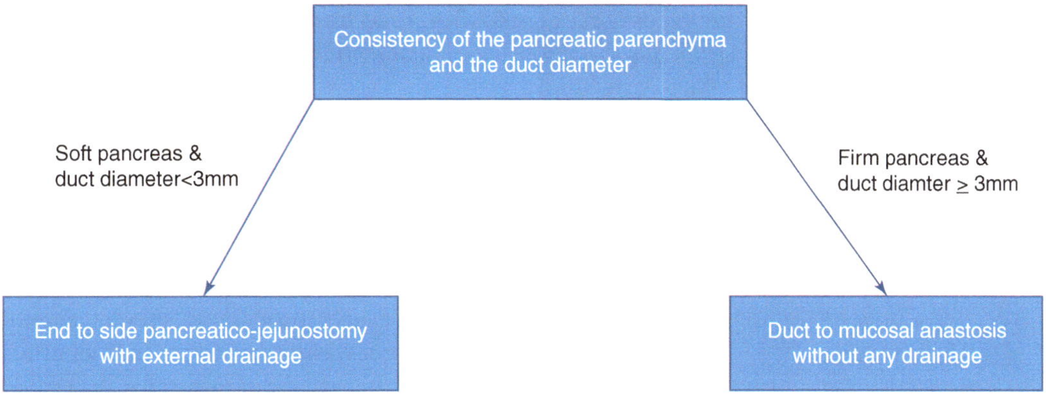

Fig. 47.10 Algorithm of pancreatico-jejunostomy according to the consistency of the pancreatic parenchyma and diameter of the duct

47.3 Pancreaticogastrostomy

Failure of pancreatic anastomosis is a major concern associated with pancreaticoenteric anastomosis. A variety of anastomotic techniques have been used to secure the postoperative pancreatic anastomosis. However, pancreaticojejunostomy is a significant risk factor, especially, in soft pancreas. Therefore, pancreaticogastrostomy is the only option to minimize the risk of failure in pancreaticoenteric anastomosis.

47.3.1 Preparation of Pancreas

Adequate bleeding control of the remnant pancreatic stump is essential prior to pancreaticoenteric anastomosis. Suture ligation using 5-0 or 6-0 monofilament suture material rather than diathermic or energy device ensures clean resection margin and minimal risk of postoperative bleeding.

Pancreatic stump should be freed from the retroperitoneal tissue at least 3 cm in length. Adequate length of pancreatic stump enables safe invagination into the anastomotic gastric lumen.

Pancreatic duct stent using a plastic tube is determined by the duct diameter and location of orifice. Pancreatic duct opening near periphery without stenting results in suture obstruction during anastomosis.

47.3.2 Preparation of Stomach

Tension at the pancreaticoenteric anastomosis is one of the major risk factors underlying anastomotic failure. Constrained sharp ventral bending over the pancreatic body to the gastric wall leads to continuous tension at the pancreaticogastric anastomosis. Adequate length of pancreatic stump and gastric antral area is essential to avoid tension at the pancreaticogastric anastomosis with organ configuration. Classical Whipple's operation involves gastric anastomosis for full mobilization of gastric body and fundic area ensuring short gastric vessel at the splenic portion.

Inadequate hemostasis at the gastric wall warrants postoperative gastroscopy for the management of bleeding focus, which increases the risk of pancreaticogastric anastomotic failure.

47.3.3 Pancreatic-Gastric Anastomosis

Secure and tension-free anastomotic conditions are a prerequisite for surgical success. Based on the elasticity of gastric wall, a relatively small opening allows invagination of pancreatic stump of at least 1 cm. Anterior wall longitudinal gastrotomy facilitates pancreaticogastric anastomosis. A full-thickness gastric interrupted suture can

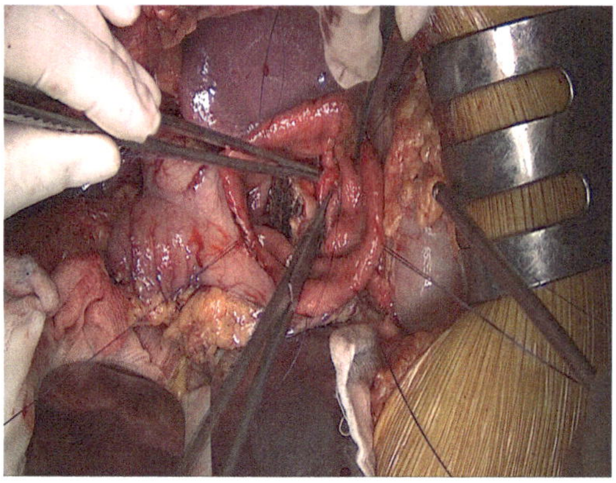

Fig. 47.11 Pancreaticogastrostomy is performed with anterior gastrotomy. A full-thickness gastric interrupted sutures are anchored to pancreas with 5-0 PDS

be obtained using 4-0 or 5-0 absorbable suture materials (Authors prefer 5-0 PDS). (Fig. 47.11).

Risk factors for pancreaticogastric anastomotic failure

1. Anastomotic tension due to excessive bend of pancreatic stump or inadequately mobilized stomach
2. Inadequate invagination of pancreatic stump to the gastric lumen
3. Excessive opening of gastric side of anastomosis
4. Imprudent suturing of the pancreatic duct area
5. Excessive strength of the knot

47.3.4 Pros and Cons of Pancreaticogastrostomy

Diminished long-term endocrine function of the pancreatic remnant is the most significant concern associated with pancreaticogastrostomy. Nevertheless pancreaticogastric reconstruction represents an appropriate option for soft pancreas and individuals with unexpected long-term cancer survival, to prevent anastomotic failure. Gastroscopy represents an effective tool to manage the postoperative pancreatic stump.

References

1. Park JH, Choi YI, Kim YH, Kang KJ, Lim TJ. The complication rate according to the method of pancreaticojejunostomy after pancreaticoduodenectomy. Kor J HBP Surg. 2009;13:42–8.
2. Kim SW, Suh KS. Hepato-biliary-pancreatic surgery. 3rd ed; 2013. p. 962–3.
3. Tani M, Kawai M, Hirono S, et al. A prospective randomized controlled trial of internal versus external drainage with pancreaticojejunostomy for pancreaticoduodenectomy. Am J Surg. 2011;199:759–64.
4. Grobmyer SR, Kooby D, Blumgart LH, et al. Novel pancreaticojejunostomy with a low rate of anastomotic failure-related complications. J Am Coll Surg. 2010;210:54–59.45.

GPSR Compliance

The European Union's (EU) General Product Safety Regulation (GPSR) is a set of rules that requires consumer products to be safe and our obligations to ensure this.

If you have any concerns about our products, you can contact us on ProductSafety@springernature.com

In case Publisher is established outside the EU, the EU authorized representative is:

Springer Nature Customer Service Center GmbH
Europaplatz 3
69115 Heidelberg, Germany

Batch number: 10732809

Printed by Printforce, the Netherlands